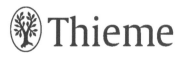

Arthroplasty in Hand Surgery

FESSH Instructional Course Book 2020

Stephan F. Schindele, MD
Orthopaedic and Hand Surgeon
Deputy Head, Department of Hand Surgery
Schulthess Klinik
Zurich, Switzerland

Grey Giddins, FRCS (Orth)
Consultant Orthopaedic and Hand Surgeon
The Royal United Hospitals;
Visiting Professor
University of Bath
Bath, UK

Philippe Bellemère, MD
Hand and Orthopaedic Surgeon
Institut de la Main Nantes-Atlantique
Nantes Saint-Herblain, France

520 illustrations

Thieme
Stuttgart • New York • Delhi • Rio de Janeiro

Library of Congress Cataloging-in-Publication Data is available from the publisher.

© 2021 Thieme. All rights reserved.

Georg Thieme Verlag KG
Rüdigerstrasse 14, 70469 Stuttgart, Germany
+49 [0]711 8931 421, customerservice@thieme.de

Cover design: © Thieme
Cover image source: Samuel Christen, MD;
St. Gallen, Switzerland
Typesetting by DiTech Process Solutions Pvt. Ltd., India

Printed in Germany by Beltz Grafische Betriebe   5 4 3 2 1

ISBN 978-3-13-243174-4

Also available as an e-book:
eISBN 978-3-13-243175-1

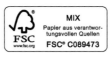

Contents

Section 2   Arthroplasty of Finger Joints

Section 2A   MCP-Arthroplasty

Preface

Dear Colleagues and Friends,

As we write this in 2021, we reflect on what a year 2020 has been. Unfortunately, for the first time in its history, the annual FESSH congress was prevented from being held due to the pandemic. It was due to be held in June 2020 in Basel, Switzerland. It was, however, replaced by a brilliant FESSH (ON)-line-week, at the beginning of September 2020, organized at short notice and in very testing circumstances.

We the Editors as well as all the authors and the publishing team worked on this book for nearly 2 years. We are very grateful to everyone involved. After considerable hard work and logistic challenges, the instructional book will be available *in printed and digital form*. We hope that all the contributions will increase the knowledge among readers about artificial joint replacement in hand surgery and that everyone can benefit from this book in their daily work.

We would like to express special thanks to our families, who supported and motivated us at all times throughout this project.

Stephan Schindele thanks Ulrike, Flurin, and Jakob for their patience. Grey Giddins thanks Jane, Imogen, Miranda, and Hugo for their support and forebearance. Philippe Bellemère thanks his family, Catherine, Olivia, Chloé, and Matthieu.

All three of us would like to express our immense thanks to all the authors who have worked so hard on their contributions, and to our colleagues for their support both during this project and for many years before.

Stephan F. Schindele, MD
Grey Giddins, FRCS (Orth)
Philippe Bellemère, MD

Contributors

Ludovic Ardouin, MD
Elsan Santé Atlantique
Institut de la Main Nantes Atlantique
Nantes, France

Philippe Bellemère, MD
Hand and Orthopaedic Surgeon
Institut de la Main Nantes-Atlantique
Nantes Saint-Herblain, France

Onur Berber, FRCS (Tr&Orth), MSc, BSc (Hons), SEM.
  UK&Ire, DipHandSurg
Department of Trauma and Orthopaedics
Whittington Health
London, UK

Michel E. H. Boeckstyns, MD, PhD
Consultant Hand Surgeon
Capio Private Hospital
Senior Researcher
Clinic for Hand Surgery
Herlev–Gentofte Hospital
University of Copenhagen
Hellerup, Denmark

Michael Brodbeck, MD
Hand Surgeon
Department of Hand Surgery
Schulthess Klinik
Zurich, Switzerland

Marion Burnier, MD
Wrist Surgery Unit
Department of Orthopaedics
Claude-Bernard Lyon 1 University
Herriot Hospital
Lyon, France

Maurizio Calcagni, MD
Division of Plastic Surgery and Hand Surgery
University Hospital Zurich
Zurich, Switzerland

Massimo Ceruso, MD
Full Professor of Orthopaedics
Past President of SICM
Past FESSH Secretary General
Florence, Italy

Kevin C. Chung, MD
Department of Surgery
Section of Plastic Surgery
University of Michigan
Ann Arbor, Michigan, USA

Gilles Dautel, MD
Centre Chirurgical Emile Gallé
Nancy Medical School
Nancy, France

David Elliot, MA (Oxon), FRCS
Consultant Hand Surgeon (Retd.)
Essex, UK

Dirck Ananos Flores, FRACS
Consultant
Sir Charles Gairdner Hospital
Perth, Western Australia

Florian S. Frueh, MD
Division of Plastic Surgery and Hand Surgery
University Hospital Zurich
Zurich, Switzerland

Lorenzo Garagnani, MD, FRCS, EBHS DipHandSurg
Department of Orthopaedics
Guy's & St Thomas' Hospitals
London, UK

Marc Garcia-Elias, MD, PhD
Consultant and Co-Founder
Kaplan Hand Institute
Barcelona, Spain
Honorary Consultant
Pulvertaft Hand Center
Derby, UK

Grey Giddins, FRCS (Orth)
Consultant Orthopaedic and Hand Surgeon
The Royal United Hospitals;
Visiting Professor
University of Bath
Bath, UK

Sam Gidwani, MBBS, FRCS (Tr & Orth), DipHand Surg
Department of Orthopaedics
Guy's and St Thomas' Hospitals
London, UK

Thomas Giesen, MD
Chirurgia della Mano
Ars Medica
Gravesano, Switzerland

Jörg Grünert, MD
Professor
Clinic for Hand, Plastic and Reconstructive Surgery
Kantonsspital St. Gallen
St. Gallen, Switzerland

Marco Guidi, MD
Division of Plastic Surgery and Hand Surgery
University Hospital Zurich
Zurich, Switzerland

Elisabet Hagert, MD, PhD
Department of Clinical Science and Education
Karolinska Institutet;
Arcademy
H. M. Queen Sophia Hospital
Stockholm, Sweden

Timothy Hardwick, MD
Hand Unit, Department of Trauma and Orthopaedics
Brighton and Sussex NHS Trust
Royal Sussex County Hospital
Brighton, UK

Daniel B. Herren, MD, MHA
Schulthess Klinik
Zurich, Switzerland

Guillaume Herzberg, MD, PhD
Professor of Orthopaedic Surgery
Lyon Claude Bernard University
Herriot Hospital
Lyon, France

Nadine Hollevoet, MD, PhD
Associate Professor
Department of Orthopaedic Surgery and
    Traumatology
Ghent University Hospital
Gent, Belgium

Tom Joyce, PhD
Professor
School of Engineering
Newcastle University
Newcastle upon Tyne, UK

Koo Siu Cheong Jeffrey Justin, MBBS (HK), FHKCOS, FHKAM (Orthopaedic Surgery), FRCSEd (Orth), MHSM (New South Wales), MScSMHS (CUHK)
Associate Consultant (Orthopaedics Traumatology)
Department of Orthopaedics & Traumatology
Alice Ho Miu Ling Nethersole Hospital
Tai Po, Hong Kong

Yngvar Krukhaug, MD, PhD
Senior Consultant Orthopaedic Surgeon
Associate Professor
Orthopaedic Clinic
Haukeland University Hospital
University of Bergen
Bergen, Norway

Nikolai Kuz, MD
Physician
Department of Hand, Plastic, and Reconstructive
    Surgery
BG Trauma Center
Frankfurt/Main, Germany

Martin Franz Langer, MD
Professor
Clinic for Trauma, Hand, and Reconstructive Surgery
University Clinic Münster
Münster, Germany

Marc Leroy, MD
Institut de la main Nantes Atlantique
Nantes, France

Bruno Lussiez, MD
Orthopaedic Surgeon
Clinique de Chirurgie orthopédique et
    traumatologique de Monaco
Principality of Monaco

Augusto Marcuzzi, MD
Department of Hand Surgery
"Policlinico di Modena" University Hospital
Modena, Italy

Miriam Marks, PhD
Department of Teaching, Research and Development
Schulthess Klinik
Zurich, Switzerland

Lawrence Stephen Moulton, MD
Consultant Orthopaedic Upper Limb Surgeon
Department of Orthopaedic Surgery
Royal Cornwall Hospitals NHS Trust
Cornwall, UK

Giovanni Munz, MD
Unit of Surgery and Reconstructive Microsurgery of
  the Hand
Azienda Ospedaliero Universitaria Careggi
Florence, Italy

Ladislav Nagy, MD
Professor
Hand Surgery Division
University Clinic Balgrist
Zurich, Switzerland

Florian Neubrech, MD
Department for Plastic, Hand and Reconstructive
  Surgery
BG Trauma Center Frankfurt am Main
Frankfurt, Germany

Michaël Y. Papaloïzos, MD
CH8-Center for Hand Surgery and Therapy
Geneva, Switzerland

Sandra Pfanner, MD
Unit of Surgery and Reconstructive Microsurgery of
  the Hand
Azienda Ospedaliero Universitaria Careggi
Florence, Italy

Lukas Pindur, MD
Resident Plastic, Hand and Reconstructive Surgery
BG Trauma Center Frankfurt
Academic Hospital of the Goethe University Frankfurt
Frankfurt, Germany

Ole Reigstad, MD, PhD
Consultant
EBHS Fellow
Hand and Microsurgery Department
Orthopedic Clinic
Oslo University Hospital
Oslo, Norway

Susanne Rein, MD, PhD, MBA
Department of Plastic and Hand Surgery, Burn Unit
Hospital Sankt Georg
Leipzig, Germany

Lisa Reissner, MD
Division of Hand Surgery
The Balgrist
Zurich, Switzerland

Martin Richter, MD
Director
Department of Hand Surgery
Malteser Hospital Seliger Gerhard
Bonn, Germany

**Matthew Ricks, BSc Hons, MBBS, MRCS, MSc Trauma
  Surgery, MSc Adv HCP, FRCS (Tr & Orth)**
Consultant Upper Limb Trauma and Orthopaedic
  Surgeon
Wrightington Hospital
Wigan, UK

Marco Rizzo, MD
Professor, Department of Orthopedic Surgery
Chair, Division of Hand Surgery
Mayo Clinic
Rochester, Minnesota, USA

Sarah E. Sasor, MD
Department of Plastic Surgery
Medical College of Wisconsin
Milwaukee, Wisconsin, USA

Michael Sauerbier, MD
Professor
Department for Plastic, Hand and Reconstructive
  Surgery
BG Trauma Center Frankfurt am Main
Frankfurt, Germany

Stephan F. Schindele, MD
Orthopaedic and Hand Surgeon
Deputy Head, Department of Hand Surgery
Schulthess Klinik
Zurich, Switzerland

Adam Sierakowski, FRCS(Plast)
Consultant Plastic and Hand Surgeon
St. Andrew's Centre for Plastic Surgery and Burns
Chelmsford, UK

Maria Sirotakova, MD
Consultant Plastic and Hand Surgeon (Retd.)
Chelmsford, UK

Sumedh C. Talwalkar, MBBS, MRCS, MS (Orth),
   MCh (Orth) Liverpool, FRCS (Tr & Orth)
Consultant Hand and Upper Limb Surgeon
Divisional Medical Director Specialist Services
WWL NHS Trust
Wigan, UK

Athanasios Terzis, MD
Orthopaedic and Trauma Surgeon, Hand Surgeon
Consultant, Department for Plastic, Hand and Recon-
   structive Surgery
BG Trauma Center Frankfurt
Academic Hospital of the Goethe University Frankfurt
Frankfurt, Germany

Ian Trail, MD, FRCS
Consultant Orthopaedic Surgeon
WWL NHS Trust
Wigan, UK

Frank Unglaub, MD
Professor
Vulpiusklinik
Bad Rappenau, Germany

Jörg van Schoonhoven, MD
Professor and Senior Consultant
Hand Center Bad Neustadt
Bad Neustadt an der Saale, Germany

David Warwick, MD, FRCSOrth, Eur Dip Hand Surg
Professor and Consultant Hand Surgeon
University Hospital Southampton
Southampton, UK

Chris Williams, FRCS(Orth)
Consultant Hand Surgeon
Trauma and Orthopaedic Department
Royal Sussex County Hospital
Brighton, UK

Claire Jane Zweifel, MD, FMH(Plast), EBOPRAS EDHS
Consultant Plastic and Hand Surgeon
St. Andrew's Centre for Plastic Surgery and Burns
Broomfield Hospital
Chelmsford, UK

Section 1

General

1 The Anatomy and Functional Importance of Finger Joints: A Short Atlas

Martin Franz Langer, David Warwick, Frank Unglaub, and Jörg Grünert

Abstract

The finger joints are incredible. They are effective and precise, mobile yet stable. This chapter presents an anatomical atlas to help the reader understand the detailed anatomy, kinematics, blood supply, and innervation of all the finger joints from the DIP to the CMC. Particular emphasis is placed on the precise structure and function of the collateral ligaments; the mechanics of the joints can be understood through the concept of two different centers of rotation of the joints: one osteocartilaginous and one ligamentous.

Keywords: finger joint, anatomy, biomechanics, innervation, kinematics, collateral ligaments, blood supply, center of rotation

1.1 Introduction

The wonderful diversity of hand function is achieved through the large freedom of movement of the fingers, which allows both stability and precise alignment of the finger joints. As Aristotle observes: "The hand is the 'tool of tools'" (Aristotle, Parts of animals IV 10, 687a: 8–10).

The anatomy, biomechanics, and mode of action of the finger and thumb joints are illustrated throughout this chapter.

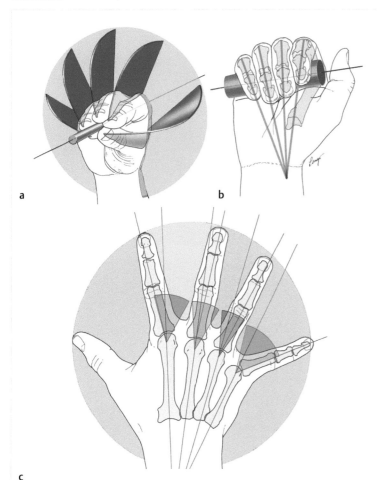

Fig. 1.1 (a) When the extended interphalangeal joints are flexed at the metacarpophalangeal joints so the finger tips are brought together, they enclose a sagittal axis that runs through the head of Metacarpal III. (b) If the fingers are bent at the interphalangeal and metacarpophalangeal joints, they enclose an axis that runs transversely in front of the metacarpal heads on the palmar side. The axes of the middle phalanges are centered on a point above the scaphoid or distal radius. (c) If the thumb and fingers are spread as far as possible, the fingers align in a circular plane. The axes of the metacarpal bones run toward a point in the radius shaft. The metacarpophalangeal joints of the fingers have the greatest lateral freedom of movement (about 40°) in this position, more toward the ulnar than the radial direction. (© Martin F. Langer)

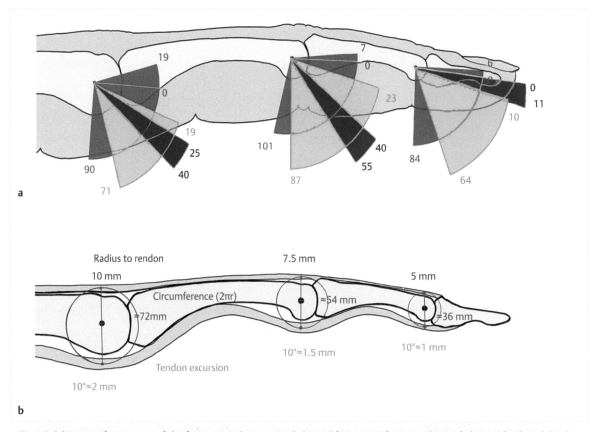

Fig. 1.2 (a) Range of movement of the finger joints (metacarpophalangeal [MP or MCP], proximal interphalangeal [PIP], and distal interphalangeal [DIP]): Red: maximum range of movement. Green: functional range of movement. Blue: recommended angle for arthrodesis. The arthrodesis angles vary from digit to digit and according to the patient's functional requirements. **(b)** Approximate distance of the flexor tendons and extensor tendons from the joint axes for simple rollover calculations. Tendon excursion with 10° joint flexion DIP 1 mm, PIP 1.5 mm, and MP 2 mm. (© Martin F. Langer)

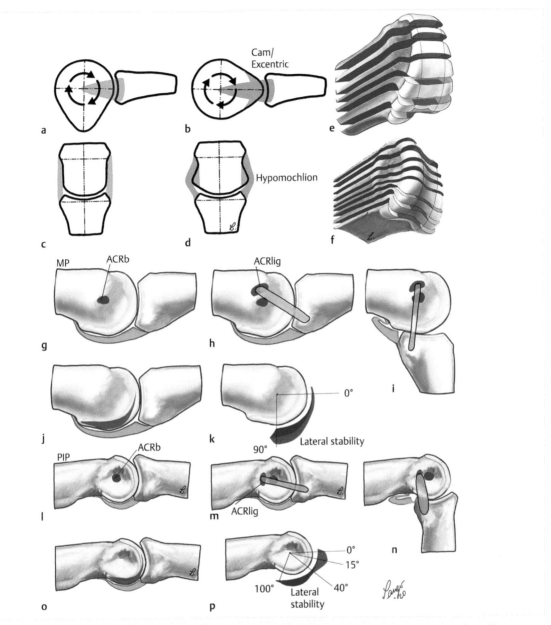

Fig. 1.3 Which mechanisms are used to stabilize the joints? There are two important mechanisms that tension the collateral ligaments: the hypomochlion (lever-arm) mechanism and the cam mechanism (eccentric position of origin of the ligaments). In addition, the bony and ligamentous structures have different centers of rotation. This is the "double eccentric rule" of the finger joints. **(a)** The collateral ligaments are not stretched with a small radius. **(b)** With an increased radius, the collateral ligaments are tensioned. **(c)** In the horizontal course distally (without the hypomochlion or lever-arm), the collateral ligaments are relaxed. **(d)** When the joint is flexed, the collateral ligaments must run over the widened base (hypomochlion) and are tensioned. **(e)** The metacarpal heads are spherical dorsally and bicondylar palmar. **(f)** The heads of the proximal phalanges are dorsal and palmar bicondylar. **(g)** Metacarpophalangeal (MP) joint: The bone does not have a precise center of rotation for the joint but an area of centers of rotation on the bone (ACRb). **(h)** The collateral ligaments have another area of centers of rotation (ACRlig). This ACRlig is in the MP joints dorsal to the ACRb. **(i)** In flexion there is a double tensioning mechanism in the collateral ligament. First, due to the larger radius in flexion, and second, due to the wider base. **(j)** The widening of the base of the metacarpal head (hypomochlion) is blue. **(k)** In the MP joint both mechanisms of ligament tensioning act in the same direction. In extension both are loose and in flexion both are tensioned: "Metacarpophalangeal (MCP) additional tensioning." **(l)** The ACRb of the proximal interphalangeal (PIP) joint. **(m)** In the PIP the ACRlig is proximal to the ACRb. The distance between ACRlig and the tubercles in extension is greater than in flexion. The collateral ligaments are tensioned. **(n)** In flexion the distance between ACRlig and the tubercle is short but the collateral ligament is tensioned by the hypomochlion of the palmar part of the head. **(o)** The widening of the palmar parts of the phalanx head (hypomochlion). **(p)** The cam mechanism (red) and the hypomochlion mechanism (blue) in the PIP are supplementary = "PIP supplementary-tensioning." (© Martin F. Langer)

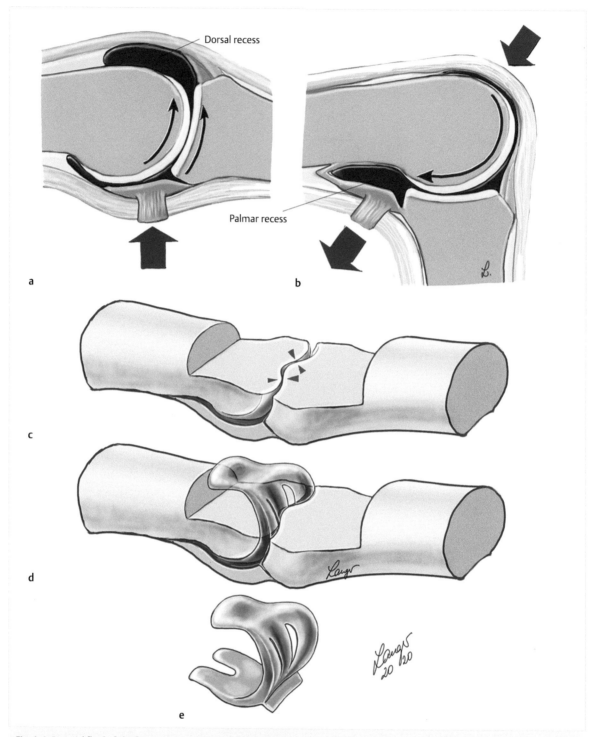

Fig. 1.4 Synovial fluid of the finger joints. **(a)** The incongruity of the joints is necessary. The greatest possible synovial flow is required to feed the cartilage. The contact areas of the adjacent cartilage are significantly smaller than the total cartilage area. When the finger is extended, the flexor tendon and the accessory collateral ligaments press the palmar plate against the joint and the synovial fluid from the palmar recess is pressed dorsally into the dorsal recess. **(b)** When the finger is flexed, the flexor tendon pulls on the palmar plate through the pulley. A suction develops that pulls the synovial fluid from the dorsal into the palmar recess. **(c–e)** The contact surfaces (red arrows) on the proximal interphalangeal (PIP) joint are on the inner sides of the condyles. The synovial cavity on the PIP joint is shown in **(d)** and **(e)**. (© Martin F. Langer)

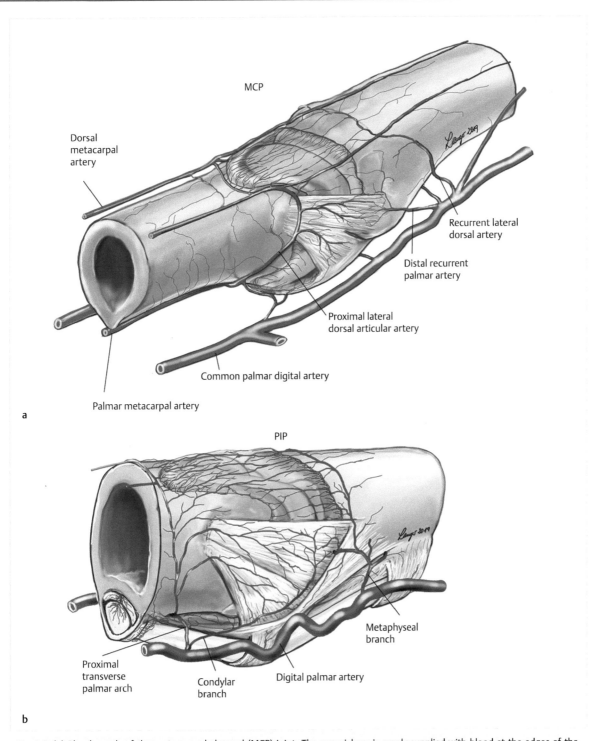

MCP

Dorsal
metacarpal
artery

Recurrent lateral
dorsal artery

Distal recurrent
palmar artery

Proximal lateral
dorsal articular artery

Common palmar digital artery

Palmar metacarpal artery

a

PIP

Metaphyseal
branch

Proximal
transverse
palmar arch

Condylar
branch

Digital palmar artery

b

Fig. 1.5 **(a)** Blood supply of the metacarpophalangeal (MCP) joint. The synovial sac is amply supplied with blood at the edges of the recess. The collateral ligaments are supplied from the proximal and distal margins. **(b)** Blood supply of the proximal interphalangeal (PIP) joint. (© Martin F. Langer)

1

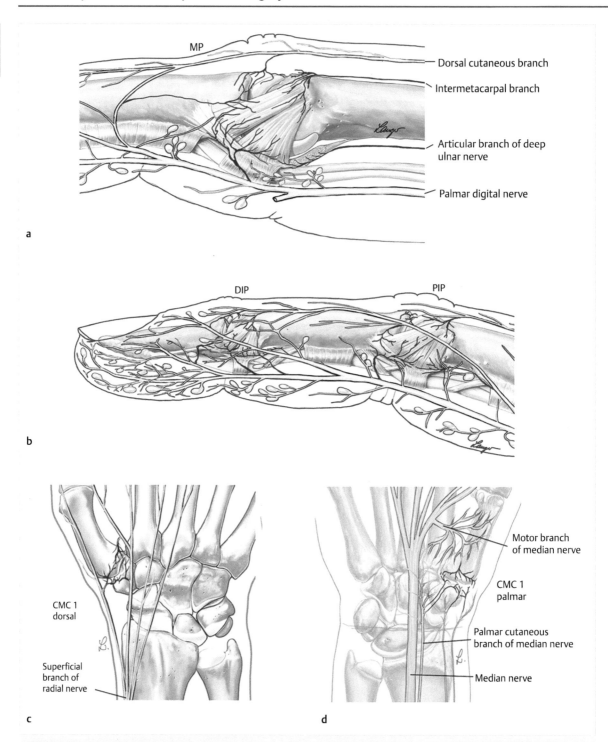

Fig. 1.6 **(a)** Nerve supply of the metacarpophalangeal (MP) joint. **(b)** Nerve supply of the proximal interphalangeal (PIP) and distal interphalangeal (DIP) joints. **(c)** Innervation of the first carpometacarpal (CMC1) joint—dorsal view. **(d)** Innervation of the CMC 1 joint—palmar view. (© Martin F. Langer)

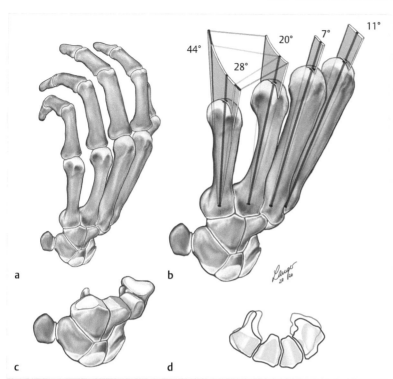

Fig. 1.7 CMC2 to CMC5 joints. **(a)** Dorsoulnar view of the hand skeleton. **(b)** Mobility of the CMC joints. Dorsopalmar mobility in metacarpal 3 (MC 3) is only 7°, in MC 4 20°, and in MC 5 28°. Together with MC 4, the MC 5 mobility is even 40°. **(c)** View of the distal articular surface of the distal carpal row. **(d)** There is very little mobility in the distal carpal row. (© Martin F. Langer)

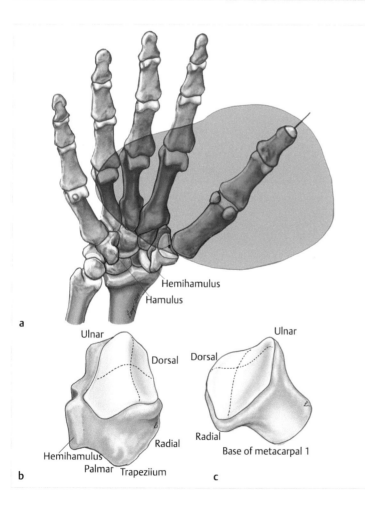

Fig. 1.8 **(a)** Area of mobility of the thumb. **(b)** CMC 1 surface of the trapezium. **(c)** CMC 1 surface of the base of MC 1. (© Martin F. Langer)

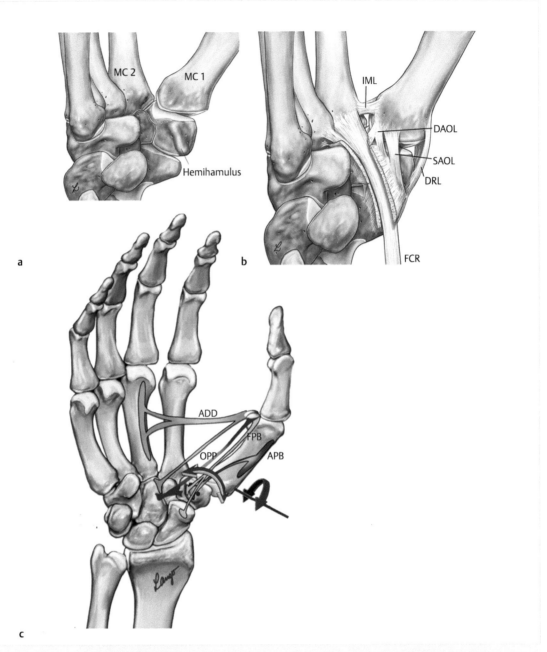

Fig. 1.9 **(a)** Palmar view of the bony structures of the CMC 1. **(b)** Palmar ligaments of the CMC 1. **(c)** Thenar muscles acting on the CMC 1. ADD, adductor pollicis muscle; APB, abductor pollicis muscle; DAOL, deep anterior oblique ligament; DRL, dorsoradial ligament; FPB, flexor pollicis muscle; IML, intermetacarpal ligament; OPP, opponens pollicis muscle; SAOL, superficial anterior oblique ligament. (© Martin F. Langer)

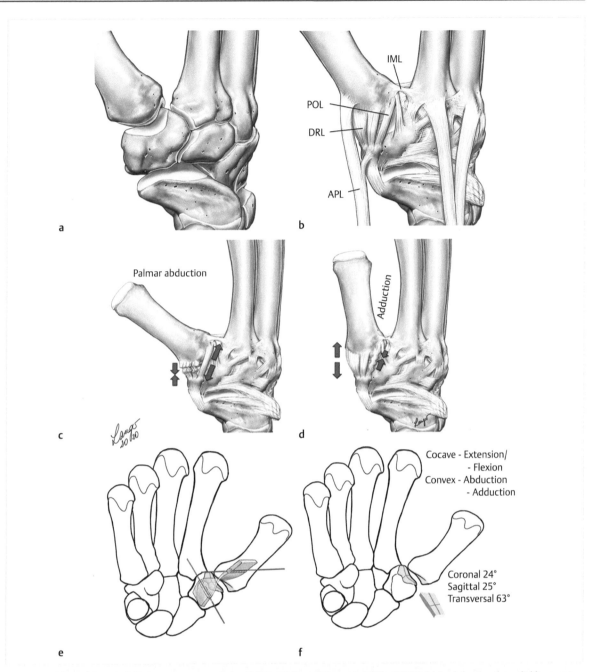

Fig. 1.10 **(a)** Dorsal view of the bony structures of the CMC 1. **(b)** Dorsal ligaments of the CMC 1. **(c)** In abduction the radial ligaments are relaxed, the ulnar under tension. **(d)** In adduction the radial ligaments are tensioned the ulnar are relaxed. **(e)** The first carpometacarpal (CMC1) joint is a universal joint (Hooke or Cardan) with two axes. **(f)** Direction and position of the CMC 1 joint. (© Martin F. Langer)

1

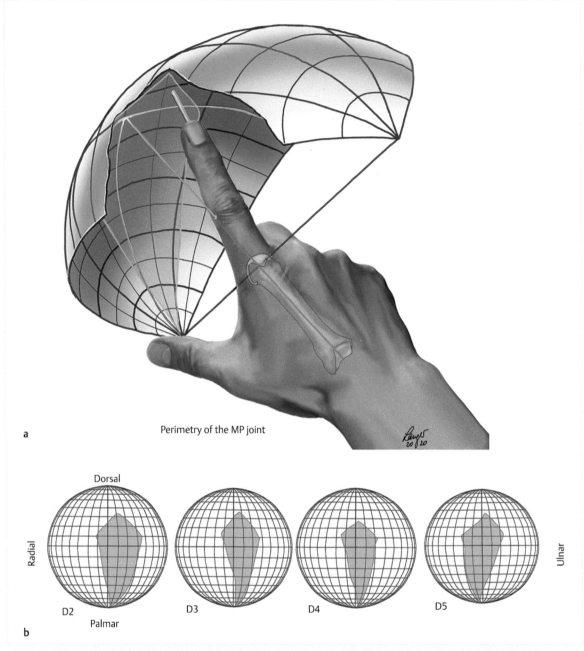

a   Perimetry of the MP joint

Dorsal

Radial   Ulnar

D2   D3   D4   D5

Palmar

b

Fig. 1.11 **(a)** Perimetry of the index MP joint. The axis of the metacarpal is the green line. **(b)** Perimetry—areas of MP 2 to MP 5. (Modified from Shiino and Fick 1925.) (© Martin F. Langer)

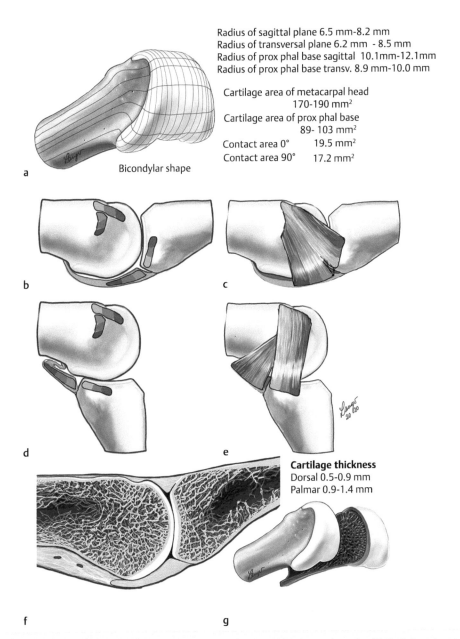

Radius of sagittal plane 6.5 mm-8.2 mm
Radius of transversal plane 6.2 mm - 8.5 mm
Radius of prox phal base sagittal 10.1mm-12.1mm
Radius of prox phal base transv. 8.9 mm-10.0 mm

Cartilage area of metacarpal head
170-190 mm²
Cartilage area of prox phal base
89- 103 mm²
Contact area 0°   19.5 mm²
Contact area 90°   17.2 mm²

a   Bicondylar shape

b

c

d

e

Cartilage thickness
Dorsal 0.5-0.9 mm
Palmar 0.9-1.4 mm

f   g

Fig. 1.12 Anatomy of the metacarpophalangeal (MP) joint. **(a)** Metacarpal head, view from distal lateral. Dorsal part of the joint is spheric and narrow, palmar part is bicondylar and wide.
(b) Origins and insertions of the collateral ligaments (red, orange, and yellow) and the accessory collateral ligaments (green, turquoise, and blue) in 0°. **(c)** MP ligaments in 0°. **(d)** Origins and insertions of the MP ligaments in 90° flexion. **(e)** MP ligaments in 90°. **(f)** Trabeculae of the metacarpal head and proximal phalanx base in sagittal section. Observe the thickness of the cartilage and of the dorsal and palmar plates. **(g)** Oblique view of the sagittal section of the metacarpal head. (© Martin F. Langer)

1

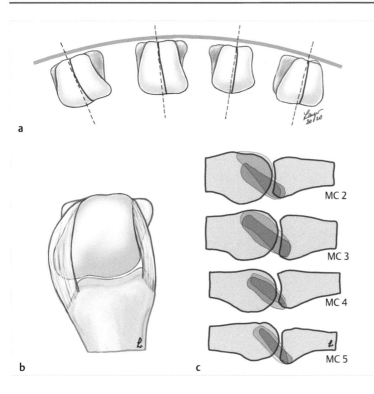

a

b

c

MC 2

MC 3

MC 4

MC 5

Fig. 1.13 Alignment of the metacarpal heads and the radial and ulnar collateral ligaments. **(a)** Normal position of the metacarpal heads in slightly arched position in the view from distal. The midline sagittal plane of the metacarpals is represented by black dotted lines; the main dorsal-palmar movement line represented in red is always ulnar. **(b)** Metacarpal head of index finger in 90° flexion shows a more prominent and more dorsal position of the radial collateral ligament. **(c)** Projection of the positions of the radial (blue) and ulnar (red) ligaments of the metacarpal heads. The radial ligaments are always more dorsal and more prominent. (© Martin F. Langer)

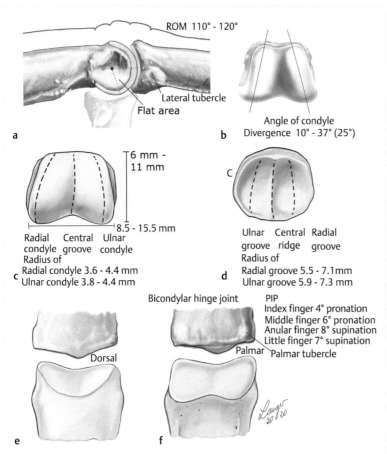

ROM 110° - 120°

Lateral tubercle
Flat area

a

b

Angle of condyle
Divergence 10° - 37° (25°)

6 mm -
11 mm

C

8.5 - 15.5 mm

Radial   Central   Ulnar
condyle   groove   condyle
Radius of
Radial condyle 3.6 - 4.4 mm
c Ulnar condyle 3.8 - 4.4 mm

Ulnar   Central   Radial
groove   ridge   groove
Radius of
Radial groove 5.5 - 7.1mm
d Ulnar groove 5.9 - 7.3 mm

Bicondylar hinge joint

PIP
Index finger 4° pronation
Middle finger 6° pronation
Anular finger 8° supination
Little finger 7° supination

Dorsal

Palmar   Palmar tubercle

e

f

Fig. 1.14 Anatomy of the proximal inter-phalangeal (PIP) joint. **(a)** Lateral view on the PIP joint in 0° and 90°. The "most accurate" center of rotation of the proximal phalanx head is the red point. The centers of rotation of the radius of the proximal phalanx base are the two blue points. They differ between 0° and 90°. Notice the central contact area of the base in 0° and the more dorsal contact area in 90°. Distal-palmar to the area of centers of rotation is a flat area of the head. This flat area is important for stretching out of the collateral ligaments in flexion by the hypomo-chlion (lever-arm) effect. **(b)** The condyles of the proximal phalanx heads have an angle of divergence of 10° to 37°. **(c)** Dimensions of the proximal phalanx head. The summits of the condyles and the lows of the central groove are in curved lines. **(d)** Dimensions of the middle phalanx base. The troughs of the ulnar and radial grooves and the summit of the central ridge form curved lines. **(e)** Dorsal aspect of the PIP joint. **(f)** Palmar aspect of the PIP joint. (© Martin F. Langer)

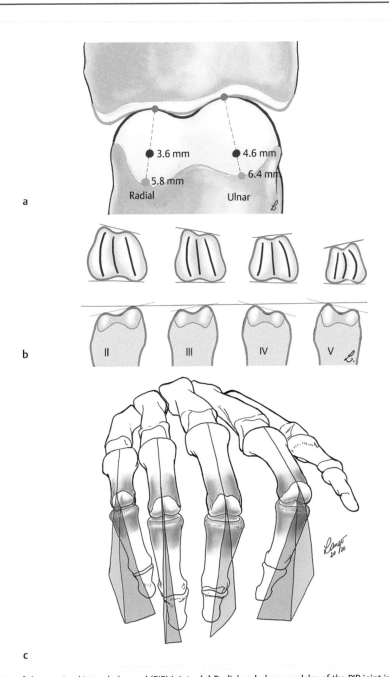

Fig. 1.15 Asymmetries of the proximal interphalangeal (PIP) joints. **(a)** Radial and ulnar condyles of the PIP joint in the view from dorsal. Blue points: small contact area. Red points: centers of rotation of radial and ulnar condyles. Green points: centers of rotation of the radial and ulnar groove of the middle phalanx base. **(b)** The "PIP paradox." Top row: axial view on the proximal phalanx heads: in most cases the radial condyles are greater than the ulnar condyles in second and third finger, and the ulnar is greater in ring and little finger. Lower row: dorsopalmar view of the proximal phalanx heads. Index and middle finger show in most cases a more prominent ulnar condyle; ring and little finger a more prominent radial condyle. So the radial condyle in index finger has the greater radius but is more proximal and the ulnar condyle is smaller but more distal. This is important for the confluence of the fingers in flexion. **(c)** Confluence of the fingertips in PIP flexion. Most radial and most ulnar fingers show a greater centralization. (© Martin F. Langer)

1

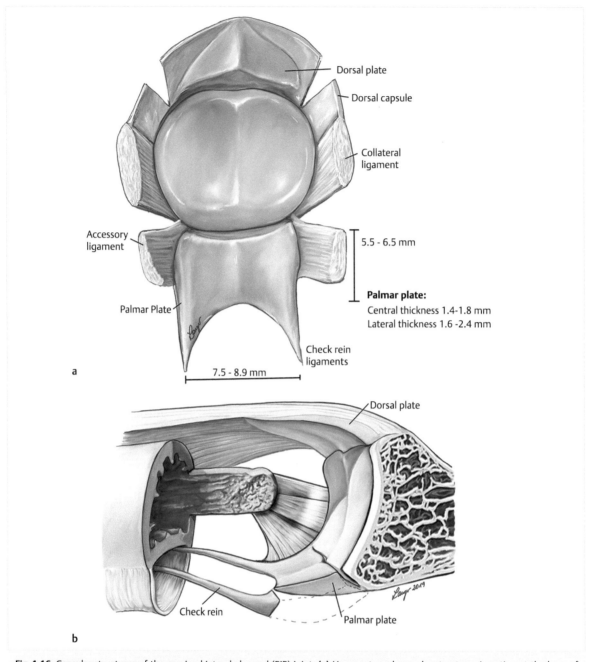

Fig. 1.16 Capsular structures of the proximal interphalangeal (PIP) joint. (a) Ligaments and capsular structures inserting at the base of the middle phalanx. (b) View inside the PIP joint with partially resected head and base. (© Martin F. Langer)

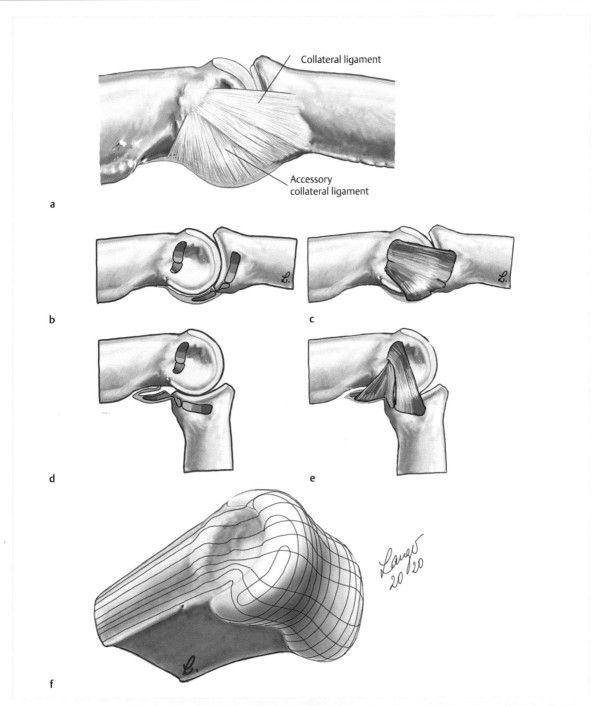

Fig. 1.17 Ligament structures of the proximal interphalangeal (PIP) joint. **(a)** Ligaments of the PIP joint. **(b)** Origins and insertions of the collateral ligaments (red, orange, and yellow) and the accessory collateral ligaments (green, turquoise, and blue) in 0°. **(c)** PIP ligaments in 0°. **(d)** Origins and insertions of the ligaments in 90°. **(e)** PIP ligaments in 90°. **(f)** The palmar parts of the condyles are most prominent laterally and form the hypomochlion parts together with the flat area. (© Martin F. Langer)

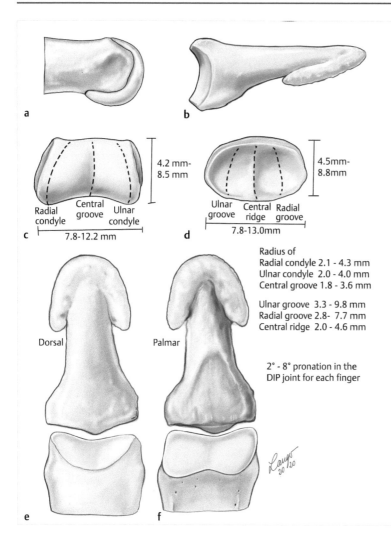

Fig. 1.18 Distal interphalangeal (DIP) joint anatomy. **(a)** Lateral view of the head of the middle phalanx. **(b)** Lateral view of the distal phalanx. **(c)** Dimensions of the head of the middle phalanx. **(d)** Dimensions of the base of the distal phalanx. **(e)** Dorsal aspect of the DIP joint. **(f)** Palmar aspect of the DIP joint. (© Martin F. Langer)

In figure:

c: 4.2 mm-8.5 mm; Radial condyle, Central groove, Ulnar condyle; 7.8-12.2 mm

d: 4.5mm-8.8mm; Ulnar groove, Central ridge, Radial groove; 7.8-13.0mm

Radius of
Radial condyle 2.1 - 4.3 mm
Ulnar condyle 2.0 - 4.0 mm
Central groove 1.8 - 3.6 mm

Ulnar groove 3.3 - 9.8 mm
Radial groove 2.8- 7.7 mm
Central ridge 2.0 - 4.6 mm

2° - 8° pronation in the DIP joint for each finger

Dorsal | Palmar

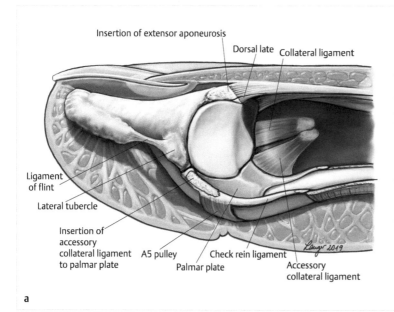

Fig. 1.19 View in the distal interphalangeal (DIP) joint after resection of the second phalanx. (© Martin F. Langer)

In figure:
Insertion of extensor aponeurosis
Dorsal late
Collateral ligament
Ligament of flint
Lateral tubercle
Insertion of accessory collateral ligament to palmar plate
A5 pulley
Palmar plate
Check rein ligament
Accessory collateral ligament

Suggested Readings

Aleksandrowicz R, Pagowski S, Seyfried A. Anatomic-geometric and kinematic analysis of the metacarpo-phalangeal articulation of the III digit of human hand. Folia Morphol (Warsz). 1974; 33(4):353–361

Allison DM. Anatomy of the collateral ligaments of the proximal interphalangeal joint. J Hand Surg Am. 2005; 30(5):1026–1031

Ash HE, Unsworth A. Proximal interphalangeal joint dimensions for the design of a surface replacement prosthesis. Proc Inst Mech Eng H. 1996; 210(2):95–108

Bade H, Schubert M, Koebke J. Functional morphology of the deep transverse metacarpal ligament. Ann Anat. 1994; 176(5):443–450

Bain GI, Polites N, Higgs BG, Heptinstall RJ, McGrath AM. The functional range of motion of the finger joints. J Hand Surg Eur Vol. 2015; 40(4): 406–411

Bogumill GP. A morphologic study of the relationship of collateral ligaments to growth plates in the digits. J Hand Surg Am. 1983; 8(1):74–79

Bowers WH, Wolf JW, Jr, Nehil JL, Bittinger S. The proximal interphalangeal joint volar plate. I. An anatomical and biomechanical study. J Hand Surg Am. 1980; 5(1):79–88

Brand PW, Hollister AM. Clinical Mechanics of the Hand. 3 rd ed. St. Louis: Mosby;1999

Burfeind H. Zur Biomechanik des Fingers unter Berücksichtigung der Krümmungsinkongruenz der Gelenkflächen. Göttingen: Cuvillier;2003

Chao EYS, An K-n, Cooney WP, Linscheid RL. Biomechanics of the Hand. World Scientific;1989

Chen J, Tan J, Zhang AX. In vivo length changes of the proximal interphalangeal joint proper and accessory collateral ligaments during flexion. J Hand Surg Am. 2015; 40(6):1130–1137

Chikenji T, Suzuki D, Fujimiya M, Moriya T, Tsubota S. Distribution of nerve endings in the human proximal interphalangeal joint and surrounding structures. J Hand Surg Am. 2010; 35(8):1286–1293

Degeorges R, Parasie J, Mitton D, Imbert N, Goubier J-N, Lavaste F. Three-dimensional rotations of human three-joint fingers: an optoelectronic measurement. Preliminary results. Surg Radiol Anat. 2005; 27(1):43–50

Dubousset J.. Les phénomènes de rotation lors de la préhension au niveau des doigts. Ann Chir. 1971; 25:19–20; C935–945

Dumont C, Albus G, Kubein-Meesenburg D, Fanghänel J, Stürmer KM, Nägerl H. Morphology of the interphalangeal joint surface and its functional relevance. J Hand Surg Am. 2008; 33(1):9–18

Dumont C, Burfeind H, Kubein-Meesenburg D, et al. Physiological functions of the human finger. J Physiol Pharmacol. 2008; 59 Suppl 5:69–74

Dumont C, Ziehn C, Kubein-Meesenburg D, Fanghanel J, Sturmer KM, Nagerl H. Quantified contours of curvature in metacarpophalangeal joints. J Hand Surg Am. 2009; 34A:317–325

Dy CJ, Tucker SM, Kok PL, Hearns KA, Carlson MG. Anatomy of the radial collateral ligament of the index metacarpophalangeal joint. J Hand Surg Am. 2013; 38(1):124–128

Dzwierzynski WW, Pintar F, Matloub HS, Yoganandan N. Biomechanics of the intact and surgically repaired proximal interphalangeal joint collateral ligaments. J Hand Surg Am. 1996; 21(4):679–683

Eaton RG. Joint Injuries of the Hand. Springfield: Charles C Thomas;1971

Fick R. Handbuch der Anatomie und Mechanik der Gelenke Band 1–3. In: Bardeleben CV, ed. Handbuch der Anatomie des Menschen. Jena: Gustav Fischer; 1904–1911

Gad P. The anatomy of the volar part of the capsules of the finger joints. J Bone Joint Surg Br. 1967; 49(2):362–367

Gigis PI, Kuczynski K. The distal interphalangeal joints of human fingers. J Hand Surg Am. 1982; 7(2):176–182

Hakstian RW, Tubiana R. Ulnar deviation of the fingers: the role of joint structure and function. J Bone Joint Surg Am. 1967; 49(2):299–316

Hendry JM, Mainprize J, McMillan C, Binhammer P. Structural comparison of the finger proximal interphalangeal joint surfaces and those of the third toe: suitability for joint reconstruction. J Hand Surg Am. 2011; 36A:1022–1027

Kaplan EB. Functional and Surgical Anatomy of the Hand. 2nd ed. Philadelphia: JB Lippincott Company;1965:39–45

Kataoka T, Moritomo H, Miyake J, Murase T, Yoshikawa H, Sugamoto K. Changes in shape and length of the collateral and accessory collateral ligaments of the metacarpophalangeal joint during flexion. J Bone Joint Surg Am. 2011A; 93(14):1318–1325

Kenesi C. Les articulations interphalangiennes des doigts. Anat Clin. 1981; 3:39–47

Kenesi C, Deroide JP. A propos de la synoviale de l'articulation méracarpophalangienne. Application chiruricale à la synovectomie par voie dorsale. Arch Anat Pathol (Paris). 1971; 19(4):409–414

Kiefhaber TR, Stern PJ, Grood ES. Lateral stability of the proximal interphalangeal joint. J Hand Surg Am. 1986; 11(5):661–669

Koebke J. A Biomechanical and Morphological Analysis of Human Hand Joints. Berlin: Springer;1983

Koo BS, Song Y, Sung Y-K, Lee S, Jun J-B. Prevalence and distribution of sesamoid bones in the hand determined using digital tomosynthesis. Clin Anat. 2017; 30(5):608–613

Kuczynski K. The proximal interphalangeal joint. Anatomy and causes of stiffness in the fingers. J Bone Joint Surg Br. 1968; 50(3):656–663

Kuczynski K. Less-known aspects of the proximal interphalangeal joints of the human hand. Hand. 1975; 7(1):31–33

Landsmeer JMF. Anatomical and functional investigations on the articulation of the human fingers. Acta Anat Suppl (Basel). 1955; 25(24) Suppl.24: 1–69

Lawrence T, Trail IA, Noble J. Morphological measurements of the proximal interphalangeal joint. J Hand Surg [Br]. 2004; 29(3):244–249

Lee SWJ, Ng ZY, Fogg QA. Three-dimensional analysis of the palmar plate and collateral ligaments at the proximal interphalangeal joint. J Hand Surg Eur Vol. 2014; 39(4):391–397

Leibovic SJ, Bowers WH. Anatomy of the proximal interphalangeal joint. Hand Clin. 1994; 10(2):169–178

Loubert PV, Masterson TJ, Schroeder MS, Mazza AM. Proximity of collateral ligament origin to the axis of rotation of the proximal interphalangeal joint of the finger. J Orthop Sports Phys Ther. 2007; 37(4):179–185

Minami A, An K-N, Cooney WP, III, Linscheid RL, Chao EYS. Ligamentous structures of the metacarpophalangeal joint: a quantitative anatomic study. J Orthop Res. 1984; 1(4):361–368

Minamikawa Y, Horii E, Amadio PC, Cooney WP, Linscheid RL, An K-N. Stability and constraint of the proximal interphalangeal joint. J Hand Surg Am. 1993; 18(2):198–204

Pagowski S, Piekarski K. Biomechanics of metacarpophalangeal joint. J Biomech. 1977; 10(3):205–209

Pang EQ, Yao J. Anatomy and biomechanics of the finger proximal interphalangeal joint. Hand Clin. 2018; 34(2):121–126

Pastrana MJ, Zaidenberg EE, Palumbo D, Cesca FJ, Zaidenberg CR. Innervation of the proximal interphalangeal joint. An anatomical study. J Hand Surg Am. 2019; 44(5):422.e1–422.e5

Podolsky D, Mainprize J, McMillan C, Binhammer P. Comparison of third toe joint cartilage thickness to that of the finger proximal interphalangeal (PIP) joint to determine suitability for transplantation in PIP joint reconstruction. J Hand Surg Am. 2011; 36(12):1950–1958

Rhee RY, Reading G, Wray RC. A biomechanical study of the collateral ligaments of the proximal interphalangeal joint. J Hand Surg Am. 1992; 17(1): 157–163

Saito S, Suzuki Y. Biomechanics of the volar plate of the proximal interphalangeal joint: a dynamic ultrasonographic study. J Hand Surg Am. 2011; 36(2):265–271

Sandhu SS, Dreckmann S, Binhammer PA. Change in the collateral and accessory collateral ligament lengths of the proximal interphalangeal joint using cadaveric model three-dimensional laser scanning. J Hand Surg Eur Vol. 2016; 41(4):380–385

Schultz RJ, Storace A, Krishnamurthy S. Metacarpophalangeal joint motion and the role of the collateral ligaments. Int Orthop. 1987; 11(2):149–155

Shiino K. (Fick R). Einiges über die anatomischen Grundlagen der Greifbewegungen. Z Anat Entw Gesch. 1925; 77:344–362

Slattery PG. The dorsal plate of the proximal interphalangeal joint. J Hand Surg [Br]. 1990; 15(1):68–73

Smith RD, Holcomb GR. Articular surface interrelationships in finger joints. Acta Anat (Basel). 1958; 32(3):217–229

SommerR. Die traumatischen Verrenkungen der Gelenke. Neue Deutsche Chirurgie Band 41. Stuttgart: Ferdinand Enke;1928

Sun YC, Sheng XM, Chen J, Qian ZW. In vivo metacarpophalanageal joint collateral ligament length changes during flexion. J Hand Surg Eur Vol. 2017; 42(6):610–615

Tamai K, Ryu J, An KN, Linscheid RL, Cooney WP, Chao EY. Three-dimensional geometric analysis of the metacarpophalangeal joint. J Hand Surg Am. 1988; 13(4):521–529

Unsworth A, Alexander WJ. Dimensions of the metacarpophalangeal joint with particular reference to joint prostheses. Eng Med. 1979; 8:75–80

Werner D, Kozin SH, Brozovich M, Porter ST, Junkin D, Seigler S. The biomechanical properties of the finger metacarpophalangeal joints to varus and valgus stress. J Hand Surg Am. 2003; 28(6):1044–1051

Williams EH, McCarthy E, Bickel KD. The histologic anatomy of the volar plate. J Hand Surg Am. 1998; 23(5):805–810

Youm Y, Gillespie TE, Flatt AE, Sprague BL. Kinematic investigation of normal MCP joint. J Biomech. 1978; 11(3):109–118

van Zwieten KJ, Kosten L, DeMunter S, et al. Het normale proximale interphalangeale gewricht van de vinger - enkele anatomische observaties. Ned Tijdsch Rheumat. 2017; 17(3):56–59

2 Biomaterials in Arthroplasty of the Hand

Koo Siu Cheong Jeffrey Justin

Abstract

Developments of hand-and-finger joint arthroplasty help to improve the quality of life for many patients suffering from rheumatoid arthritis, osteoarthritis, and posttraumatic conditions. Extensive research has been performed in the past few decades on biomaterials to replace damaged joints. Biomaterials are either used in their native form, altering their formulations, or combined with others materials such as for arthroplasties. We need to understand the mechanical properties of the biomaterials so that we can use the materials appropriately. The limitations of current materials and future research avenues will be discussed.

Keywords: Biomaterials, biocompatibility, hand, polymers, silicone elastomers, metal alloys, calcium hydroxyapatite, pyrolytic carbon

2.1 Introduction

Since 1890, when Themistocles Gluck performed the first wrist replacement using an ivory prosthesis, substantial effort has been directed onto the development of small joint prostheses for the hand. Success in arthroplasty relies upon a thorough understanding of joint mechanics, and implant design and materials employed for manufacturing the implant.

In 1969, Alfred Swanson defined the criteria for ideal joint arthroplasty (▶ Table 2.1). He also pointed out that the materials used for manufacturing the implant component should be able to provide durable fixation to the host tissue and survive the stresses involved in joint movement. Moreover, the implant(s) should be biologically and mechanically acceptable to the host and should be easy to manufacture, sterile, and use.[1]

Any material that has been engineered to interact with biological systems for a medical purpose is collectively known as biomaterials. According to the definition proposed by the European Society for Biomaterials Consensus Conference II, a biomaterial is "a material intended to interface with biological system to evaluate, augment, or replace any tissue, organ, or function of the body."[2]

I will provide an introduction to the basic concepts related to biomaterials science and review the main classes of biomaterials that are currently used in small joint and hand arthroplasty.

2.2 Behavior of Biomaterials

When an implant is inserted into the body, they are immersed into an environment that is more hostile than in air at room temperature. The higher temperature and sodium chloride content in the body as well as high stress concentrations lead to accelerated metal corrosion and degradation of polymers. At the same time, depending upon the types of material the human body will initiate a foreign body reaction. In order to allow the implant to perform the intended function for a sufficient period of time, the selection of biomaterials and their design must comply with the following basic requirements.

2.2.1 Biocompatibility

The definition of biocompatibility has been evolved over the years. In the 1960s and 1970s, the first-generation biomaterials tried to match the chemical and physical properties to those of the replaced tissue with a minimal host/foreign body response in order to minimize any biological rejection.[3] "Bioinertness" was the underlying principle for these biomaterials and still holds true today for many implants.

With better understanding on the foreign body response in the 1980s and 1990s, there was a paradigm shift to develop bioactive components that can elicit biological bonding response at the bone–implant interface to improve implant fixation.[4] The ability to form an adherent interface with the living tissues has been defined as bioactivity.[5] Currently biocompatibility is the "ability of a material to perform with an appropriate host response in a specific application"; the "appropriate host response" refers to acceptable levels of toxicity and immune response, a lack of foreign body reactions, and promotion of normal healing.[6]

2.2.2 Nontoxicity

Materials that are embedded into the body should not have any toxic effect due to release of ions or other harmful products that can develop unnecessary allergies, inflammatory, tissue necrosis, calcification, or even neoplastic hazards.[7] Examples of the failure of this are silicone synovitis[8,9,10,11] or metallosis in hip joint replacements.[12,13]

Table 2.1 Criteria for ideal joint arthroplasty suggested by Swanson

- To maintain joint space
- To allow joint motion with stability
- To be of simple and efficient design
- To provide simple and durable fixation
- To be resistant to stress and deterioration
- To be biologically and mechanically acceptable to the host
- To be easy to manufacture, sterilize, and use
- To facilitate rehabilitation

2

2.2.3 Corrosion Resistance

Corrosion is unwanted degradation of metal immersed inside solution, which may result from electrochemical dissolution phenomenon, wear, or both. This property determines the metallic implant durability and should be very high if the implant is intended to be permanent. Passivation helps to protect metal from corrosion by forming a thin layer of oxide layer.[14]

2.2.4 Strength

Strength describes the magnitude of stress at which the materials begin to fracture and correspond to implant durability. It depends on the type and vector of the force applied to the material. It can be described by multiple values, for example, compressive strength, tensile strength, and yield strength.[15]

2.2.5 Modulus of Elasticity

The modulus of elasticity describes the ability of a material to undergo elastic deformation under stress. ▶ Table 2.2 provides the data of common biomaterials used in hand-and-finger joint arthroplasty.[16,17,18] A favorable value for implant anchorage or the intramedullary stem of an implant should be as close to that of cortical bone as possible. Otherwise, it will lead to stress shielding with bone resorption around the implant and the potential for bone–implant interface failure.[15,19]

2.2.6 Fatigue Resistance

Fatigue is caused by a repetitive cyclic load below that of ultimate tensile strength of a material eventually causing deformations and fatigue fracture. For metallic biomaterials, this is strongly related to the type of processing and heat treatment used during manufacturing.[20]

2.2.7 Wear Resistance

Low wear resistance is undesirable as it will produce wear particles into the articular or bone–implant interface, leading to an inflammatory reaction, osteolysis, and eventually implant loosening. Furthermore, corrosion will be accelerated and increase release of cytotoxic metal ions from worn implants.[21]

2.2.8 Creep Resistance

Creep refers to plastic deformation of a material over a long period of time under constant pressure. High resistance to creep is important to decrease the deformation and wear of the articular component of arthroplasty.[22] Creep is a material feature of bone cement and used by some implants such as the Exeter stem to optimize outcomes.

2.2.9 Osteointegration

Osteointegration refers to a direct structural and functional connection between living bone and the surface of a load-carrying part of the implant. It may depend on the surface topography of the implant.[23] It can be critical for prosthesis longevity. Many methods of surface treatment have been developed to promote osteointegration, including trying to produce an optimal surface roughness or adding osteoconductive coating to promote bone ingrowth.[24]

2.3 Classical Biomaterials

Four main types of biomaterials are currently used in clinical practice: polymers; metal alloys; ceramics; and pyrolytic carbon. Most of them were developed for the first generation of biomaterials typically developed from industrial purposes.

2.3.1 Polymers

Numerous classes of polymers have been used, e.g., silicone, polyethylene (PE), and polymethyl methacrylate (PMMA; bone cement).

Silicone

Swanson marked the start of modern era of small joint arthroplasty with the development of the silicon spacer in 1966.[1,25,26,27] Silicones also known as polysiloxanes are polymers composed of repeating siloxane units forming chains of alternating silicon and oxygen atoms (▶ Fig. 2.1). Silicone elastomers are created by three-dimensional (3D) cross-linking of linear silicone polymer chains. Chemical inertness, heat stability, and durability have led to its widespread use in medicine. Good biotolerance, high hydrophobic capacity, and ability to withstand various

Table 2.2 Modulus of elasticity of common biomaterials[10,11,12]

Material	Modulus of elasticity (GPa)
Cancellous bone	0.5–1.5
Cortical bone	7–30
Silicone elastomer	0.08
Ultrahigh-molecular-weight polyethylene	1.2
Polymethyl methacrylate bone cement	2.2
Titanium alloy (Ti6Al4V)	110
Stainless steel 316L	190
Cobalt chrome alloy	210
Pyrolytic carbon	13.7

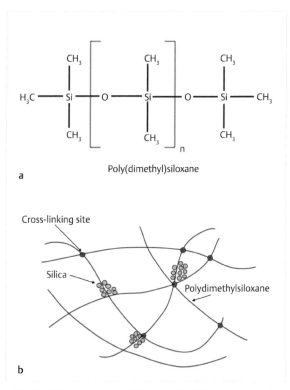

a
Poly(dimethyl)siloxane

b

Fig. 2.1 (a) Chemical structure of silicone. **(b)** Silicone elastomer matrix.

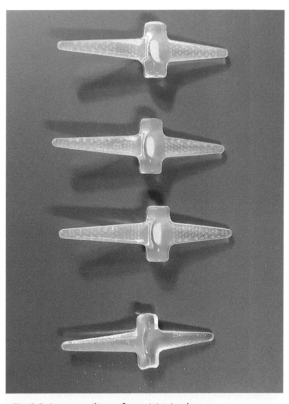

Fig. 2.2 Swanson silicone finger joint implants.

sterilization process are further benefits allowing use of silicone elastomers in implant arthroplasty.[26,28,29,30,31,32,33]

Hardening of silicone elastomers is by curing, a chemical process which adds curatives to induce polymer cross-linking.[29] Tensile strength is further enhanced by incorporation of "filler." Silicone elastomers for medical applications normally utilize amorphous silica filler to reinforce the cross-linked matrix. While mixing the silica with the silicone polymers, a hydrogen bond is formed between hydroxyl groups on the filler's surface and silicone polymer, resulting in higher tensile strength and better capacity to resist elongation (▶ Fig. 2.1).[34]

The original Swanson prosthesis was made from heat-vulcanized, medical-grade silicone elastomer stock. The prostheses are single-piece and formed in a mold at 121.1 °C under 22.8 kg/cm² of pressure.[1] Most silicone finger prostheses consist of intramedullary stems bridged by a hinge[26] (▶ Fig. 2.2). The inherent flexibility of the silicone elastomer allows flexion and extension at the hinge and provides dampening effect on the bone. At the same time, it is stiff enough to maintain some joint alignment. The long-term functional stability of silicone prostheses occurs by development of well-encapsulated fibrous capsule which starts to develop within 3 days of implantation.[32]

However, there are problems with the silicone elastomer implant. These include implant fracture, wear debris generation, and particulate synovitis.

Joyce et al analyzed the cause of silicone implant fracture by retrieving 12 Sutter metacarpophalangeal (MCP) prostheses from three patients.[35] They found that fractures generally occurred at the junction of the distal stem and hinge as a result of subluxing forces concentrated on MCP joint and flexion occurring at the stem rather than the hinge. In addition, the cortical bone of the proximal phalanx impinges on the dorsal surface of the distal stem of prosthesis. It is presumed that sharp spurs from the proximal phalangeal bone will produce small cuts over dorsal surface of the prostheses. With time, the crack propagates resulting in a fatigue fracture (▶ Fig. 2.3).[35,36] Two-thirds of silicone MCP joint prostheses fracture by 14 to 17 years after implantation.[37,38] Fortunately, by the time a fracture occurs, a fibrous pseudojoint is formed. The finger joint has some stability and often do not require revision surgery.[26]

During the process of abrasion and fatigue fracture, microscopic wear particles shed around the joint. This will stimulate proliferation and accumulation of mononuclear cells which will secrete cytokines and proteolytic enzymes, causing swelling and inflammation of pseudosynovial and synovial membranes. Persistent chronic synovitis can lead to fibrosis, osteolysis, and bone necrosis surrounding the prosthesis. Despite these downsides, silicone arthroplasty remains popular options in finger joint arthroplasty.

2

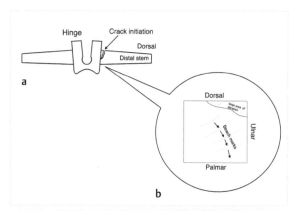

Fig. 2.3 Illustration showing the fatigue fracture site over the retrieved Sutter metacarpophalangeal prosthesis. **(a)** Site of fatigue fracture; **(b)** end on view over fatigue fracture site showing abrasion over dorsal site and crack propagation with beach mark. (See also Joyce et al 2003.[35])

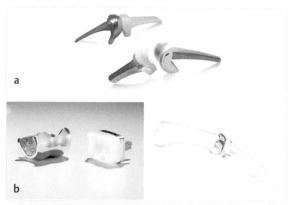

Fig. 2.4 Various designs for proximal interphalangeal (PIP) joint surface replacement implant: **(a)** SR MCP and PIP arthroplasty system (with courtesy of Stryker Corporation, USA). **(b)** CapFlex-PIP arthroplasty system (with courtesy of KLS Martin Group, Tuttlingen, Germany).

2.3.2 "Nouvelle Vague" for Hand Arthroplasty Development

Successes in total hip-and-knee arthroplasty were eye-catching. This led to the introduction of surface replacement into hand arthroplasty pioneered by Linscheid and Dobyns in 1979.[39]

The concept was trying to reproduce a physiological articulation and retain the collateral ligaments to improve stability and in turn minimize osteolysis and subsidence.[40] There is no single biomaterial that can replicate all the biomechanical properties of different structures inside the joint. By using two or more biomaterials with different characteristics in various parts of implant, it can more closely match the natural material properties. This resulted in a new surface replacement design with a cobalt-chrome proximal component and an ultrahigh-molecular-weight polyethylene (UHMWPE) distal component for a proximal interphalangeal (PIP) joint surface replacement implant (▶ Fig. 2.4).[39]

Ultrahigh Molecular Weight Polyethylene (UHMWPE)

Polyethylene (PE) has the advantage of easily being formed into many different shapes. It is mainly used coupled with a metallic component. It is formed from ethylene gas and is polymerized by Ziegler–Natta catalyst (titanium(III) chloride) into UHMWPE powder. The powder is consolidated under high temperatures and pressure. Because of its high melt viscosity, the final product is produced by compression molding and ram extrusion.[41]

UHMWPE is a high-density PE having a semicrystalline structure with a molecular mass more than 2,000,000 amu. The macromolecules consist of local ordered sheet-like crystalline lamellae embedded within amorphous regions and communicate with surrounding lamellae by tie molecules (▶ Fig. 2.5).[42] It has been extensively used in large joint arthroplasty because of its low friction, high resistance to wear, and high toughness.[43]

Medical-grade UHMWPE is free of calcium stearate and requirements are set according to the American Society for Testing and Materials (ASTM) 648–14.[44] Since the polymerization of UHMWPE requires a specialized production plant to handle the dangerous chemicals, there are only two companies capable of making these resins (▶ Table 2.3). Despite identical manufacturing methods, there are slight variations in molecular weight and resin morphology which affects their mechanical properties and wear abrasion resistance.[45]

The main factor responsible for UHMWPE failure in joint replacement is oxidative degradation. The presence of oxidation is related to the sterilization and storage methods. High-energy radiation such as gamma or electron beam radiation are the most commonly used sterilization methods for PE components.[46] A nominal dose of 25 to 40 kGy gamma radiation is commonly used, which will emit energy higher than that of the polymeric chemical bonds. This would generate the scission of some chemical bonds of the UHMWPE, and decrease its molecular mass. In the presence of oxygen, this will lead to the formation of free radicals, causing worsening of some chemical and physical material characteristics.[47,48,49] The oxidation process continues as long as there is an oxygen supply. This phenomenon is known as post-irradiation aging. It has been shown to occur in UHMWPE implants that were gamma sterilized in air and packaged in air-permeable packaging.[50,51,52] Decreased abrasive wear resistance, due to oxidation, leads to a decrease in mechanical properties such as abrasive wear resistance which results in the formation of wear debris and consequently osteolysis, which has been recognized as being the main cause of failure in orthopaedic implants.[53]

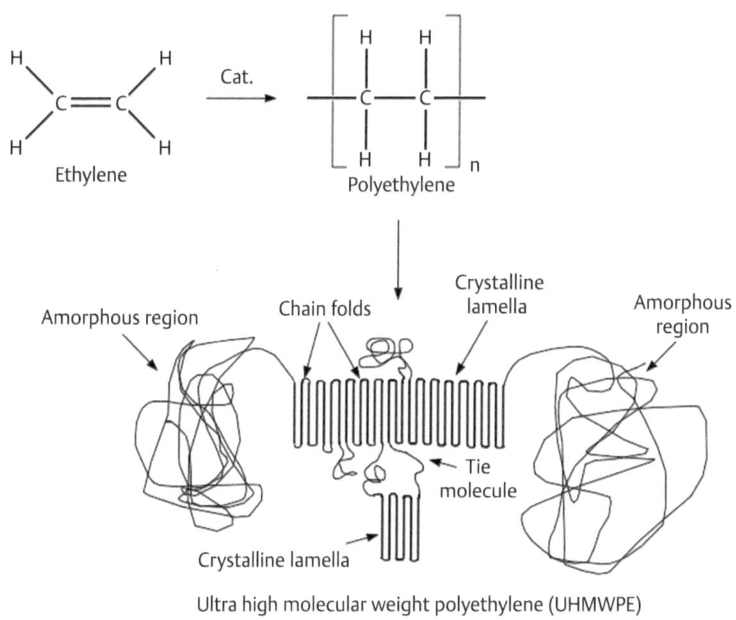

Fig. 2.5 Chemical structure of ultrahigh-molecular-weight polyethylene (UHMWPE).

Table 2.3 Physical properties of medical-grade ultrahigh-molecular-weight polyethylene resins

Properties	Type 1 GUR 1050	Type 2 GUR 1020	Type 3 1900[a]
Mean molecular weight ($\times 10^6$, g/mol)	3.5	5–6	>4
Particle size (mm)	140	140	300
Tensile modulus (MPa)	720	680	750
Impact strength (kJ/m^2)	>210	>130	>65
Yield stress (MPa)	>17	>17	19

[a]Type 3 1900 resin is no longer in the market.

To decrease the effect of oxidation on wear and the mechanical properties of UHMWPE, orthopaedic implant manufacturers modified their sterilization protocols aiming to reduce the amount of oxygen exposure during storage. These include gamma radiation sterilization in vacuum-packaging or inert-gas packaging. However, free radicals that are already present cannot be eliminated and in vivo oxidation is still possible.[54] Therefore, several methods have been attempted to improve the wear resistance of UHMWPE, including cross-linking, thermal treatment, and the addition of antioxidant vitamin E.

Cross-linking is achieved by formation of active sites at the chain ends, which can recombine to form trans-vinylene bonds.[55] This can be achieved by gamma radiation and the peroxide method. The wear rate of highly cross-linked UHMWPE is six times less than conventional UHMWPE.[56] These should allow manufacturers to produce thinner inserts that could be applied in hand arthroplasty. However, as the cross-linking density increases, elastic modulus, ultimate tensile strength, yield strength, and ductility reduce, which reflect the reason why cross-linked UHMWPE has less resistance to fatigue crack propagation.[56] Therefore, it is preferable to have optimal cross-linking density and keep it local to the surface to retain the bulk mechanical properties.[57]

To remove free radicals formed during the cross-linking or sterilization of UHMWPE, thermal treatment has been employed. Two common thermal treatments are remelting and annealing. Remelting is when the temperature is elevated above the melting point (150 °C), which allows free radicals trapped inside the crystalline region to diffuse out. Typically, the residual free radicals drop to undetectable level with this method.[54] But remelting has been shown to significantly reduce the degree of crystallinity, which affect the mechanical properties.[58,59] During annealing the temperature does not exceed the melting point, so the crystalline region does not undergo dissolution but this leaves measurable amounts of free radicals inside processed UHMWPE, which is still susceptive to in vivo oxidative degradation.[60,61]

Vitamin E is a natural antioxidant, which is able to consume the free radicals and improve wear resistance. Two methods of incorporation are currently used: one is to blend vitamin E (concentration less than 0.3 wt.-%) with UHMWPE powder before consolidation; and the other is to allow vitamin E to diffuse into the bulk UHMWPE. Vitamin E–containing UHMWPE has shown superior oxidative stability with greater mechanical and fatigue strength; these are now used clinically.[62,63,64]

Polymethylmethacrylate (PMMA)

Polymethylmethacrylate (PMMA) is commonly known as bone cement. It has been the material of choice for implant fixation to the host bone over 50 years, after being popularized by John Charnley in 1958.[65] The primary function of PMMA is transfer of weight-bearing forces from bone-toimplant and vice versa. The term "cement' is a misnomer because PMMA has no adhesive properties. Rather, it acts as a space-filler to create a close mechanical interlock between the rough medullary canal and the implant. This close association leads to optimal stress and interface strain energy distribution which are paramount in longevity of the implant. If the extreme stresses generated exceed the capability of the bone cement to transfer and absorb forces, fatigue fracture will result.

PMMA is an acrylic polymer that is formed by mixing liquid methyl methacrylate (MMA) monomer and a powdered MMA-styrene co-polymer. Benzoyl peroxide (BPO) in polymer powder acts as initiator while N,N-dimethyl *para*-toluidine (DMPT) or dimethyl *para*-toluidine (DMpt) in liquid monomer act as an accelerator for the free-radical polymerization reaction at room temperature (cold curing). To avoid premature polymerization of the liquid component during storage, hydroquinone is added as stabilizer (▶ Table 2.4).

Most of the commercial bone cements have a polymer powder/liquid monomer ratio of 2:1 (weight in g/volume in mL) in order to decrease the shrinkage level due to the density change in MMA-to-PMMA conversion during the polymerization. When mixed together, the reaction starts to take place between BPO initiator and the DMPT accelerator forming benzoyl free radicals at room temperature. These unstable free radicals start the initiation step of polymerization by forming a new chemical bond between the initiator fragment and one of the double carbon bonds of the monomer molecule. A new free radical is created on the activated monomer molecule which can react with the double carbon bond of a new monomer

molecule in the same way as the initiator fragment did. This process, known as propagation, takes place over and over again to form a long chain of monomeric units. Polymerization ceases when there is regrouping of the two radical chains leading to depletion of free radicals (▶ Fig. 2.6).[66]

The free-radical polymerization process of PMMA bone cement is a highly exothermic chemical reaction as a result of energy released from the breaking down of $C = C$ double bonds during polymer chain propagation. The invitro peak temperature can reach 110 °C. It is particularly influenced by the liquid monomer composition, the polymer powder/liquid monomer ratio, and the radioopacifier content.[67] Bone necrosis can occur when exposed to temperature of 50 °C for 1 minute or 47 °C for 5 minutes.[68] Although clinical studies have showed lower peak temperatures (40–47 °C) has detected at the bone interface, which may be due to a thinner cement coating and heat dissipation through the broad implant surface and local blood circulation.[69,70] However, thermal-induced bone necrosis has been shown in animal model study and the possibility of leading to early loosening and subsequent implant failure are still the concern.[71]

Various additives improve the workability of the polymer (▶ Table 2.4). To make the cement radiopaque, contrast agents such as barium sulfate ($BaSO_4$) or zirconia dioxide (ZrO_2) are added. Chlorophyll dye helps to distinguish bone cement from native bone and facilitate removal when performed revision surgery. Antibiotic-loaded bone cements are often used as drug-delivery systems. Implants are more susceptible to bacterial colonization on their surfaces because the bacteria can form a glycocalyx-blocking immune scrutiny by the body and leading to periprosthetic infection. The local active antibiotic levels are often not sufficient to reach a therapeutic dose when delivered by the intravenous route alone. When loaded with antibiotics, bone cement functions as carrier matrix and offers a synergistic effect with systemic antibiotics.[72] Many antibiotics has been added to PMMA bone cement clinically but

Table 2.4 Constituents of bone cement

Powder component		Liquid component	
Polymer	Polymethyl methacrylate	Monomer	Methyl methacrylate (MMA)
Initiator	Benzoyl Peroxide	Accelerator	N,N-Dimethyl *para*-toluidine (DMPT)/ Dimethyl *para*-toluidine (DMpt)
Radio-opacifier	Barium sulfate ($BaSO_4$)/Zirconia dioxide (ZrO_2)	Stabilizer	Hydroquinone
Antibiotics	Gentamicin sulfate Clindamycin hydrochloride Tobramycin Erythromycin-glucoheptonate Colistin-methane-sulfonate-sodium		
Additives	Dye (chlorophyll) Plasticizer (di-cyclo-hexyl phthalate)		

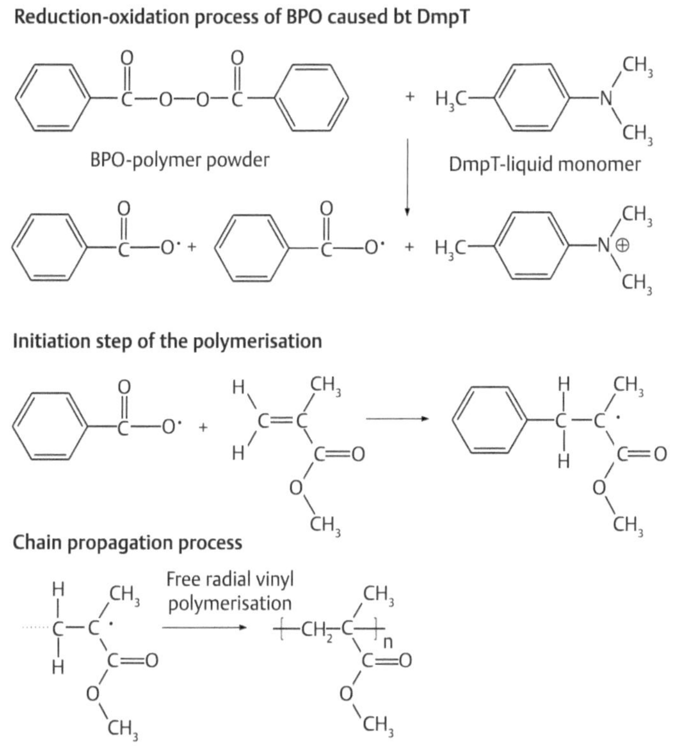

Reduction-oxidation process of BPO caused bt DmpT

Fig. 2.6 Chemical structure of polymethyl methacrylate (PMMA) and polymerization process of methyl methacrylate (MMA).

BPO-polymer powder   DmpT-liquid monomer

Initiation step of the polymerisation

Chain propagation process

Free radial vinyl polymerisation

Table 2.5 Factors that should be taken into account when selecting an antibiotic to incorporate into polymethyl methacrylate bone cement

Board antibacterial spectra

Good bactericidal effect at low concentrations

Low frequency of primary resistant bacteria

Low rate of developing bacteria resistance

Low protein bonding

Low probability of allergic reaction

Insignificant effect on cement performance

Chemically and thermally stable

Good solubility in water

Good rate of antibiotic release from bone cement

many factors including bacteriologic, physical, and chemical aspects need be assessed to optimize outcomes (▶ Table 2.5).[73]

During different stages of PMMA bone cement polymerization, the appearance and handling characteristics change. There are four different phases. The mixing phase is the period when thorough mixing of the powder and liquid component takes place. It can be mixed manually or with a commercially available mixing system with the ability to apply a vacuum to minimize the number of pores; this phase lasts around 1 minute. In the next (waiting) phase the viscosity of bone cement progressively increases to a condition that can be handled without sticking to surgical gloves; it lasts for several minutes. The bone cement surface often shows the distinctive change from a gloss to a matt appearance. The working phase is the period during which the surgeon can apply the cement and insert the prosthesis; this lasts around 2 to 4 minutes. The viscosity should be high enough to withstand the bleeding pressure but fluid enough to allow cement interdigitation into the surrounding cancellous bone. These two phases often depend on the type of cement and the handling temperature. Bone cement hardens when reaching the setting phase; this is the exothermic period with peak temperatures. The overall setting time, starts from the time of mixing liquid and powder to the time when the cement temperature drops to halfway between the ambient and maximum temperature; it usually lasts 8 to 10 minutes. Many factors can affect the setting time (▶ Table 2.6).[74,75,76]

Some of the designs of MCP and PIP joint surface replacement require cement to help to accommodate the variations in endosteal canal configuration and to restore proper alignment.[40] PMMA bone cement serves as a suitable material to fill up the defect between the implant and bone because of its excellent intraoperative workability. However, hand joint arthroplasty systems do not have any cement restrictor or cement gun to achieve pressurization, meaning there will be a less uniform and so weaker cement mantle that is prone to developing overstress. This may lead to cement fracture with release

Table 2.6 Various factors affecting mechanical properties of polymethyl methacrylate

Environmental temperature and humidity	An increase in the temperature or humidity leads to a decrease in the working phase
Powder(P)/Liquid(L) component ratio	A decrease in P/L ratio (i.e., more liquid added) leads to increased setting time
Mixing process	Vigorous mixing accelerates the dough time Vacuum mixing accelerates the setting time
Methods of application	Manual handling reduces the setting time

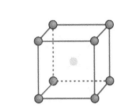 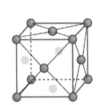 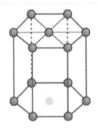

Fig. 2.7 Common metal crystalline arrangements: cubic body centered, cubic face centered, hexagonal.

Cubic body centered (bcc)
Fe,V, Nb, Cr

Cubic face centered (fcc)
Al,Ni, Ag, Cu, Au

Hexagonal
Ti, Zn, Mg, Cd

of cement particles which would induce a local inflammatory reaction and possibly periprosthetic osteolysis.[77]

Metals Alloys

Metals alloys are constituted from metallic and nonmetallic elements which are frequently used because of their mechanical strength. Most of the metals used for biomedical applications comply with the ISO 5832 standard. They mainly include three families of metals: stainless steel; cobalt chromium (CoCr) alloys; and titanium (Ti) alloys.[19] They have different mechanical properties and corrosion responses. All metal alloys are stiff, ductile, and hard. Appropriate metal selection for a specific application requires consideration of a variety of parameters.

Pure metal forms a crystalline lattice microstructure, i.e., a repeating 3D unit with a closely packed, high-density arrangement of metal atoms. They are packed into one of three crystalline arrangements: body-centered cubic, face-centered cubic, or hexagonal close packed (▶ Fig. 2.7). However, the units often do not combine perfectly and form clusters of grains, imprecisely aligned with each other. This causes imperfections within grain microstructure and defects in macrostructure known as scratches and voids. The size of the grains affects the mechanical properties of strength and isotropy on the materials. Biomechanically the larger the grain size, the earlier material fatigue and failure.[14]

Alloys are usually formed by adding the alloying metal elements to the principalmetal element in the molten state. When it solidifies, the metallic alloying elements, such as chromium and nickel in stainless steel, substitute for iron atoms in the crystalline lattice because of similar atomic sizes. When nonmetallic alloying elements are added, they are smaller and so fit in the spaces among the metal atoms. Deformation of the crystalline lattice occurs, which, in turn, causes resistance to the flow between crystal units leading to increase in resistance to plastic deformation and yield stress.[14]

Several steps are required to turn raw metal alloys into metallic components for joint prostheses. Casting is regularly used in manufacturing orthopaedic implants as it provides an efficient way for mass production that is difficult to achieve by machining. But the casting process produces large grains and metallurgical imperfections so they have lower mechanical properties than wrought or forged alloys. Forging is a manufacturing process to optimize material properties under pressure and classified as cold or hot working relative to its recrystallization temperature. Cold working increases the number and density of strains by plastic deformation at room temperature which makes it difficult to deform further. The yield strength increases but ductility decreases. Hot working is plastic deformation above the recrystallization temperature; it allows an increase in grain size which increases homogeneity and ductility. Sintering is the process of compacting and forming a solid mass of material by heat or pressure without reaching the melting point of the material. It can increase the mechanical strength of the material and is used for the shaping process of materials that have extremely high temperature. A summary of different techniques producing the metallic parts of joint prostheses from various alloys are listed in ▶ Table 2.7.[14,78,79,80]

Table 2.7 Techniques used to produce metallic biomaterials for arthroplasty

Technique	Stainless steels	COCr-based alloys	cP-Ti	Ti-based alloys
Casting	Not used	Investment casting	Difficult	Difficult
Machining	Possible	Difficult	Possible	Possible
Cold working	Rolling	Difficult	Rolling	Difficult
Hot working	Wrought, forged	Wrought, forged	Not used	Wrought, forged
Sintering	Possible	Hot isostatic pressing	Not used	Not used
Thermal treatments	Recrystallization	Precipitation hardening	Recrystallization	Precipitation hardening

Stainless Steel

Stainless steel was the first metal alloy used for orthopaedic implants. It normally comprises carbon and iron. If chromium is added, it will form a corrosion-resistant coating of oxide of CrO_3.[80] AISI 316 L is the mostly commonly used stainless steel in orthopaedics. The number 316 stands for 3% molybdenum and 16% of nickel added into the alloy and the letter "L" refers to low carbon content (less than 0.03%). The low carbon content improves corrosion resistance as carbon reacts with chromium to form brittle carbides, which exposes the metal to corrosion and subsequent failure.[14] Its superior fatigue strength at a relatively low cost and easy processing means it is used in many orthopaedic implants, e. g., plates and screws in trauma surgery. AISI 316 L stainless steel had relatively good corrosion resistance but when compared with CoCr and Ti alloys, it still has the disadvantage of being susceptible to crevice and pit corrosion. In addition, stainless steel has 200 GPa modules of elasticity, which is ten times stiffer than cortical bone. This modulus mismatch leads to peri-implant bone resorption and weakening of the implant bone interface, a phenomenon called stress shielding.[13,81,82] Currently, stainless steel is out of favor in manufacturing metallic components in joint arthroplasties.

Titanium Alloys

Titanium alloys were originally used in aeronautics and are now widely used in orthopaedic implants. Titanium 6Al4V is the most commonly used titanium alloy in orthopaedics. The number 6Al4V refers to the proportions of the alloying elements: aluminum (6%) and vanadium (4%). It has excellent corrosive resistance as it forms an oxide layer (TiO_2) on the surface by passivation. The modulus of elasticity is about 50% of stainless steel, making it less rigid so lessening the effect of stress shielding.[14] Moreover, titanium implants can osteointegrate into bone, which greatly increases the biocompatibility and long-term survival of the implant device.[83] However, titanium has the disadvantage of notch sensitivity, i. e., scratches or notching of the surface can lead to fatigue failure. It is also less resistant to particle-induced wear and cytotoxic vanadium ion release occurs; hence, titanium alloy cannot be used as a bearing surface.[80,84]

Cobalt Chrome Alloys

Cobalt chrome (CoCr) alloys contain cobalt (30–60%), significant amounts of chromium (20–30%) to improve the corrosion resistance, minor amounts of molybdenum which can decrease grain size in order to improve mechanical strength, as well as some carbon and nickel.[14,79] CoCr alloys exhibit excellent corrosion resistance, higher stiffness due to a higher modulus of elasticity (▶ Table 2.2), and good wear resistance which is suitable for manufacturing joint bearing surfaces as well as the stem of the prosthesis. However, on direct contact with bone, the CoCr implant will take up most of the load due to their high modulus of elasticity; the stress shielding effect will lead to bone resorption and failure of implant fixation.[83,84] In order to overcome the mismatch in modulus of elasticity between the alloy and cortical bone, PMMA bone cement is used to fix the CoCr implant to bone since the modulus of elasticity of PMMA bone cement is lower than that of CoCr alloy. Nonetheless there are problems with long-term implant stability as no bone ingrowth occurs onto the implant and loosening can occur when the cement mantle breaks down. In the view of this, cementless options have been developed that require a special surface treatment for the metallic implant surface.

2.3.3 Surface Treatment to Improve Bone Bonding

The need to improve the rate and area of cementless implant osteointegration has led to development of surface treatments. Two methods had been developed: porous coating and osteoconductive coating.

Application of porous coating onto cementless implants was introduced in the 1970s and may give better results than cemented implants due to superior osteophilicity and the osteointegration which leads to bone ingrowth onto the coated implants.[85,86] Based on the experiences borrowed from total hip-and-knee arthroplasty, there are several established methods to produce porous metallic coatings (▶ Table 2.8).

The roughness of the implant surface affects osteoblast adhesion and differentiation. Osteoblast-like cells grown

2

Table 2.8 Methods to create porous coating in cementless implant

Methods	Descriptions
Sintering	Placing powder or fines on the implant surface followed by heating up sufficient (90–95 % of melting point) to cause adherence of the coating material to implant surface. Mechanical properties can be impaired by high temperature and lead to low bond strength between the coating and implant.
Diffusion bonding	Similar to sintering but can be done at lower temperature (65–75 %) with application of pressure. So the changes in mechanical properties can be avoided. The welding process is achieved through migration of atoms across the joint due to concentration gradients.
Thermal spraying	Melted materials are sprayed onto a surface. It is an economical way to provide a high deposition rate and offer a wide range of coating thickness. However, this method is difficult to coat undercut and complex surfaces and induces decomposition as thermal spraying requires high temperatures and rapid cooling leads to amorphous coatings.
Plasma spraying	A type of thermal spraying that uses molten or heat softened metal powder or wire, injected into a very high temperature plasma flame and accelerated toward the implant in a high velocity. It can spray very high melting point materials such as refractory metals like tungsten and ceramics like zirconia unlike combustion processes. The hot material impacts on the substrate surface and rapidly cools forming a coating. The advantage of plasma spraying is that the coatings are generally much denser, stronger, and cleaner than the other thermal spray processes and the implant can be kept at low temperature during processing to avoid damage, metallurgical changes, and distortion to the substrate material.
Electron beam deposition	Form of physical vapor deposition in which the target is bombarded with an electron beam under high vacuum and the additive is normally brought under the beam spot as metal wire. This can produce a dense uniform film on the implant surface at low temperatures.

on rough titanium surfaces show reduced proliferation and enhanced osteogenic differentiation with upregulation of alkaline phosphatase (ALP) activity and the osteogenic differentiation marker osteocalcin.[87,88,89,90,91,92,93] This is likely to be mediated by integrin α2β1 with upregulation of a range of osteogenic growth factors including transforming growth factor 1 (TGF-1), prostaglandin E2 (PGE2), Wnt pathway agonist Dickkopf-related protein 2 (Dkk 2), vascular endothelial growth factor (VEGF), epidermal growth factor (EGF), and fibroblast growth factor (FGF).[93,94,95,96] In addition to their effect on osteoblasts, microrough surfaces also inhibit osteoclast activity by upregulating receptor activator of nuclear factor kappa-B ligand (RANKL) and decoy receptor osteoprotegerin (OPG) on osteoblasts which indirectly promote net bone deposition.[92,97]

Surface porosity allows direct osteogenic cells ingrowth onto the implant, strengthening the bone–implant interface. A number of research groups have investigated the effect of pore morphology and dimension, showing that pore size (50–400 µm), pore interconnectivity (75–100 µm), particle interconnectivity, volume fraction porosity (3–40 % for spherical beads), and the percentage area coated are factors that are important for porous coating fixation.[79]

Another method to promote osteointegration is to introduce osteoconductive materials onto the implants. This has developed around second-generation biomaterials. Bioactive materials have been added to uncemented components to enhance the fixation; calcium hydroxyapatite (HA) is the most popular additive biomaterial.

Calcium hydroxyapatite (HA)

Calcium hydroxyapatite is a ceramic. Ceramics are compounds of metallic elements bound ionically and covalently with nonmetallic elements. The calcium-to-phosphate ratio of HA resembles the minimal phase of bone, which accounts for their osteoconductive features.[98] Once HA is implanted in vivo, a layer of carbonate-hydroxyapatite (CO-HA) will develop on its surface as a result of ion exchange with the surroundings.[99,100,101,102] The resulting coating layer on the HA is known as carbonate-hydroxyapatite (CO-HA); it resembles the apatite present in normal bone.[103] The new apatite layer acts as a scaffold for osteoblasts and with time, it is further resorbed by osteoclasts and replaced by new bone.[101] Some studies have shown that HA-coated implants reduce the migration of components and have higher survival rate of comparable press-fit implants.[104] However, because of its low interface bonding strength and low toughness of the HA layer, it can result in fracture and delamination from the stem surface leading to osteolysis or third-body wear if the debris migrate into the joint space.[105] A different coating technique has been investigated with the aim to improve the interface bonding strength of the HA layer (▶ Table 2.8).[79]

2.3.4 Pyrolytic Carbon

Carbon is a nonmetallic tetravalent chemical element. The bonding pattern determines its physical form and differs widely. The best known allotropes include diamond, graphite, and amorphous carbon. Physical properties of carbon compounds vary as the flexibility of its valence electrons allows it to exhibit a spectrum of structural organization from haphazard carbon array stacking to complex but yet precise sequences.[106]

Pyrolytic carbon is a synthetic material and belongs to a group of carbon compounds known as turbostratic carbon. It lacks structural organization; it is formed by parallel layers of carbon without any particular spatial relationship. This arrangement provides pyrolytic carbon with a low modulus of elasticity whilst possessing high strength (▶ Fig. 2.8).

"Pyrolytic" derives from "Pyrolysis," which is the thermal decomposition of organic materials. Pyrolytic carbon is formed from pyrolysis of a hydrocarbon such as propane in the absence of oxygen. It is normally carried out in a fluidized-bed reactor under high temperatures (1000 °C; ▶ Fig. 2.9).[107] Without oxygen, hydrocarbon cannot decompose into carbon dioxide and water but breaks down into gas phase os nucleated droplets of carbon and hydrogen atoms. The carbon gas condenses and deposits as a thin coat over the implant. The resulting components are layered structures with pyrolytic carbon forming the outer shell of 0.5 mm thickness encasing an inner refractory substrate such as fine-grained graphite (▶ Fig. 2.9).

The choice of the implant substrate is very limited as the pyrolysis process takes place at a high temperature which would affect the mechanical properties of most metals. In addition, the thermal expansion coefficient of the implant substrate and pyrolytic carbon must be matched. Otherwise, upon cooling down to room temperature, the coating will be subjected to high stresses and

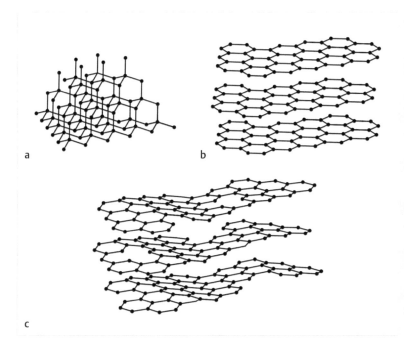

Fig. 2.8 Structures of different allotropes of carbon: **(a)** diamond, **(b)** graphite, **(c)** turbostratic pyrolytic carbon.

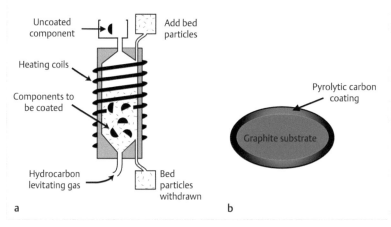

Fig. 2.9 (a) Fluidized-bed reactor schematics of pyrolytic carbon. **(b)** Cross-section of pyrolytic carbon implant.

2

cracks will develop. The articulating surfaces are polished to improve wear resistance; the stems are left unpolished to try to enhance bone apposition.[108]

Pyrolytic carbon was used initially in nuclear plants to coat the nuclear fuel kernels. Its use in orthopaedic implants started in 1983 as MCP joint arthroplasty after successful use in mechanical heart valves.[109,110] Many mechanical properties of pyrolytic carbon make it suitable for a variety of implant applications. The modulus of elasticity is similar to bone providing biomechanical compatibility and minimizing stress shielding at the bone–implant interface.[108,111] Fracture-crack initiation that occurs in metals does not exist in pyrolytic carbon. It is remarkably fatigue resistant such that the existence of a fatigue threshold is very nearly the single-cycle fracture strength; there are only a few pyrolytic carbon components that have fractured.[110,112,113,114] The wear resistance of pyrolytic carbon is excellent. Unlike metals and polymers, pyrolytic carbon will not develop degradation after cyclic loading and is able to bear large amount of elastic strain without deformation. In vivo testing for pyrolytic carbon bearing wear in PIP joint is negligible after 5 million cycles and ex vivo implant assessment showed similar findings.[115,116] Also, pyrolytic carbon shows excellent biocompatibility with cartilage. An animal study on assessment of cartilage wear with a different articulating surface material shows significantly lower gross cartilage wear, fibrillation, eburnation, glycosaminoglycan loss, and subchondral change with pyrolytic carbon than metallic surfaces.[117] Fibrocartilage regeneration of an opposing articular surface is seen in 86 % with pyrolytic carbon implants but only 25 % with CoCr alloy implants.[118] It is postulated that graphite-like pyrocarbon absorbs phospholipids on their surface without disrupting them. Surface active phospholipids produced by type-B synoviocytes act as cartilage lubricant and can act as an antiwear agent. One of the major components, dipalmitoylphosphatidylcholine has a strong affinity for pyrolytic carbon and explains its remarkable tribological properties in terms of lubrication and friction reduction between joint cartilage and its surface.[119] The excellent biocompatibility to cartilage has led to development of hemiarthroplasties and interpositional arthroplasty made by pyrolytic carbon.[118]

Unfortunately, there is no osteointegration or osteoinduction with pyrolytic carbon stems.[120] Bone fixation is made by means of apposition matching the stem of implant with the prepared medullary cavity. In theory, careful bone preparation to achieve optimal alignment to decrease stress and to maximize bone contact is needed to achieve long-lasting primary fixation. Around 80 % of cases result in mechanically less solid but macroscopically stable bone fixation by surrounding the implant with a fibrocartilage membrane.[121] High complication rate has been seen with pyrolytic carbon implants with radiographic lucency, loosening, and subsidence. One study has suggested that there is potential risk that the cancellous-bone support suffers fatigue failure in in the mid-to-longterm due to the strain increase with cyclic loads in daily hand activities. This risk appears much more important than the risk of bone resorption due to strainshielding.[122]

2.4 The Limitations of Current Materials

Despite better designs for hand joint arthroplasty, these implants still have limited ability to integrate with the surrounding bone. Thus the anchorage of implants may not be strong enough to stably hold the implants. Together with a large mismatch in the modulus of elasticity between bone and implant material, stress shielding can lead to peri-implant bone resorption. This will affect the longevity of the implanted arthroplasty.[123] For some implant materials, wear debris development is still a problem as it will elicit a foreign body reaction leading to osteolysis and aseptic loosening, although this is much less of a problem in the wrist and hand than for lower limb arthroplasties. If a perioperative infection occurs, bacterial colonization with adhesion to the implant surface covered by the glycocalyx often makes it impossible to eradicate the infection without removal of the infected implant.

2.5 Future of Biomaterials in Hand Arthroplasty

Since the introduction of joint arthroplasty in the hand, newer concepts and technology have developed. We see a paradigm shift in methods dealing with damaged hand joint, from replacing damaged tissue with permanent bioinert implants to a more biological approach by introducing bioactive components to elicit specific biological responses at the bone–implant interface. Newer third-generation biomaterials are now being developed, designed to encourage the responses at cellular and molecular levels.[124] Development of biodegradable 3D porous scaffolds in order to stimulate bone ingrowth by cell invasion and attachment is on the horizon.[125] Precise control of pore size, structural geometry, and composition requires advanced computer-aided design and 3D printing manufacturing techniques to generate highly defined hierarchical structure ideal for cell invasion.[126,127] Incorporation of growth factors, such as TGF-β2 and bone morphogenetic protein-2 (BMP-2), into the implant stem coating helps to trigger the body's inherent healing and repair capacity, which, in turn, should improve implant osteointegration.[128] Animal studies have demonstrated that biodegradable, drug-loaded chitosan-tripolyphosphate nanoparticles can successfully deliver biologically active BMP-2 on common implant materials like Ti6Al4V.[129] Manipulating the composition of the coating can offer new properties such as improving the antimicrobial efficacy. HA coatings can be altered by antibiotics or silver coverings to improve their antimicrobial efficacy and osseointegrative properties.[129,130,131]

2.6 Conclusion

Over the years, many different materials have been employed from different industrial applications into the development of hand joint arthroplasty. Greater understanding of the host response to implanted materials helps us to develop materials with better ability to interact with the biological environment. Interest in developing new biomaterials for orthopaedic implants will continue, either using novel materials, altering the formulations of existing materials, or finding new applications for existing materials. But we need to remain cautious in translating the invitro laboratory evaluation and animal studies results into clinical use.

References

[1] Swanson AB. Finger joint replacement by silicone rubber implants and the concept of implant fixation by encapsulation. Ann Rheum Dis. 1969; 28(5) Suppl:47–55

[2] Williams DF, Black J, Doherty PJ. Second consensus conference on definitions in biomaterials, Chester, England. In: Doherty PJ, Williams RF, Williams DF, Lee AJC, eds. Biomaterial–Tissue Interfaces. Advances in Biomaterials, Vol. 10. Amsterdam: Elsevier; 1992

[3] Hench LL. Biomaterials. Sci. 1980; 208:826–831

[4] Hench LL, Thompson I. Twenty-first century challenges for biomaterials. J R Soc Interface. 2010; 7 Suppl 4:S379–S391

[5] Shi D, ed. Introduction to Biomaterials. Beijing, China; Singapore; Hackensack, NJ: Tsinghua University Press; 2006

[6] Williams DF, ed. Definitions in Biomaterials. Proceedings of a Consensus Conference of the European Society for Biomaterials, Vol. 4. Chester, England, March 3–5, 1986. New York:Elsevier; 1987

[7] Adamovic D,Ristic B,Zivic F. Review of existing biomaterials—Method of material selection for specific applications in orthopedics. In: Zivic F, Affatato S, Trajanovic M, Schnabelrauch M, Grujovic N, Choy K, eds. Biomaterials in Clinical Practice. Cham: Springer; 2018: 47–99

[8] Peimer CA, Medige J, Eckert BS, Wright JR, Howard CS. Reactive synovitis after silicone arthroplasty. J Hand Surg Am. 1986; 11(5):624–638

[9] Atkinson RE, Smith RJ. Silicone synovitis following silicone implant arthroplasty. Hand Clin. 1986; 2(2):291–299

[10] Khoo CTK. Silicone synovitis:the current role of silicone elastomer implants in joint reconstruction. J Hand Surg [Br]. 1993; 18(6):679–686

[11] Foliart DE. Swanson silicone finger joint implants: a review of the literature regarding long-term complications. J Hand Surg Am. 1995; 20(3):445–449

[12] Korovessis P, Petsinis G, Repanti M, Repantis T. Metallosis after contemporary metal-on-metal total hip arthroplasty. Five to nine-year follow-up. J Bone Joint Surg Am. 2006; 88(6):1183–1191

[13] Ollivere B, Darrah C, Barker T, Nolan J, Porteous MJ. Early clinical failure of the Birmingham metal-on-metal hip resurfacing is associated with metallosis and soft-tissue necrosis. J Bone Joint Surg Br. 2009; 91(8):1025–1030

[14] Chatterjee S, Blunn G. Biomaterials. In: Ramachandran M, ed. Basic Orthopaedic Sciences: The Stanmore Guide. London: Hodder Education; 2006: 154–163

[15] Hudecki A, Kiryczyński G, Łos MJ. Biomaterials, definition, overview. In: Łos MJ, Hudecki A, Wiecheć E, eds. Stems Cells and Biomaterials for Regenerative Medicine. London, UK: Academic Press; 2019:85–98

[16] Li Y, Yang C, Zhao H, Qu S, Li X, Li Y. New developments of Ti-based alloys for biomedical applications. Materials (Basel). 2014; 7(3): 1709–1800

[17] Overview of Materials for Silicon Rubber. http://www.matweb. com/search/datasheettext.aspx?matguid = cbe7a469897a47eda563 816c86a73520. Accessed June 15, 2019

[18] Tian CL, Hetherington VJ, Reed S. A review of pyrolytic carbon: application in bone and joint surgery. J Foot Ankle Surg. 1993; 32(5): 490–498

[19] Mc Tighe T, Brazil D, Bruce W. Metallic alloys in total hip arthroplasty. In: Cashman J, Nitin G, Parvizi, eds. The Hip: Preservation, Replacement, and Revision. Data Trace Publishing Company; 2015:14.1–14.12

[20] Boretos JW, Eden M. Contemporary Biomaterials, Material and Host Response, Clinical Applications, New Technology and Legal Aspects. Park Ridge, NJ: Noyes Publications; 1984:232–233

[21] Singh R, Dahotre NB. Corrosion degradation and prevention by surface modification of biometallic materials. J Mater Sci Mater Med. 2007; 18(5):725–751

[22] Ashby MF, Jones DRH. Engineering Materials 1: An Introduction to Their Properties and Applications. Pergamon Press; 1980

[23] Brånemark PI. Osseointegration and its experimental background. J Prosthet Dent. 1983; 50(3):399–410

[24] Rigo ECS, Boschi AO, Yoshimoto M, Allegrini SJ, Konig BJ, Carbonari MJ. Evaluation in vitro and in vivo of biomimetic hydroxyapatite coated on titanium dental implants. Mater Sci Eng C. 2004; 24: 647–651

[25] Swanson AB. Silicone rubber implants for replacement of arthritis or destroyed joints in the hand. Surg Clin North Am. 1968; 48(5): 1113–1127

[26] Swanson AB. Flexible implant arthroplasty for arthritic finger joints: rationale, technique, and results of treatment. J Bone Joint Surg Am. 1972; 54(3):435–455

[27] Swanson AB. Implant resection arthroplasty of the proximal interphalangeal joint. Orthop Clin North Am. 1973; 4(4):1007–1029

[28] Murray PM. New-generation implant arthroplasties of the finger joints. J Am Acad Orthop Surg. 2003; 11(5):295–301

[29] Jerschow P. Silicone Elastomers. Shawbury, UK: Smithers Rapra; 2001

[30] Nalbandian RM, Swanson AB, Maupin BK. Long-term silicone implant arthroplasty:implications of animal and human autopsy findings. JAMA. 1983; 250(9):1195–1198

[31] Swanson AB, Nalbandian RM, Zmugg TJ, et al. Silicone implants in dogs:a ten-year histopathologic study. Clin Orthop Relat Res. 1984 (184):293–301

[32] DeHeer DH, Owens SR, Swanson AB. The host response to silicone elastomer implants for small joint arthroplasty. J Hand Surg Am. 1995; 20(3 Pt 2):S101–S109

[33] Poitout DG. Biomaterials used in orthopaedics. In: DG Poitout, ed. Biomechanics and Biomaterials in Orthopaedics. London: Springer-Verlag; 2016:13–19

[34] Lynch W. Handbook of Silicone Rubber Fabrication. New York, NY: Van Nostrand Reinhold; 1978

[35] Joyce TJ, Milner RH, Unsworth A. A comparison of ex vivo and in vitro Sutter metacarpophalangeal prostheses. J Hand Surg [Br]. 2003; 28(1):86–91

[36] Gillespie TE, Flatt AE, Youm Y, Sprague BL. Biomechanical evaluation of metacarpophalangeal joint prosthesis designs. J Hand Surg Am. 1979; 4(6):508–521

[37] Trail IA, Martin JA, Nuttall D, Stanley JK. Seventeen-year survivorship analysis of silastic metacarpophalangeal joint replacement. J Bone Joint Surg Br. 2004; 86(7):1002–1006

[38] Goldfarb CA, Stern PJ. Metacarpophalangeal joint arthroplasty in rheumatoid arthritis:a long-term assessment. J Bone Joint Surg Am. 2003; 85(10):1869–1878

2

[39] Linscheid RL, Dobyns JH. Total joint arthroplasty:the hand. Mayo Clin Proc. 1979; 54(8):516–526

[40] Linscheid RL, Murray PM, Vidal MA, Beckenbaugh RD. Development of a surface replacement arthroplasty for proximal interphalangeal joints. J Hand Surg Am. 1997; 22(2):286–298

[41] Kurtz SM. From ethylene gas to UHMWPE component: the process of producing orthopedic implants. Ultra-high molecular weight polyethylene in total joint replacement. In: Kurtz SM, ed.The UHMWPE Handbook. San Diego, CA: Academic Press; 2004:13–36

[42] Turell MB, Bellare A. A study of the nanostructure and tensile properties of ultra-high molecular weight polyethylene. Biomaterials. 2004; 25(17):3389–3398

[43] Zaribaf FP. Medical-grade ultra-high molecular weight polyethylene: past, current and future. Mater Sci Technol. 2018; 34(16):1940–1953

[44] American Society for Testing and Materials. ASTM F648-14 Standard Specification for Ultra-high-molecular Weight Polyethylene Powder and Fabricated Form for Surgical Implants. ASTM International; 2012

[45] Lancin P, Essner A, Yau SS, Wang A. Wear performance of 1900 direct compression molded, 1020 direct compression molded, and 1020 sheet compression molded UHMWPE under knee simulator testing. Wear. 2007; 263(7–12):1030–1033

[46] Bruck SD, Mueller EP. Radiation sterilization of polymeric implant materials. J Biomed Mater Res. 1988; 22(A2) Suppl:133–144

[47] McKellop H, Shen FW, Lu B, Campbell P, Salovey R. Effect of sterilization method and other modifications on the wear resistance of acetabular cups made of ultra-high molecular weight polyethylene:a hip-simulator study. J Bone Joint Surg Am. 2000; 82(12):1708–1725

[48] Costa L, Jacobson K, Bracco P, Brach del Prever EM. Oxidation of orthopaedic UHMWPE. Biomaterials. 2002; 23(7):1613–1624

[49] Brach del Prever E, Crova M, Costa L, Dallera A, Camino G, Gallinaro P. Unacceptable biodegradation of polyethylene in vivo. Biomaterials. 1996; 17(9):873–878

[50] Costa L, Bracco P. Mechanisms of crosslinking and oxidative degradation of UHMWPE. In: Kurtz SM,ed. The UHMWPE Handbook. Oxford, UK: William Andrew Publishing;2016:467–487

[51] Bracco P, Brunella V, Luda MP, del Prever EB, Zanetti M, Luigi C. Oxidation behaviour in prosthetic UHMWPE components sterilised with high-energy radiation in the presence of oxygen. Polym Degrad Stabil. 2006; 91(12):3057–3064

[52] Rimnac CM, Klein RW, Betts F, Wright TM. Post-irradiation aging of ultra-high molecular weight polyethylene. J Bone Joint Surg Am. 1994; 76(7):1052–1056

[53] Shaw JH. The Effect of Gamma Irradiation on Ultra High Molecular Weight Polyethylene. London:Medical Devices Agency, UK Department of Health;1997

[54] Kurtz SM, Muratoglu OK, Evans M, Edidin AA. Advances in the processing, sterilization, and crosslinking of ultra-high molecular weight polyethylene for total joint arthroplasty. Biomaterials. 1999; 20(18):1659–1688

[55] Muratoglu OK, Bragdon CR, O'Connor DO, Jasty M, Harris WH. A novel method of cross-linking ultra-high-molecular-weight polyethylene to improve wear, reduce oxidation, and retain mechanical properties. Recipient of the 1999 HAP Paul Award. J Arthroplasty. 2001; 16(2):149–160

[56] Muratoglu OK, Bragdon CR, O'Connor DO, et al. Unified wear model for highly crosslinked ultra-high molecular weight polyethylenes (UHMWPE). Biomaterials. 1999; 20(16):1463–1470

[57] Gul RM, Oral E, Muratoglu OK. Oxidation resistant peroxide crosslinked UHMWPE produced by blending and surface diffusion. In: IOP Conference Series: Materials Science and Engineering. IOP Publishing;2014;60(1):012015

[58] Slouf M, Synkova H, Baldrian J, et al. Structural changes of UHMWPE after e-beam irradiation and thermal treatment. J Biomed Mater Res B Appl Biomater. 2008; 85(1):240–251

[59] Jahan MS, Wang C, Schwartz G, Davidson JA. Combined chemical and mechanical effects on free radicals in UHMWPE joints during implantation. J Biomed Mater Res. 1991; 25(8):1005–1017

[60] Muratoglu OK, Bragdon CR. Highly cross-linked and melted UHMWPE. In: Kurtz SM,ed. The UHMWPE Handbook. Oxford, UK: William Andrew Publishing;2016:264–273

[61] Shen FW, McKellop HA. Interaction of oxidation and crosslinking in gamma-irradiated ultrahigh molecular-weight polyethylene. J Biomed Mater Res. 2002; 61(3):430–439

[62] Shibata N, Kurtz SM, Tomita N. Recent advances of mechanical performance and oxidation stability in ultrahigh molecular weight polyethylene for total joint replacement: highly crosslinked and α-tocopherol doped. J Biomechan Sci Eng. 2006; 1(1):107–123

[63] Bracco P, Oral E. Vitamin E-stabilized UHMWPE for total joint implants: a review. Clin Orthop Relat Res. 2011; 469(8):2286–2293

[64] Oral E, Wannomae KK, Hawkins N, Harris WH, Muratoglu OK. α-Tocopherol-doped irradiated UHMWPE for high fatigue resistance and low wear. Biomaterials. 2004; 25(24):5515–5522

[65] Charnley J. Anchorage of the femoral head prosthesis to the shaft of the femur. J Bone Joint Surg Br. 1960; 42-B:28–30

[66] Dunne N, Clements J, Wang JS. Acrylic cements for bone fixation in joint replacement. In: Revell PA, ed. Joint Replacement Technology. Cambridge, UK: Woodhead Publishing; 2014:212–256

[67] Dunne NJ, Orr JF. Curing characteristics of acrylic bone cement. J Mater Sci Mater Med. 2002; 13(1):17–22

[68] Lundskog J. Heat and bone tissue:an experimental investigation of the thermal properties of bone and threshold levels for thermal injury. Scand J Plast Reconstr Surg. 1972; 9:1–80

[69] Toksvig-Larsen S, Franzen H, Ryd L. Cement interface temperature in hip arthroplasty. Acta Orthop Scand. 1991; 62(2):102–105

[70] Kuehn KD, Ege W, Gopp U. Acrylic bone cements: composition and properties. Orthop Clin North Am. 2005; 36(1):17–28, v

[71] Berman AT, Reid JS, Yanicko DR, Jr, Sih GC, Zimmerman MR. Thermally induced bone necrosis in rabbits:relation to implant failure in humans. Clin Orthop Relat Res. 1984(186):284–292

[72] Hendriks JGE. Antibiotic Release from Bone Cement under Simulated Physiological Conditions. University Library Groningen; 2003

[73] Breusch SJ, Kühn KD. Bone cements based on polymethylmethacrylate. Orthopade. 2003; 32(1):41–50

[74] Hosseinzadeh HRS, Emami M, Lahiji F, Shahi AS, Masoudi A, Emami S.The acrylic bone cement in arthroplasty. In: Kinov P, ed. Arthroplasty-Update. IntechOpen; 2013

[75] Ranjan RK, Kumar M, Kumar R, Ali MF. Bone cement. Int J Orthopaed Sci. 2017; 3(4):79–82

[76] Vaishya R, Chauhan M, Vaish A. Bone cement. J Clin Orthop Trauma. 2013; 4(4):157–163

[77] Goldring SR, Jasty M, Roelke MS, Rourke CM, Bringhurst FR, Harris WH. Formation of a synovial-like membrane at the bone-cement interface:its role in bone resorption and implant loosening after total hip replacement. Arthritis Rheum. 1986; 29(7):836–842

[78] del Prever EMB, Costa L, Baricco M, Piconi C, Massé A. Biomaterials for total joint replacements. In: Poitout DG, ed. Biomechanics and Biomaterials in Orthopedics. London, UK: Springer; 2016:59–70

[79] Kaivosoja E, Tiainen VM, Takakubo Y,et al. Materials used for hip and knee implants. In: Affatato S, ed. Wear of Orthopaedic Implants and Artificial Joints. Woodhead Publishing Series in Biomaterials. Woodhead Publishing; 2013: 178–218

[80] Navarro M, Michiardi A, Castaño O, Planell JA. Biomaterials in orthopaedics. J R Soc Interface. 2008; 5(27):1137–1158

[81] Bauer TW, Schils J. The pathology of total joint arthroplasty.II. Mechanisms of implant failure. Skeletal Radiol. 1999; 28(5):483–497

[82] Huiskes R, Weinans H, van Rietbergen B. The relationship between stress shielding and bone resorption around total hip stems and the effects of flexible materials. Clin Orthop Relat Res. 1992(274):124–134

[83] Breine U, Johansson B, Roylance PJ, Roeckert H, Yoffey JM, Yoffey JM. Regeneration of bone marrow: a clinical and experimental study following removal of bone marrow by curettage. Acta Anat (Basel). 1964; 59:1–46

[84] Brown RP, Fowler BA, Fustinoni S, Nordberg M. Toxicity of metals released from implanted medical device. In: Nordberg GF, Fowler BA, Nordberg M, eds. Handbook on the Toxicology of Metals. London, UK: Academic Press; 2014:113–122

[85] Froimson MI, Garino J, Machenaud A, Vidalain JP. Minimum 10-year results of a tapered, titanium, hydroxyapatite-coated hip stem: an independent review. J Arthroplasty. 2007; 22(1):1–7

[86] Junker R, Dimakis A, Thoneick M, Jansen JA. Effects of implant surface coatings and composition on bone integration: a systematic review. Clin Oral Implants Res. 2009; 20 Suppl 4:185–206

[87] Schwartz Z, Lohmann CH, Oefinger J, Bonewald LF, Dean DD, Boyan BD. Implant surface characteristics modulate differentiation behavior of cells in the osteoblastic lineage. Adv Dent Res. 1999; 13:38–48

[88] Lincks J, Boyan BD, Blanchard CR, et al. Response of MG63 osteoblast-like cells to titanium and titanium alloy is dependent on surface roughness and composition. Biomaterials. 1998; 19(23):2219–2232

[89] Batzer R, Liu Y, Cochran DL, et al. Prostaglandins mediate the effects of titanium surface roughness on MG63 osteoblast-like cells and alter cell responsiveness to 1 α,25-(OH)2D 3. J Biomed Mater Res. 1998; 41(3):489–496

[90] Boyan BD, Batzer R, Kieswetter K, et al. Titanium surface roughness alters responsiveness of MG63 osteoblast-like cells to 1 α,25-(OH) 2D 3. J Biomed Mater Res. 1998; 39(1):77–85

[91] Kieswetter K, Schwartz Z, Hummert TW, et al. Surface roughness modulates the local production of growth factors and cytokines by osteoblast-like MG-63 cells. J Biomed Mater Res. 1996; 32(1):55–63

[92] Lossdörfer S, Schwartz Z, Wang L, et al. Microrough implant surface topographies increase osteogenesis by reducing osteoclast formation and activity. J Biomed Mater Res A. 2004; 70(3):361–369

[93] Olivares-Navarrete R, Hyzy SL, Hutton DL, et al. Direct and indirect effects of microstructured titanium substrates on the induction of mesenchymal stem cell differentiation towards the osteoblast lineage. Biomaterials. 2010; 31(10):2728–2735

[94] Raines AL, Olivares-Navarrete R, Wieland M, Cochran DL, Schwartz Z, Boyan BD. Regulation of angiogenesis during osseointegration by titanium surface microstructure and energy. Biomaterials. 2010; 31 (18):4909–4917

[95] Olivares-Navarrete R, Raz P, Zhao G, et al. Integrin α2β1 plays a critical role in osteoblast response to micron-scale surface structure and surface energy of titanium substrates. Proc Natl Acad Sci U S A. 2008; 105(41):15767–15772

[96] Wang L, Zhao G, Olivares-Navarrete R, et al. Integrin β1 silencing in osteoblasts alters substrate-dependent responses to 1,25-dihydroxy vitamin D 3. Biomaterials. 2006; 27(20):3716–3725

[97] Khosla S. Minireview: the OPG/RANKL/RANK system. Endocrinology. 2001; 142(12):5050–5055

[98] Murshed M, Harmey D, Millán JL, McKee MD, Karsenty G. Unique coexpression in osteoblasts of broadly expressed genes accounts for the spatial restriction of ECM mineralization to bone. Genes Dev. 2005; 19(9):1093–1104

[99] Wongwitwichot P, Kaewsrichan J, Chua KH, Ruszymah BH. Comparison of TCP and TCP/HA hybrid scaffolds for osteoconductive activity. Open Biomed Eng J. 2010; 4:279–285

[100] Daculsi G, LeGeros RZ, Nery E, Lynch K, Kerebel B. Transformation of biphasic calcium phosphate ceramics in vivo: ultrastructural and physicochemical characterization. J Biomed Mater Res. 1989; 23(8):883–894

[101] Daculsi G, Laboux O, Malard O, Weiss P. Current state of the art of biphasic calcium phosphate bioceramics. J Mater Sci Mater Med. 2003; 14(3):195–200

[102] Heughebaert M, LeGeros RZ, Gineste M, Guilhem A, Bonel G. Physicochemical characterization of deposits associated with HA ceramics implanted in nonosseous sites. J Biomed Mater Res. 1988; 22(3) Suppl:257–268

[103] Barrère F, van Blitterswijk CA, de Groot K. Bone regeneration: molecular and cellular interactions with calcium phosphate ceramics. Int J Nanomedicine. 2006; 1(3):317–332

[104] Søballe K, Toksvig-Larsen S, Gelineck J, et al. Migration of hydroxyapatite coated femoral prostheses:a Roentgen Stereophotogrammetric study. J Bone Joint Surg Br. 1993; 75(5):681–687

[105] D'Angelo F, Molina M, Riva G, Zatti G, Cherubino P. Failure of dual radius hydroxyapatite-coated acetabular cups. J Orthop Surg Res. 2008; 3:35

[106] Bokros JC. Carbon biomedical devices. Carbon. 1977; 15(6):353, 355–371

[107] Stanley J, Klawitter J, More R. Replacing joints with pyrolytic carbon. In: Revell PA, ed. Joint Replacement Technology. Cambridge, UK: Woodhead Publishing; 2008:631–656

[108] More RB, Haubold AD, Bokros JC. Pyrolytic carbon for long-term medical implants. In: Ratner B, Hoffman A, Schoen F, Lemons J, eds. Biomaterials Science: An Introduction to Materials in Medicine. London, UK: Elsevier Academic Press; 2004:170–180

[109] Beckenbaugh RD. Preliminary experience with a noncemented noncontrained total joint arthroplasty for the metacarpophalangeal joints. Orthopedics. 1983; 6(8):962–965

[110] Haubold AD. On the durability of pyrolytic carbon in vivo. Med Prog Technol. 1994; 20(3–4):201–208

[111] Reilly DT, Burstein AH. Review article:the mechanical properties of cortical bone. J Bone Joint Surg Am. 1974; 56(5):1001–1022

[112] Gilpin CB, Haubold AD, Ely JL. Fatigue crack growth and fracture of pyrolytic carbon composites. In: Ducheyne P, Christiansen D, eds. Bioceramics.1993;6(1):217–223

[113] Ma L, Sines G. Fatigue behavior of a pyrolytic carbon. J Biomed Mater Res. 2000; 51(1):61–68

[114] Beavan LA, James DW, Kepner JL. Evaluation of fatigue in pyrolite carbon. In: Ducheyne P, Christiansen D, eds. Bioceramics. 1993;6 (1):205–210

[115] Naylor A, Bone MC, Unsworth A, Talwalkar SC, Trail IA, Joyce TJ. In vitro wear testing of the PyroCarbon proximal interphalangeal joint replacement: five million cycles of flexion and extension. Proc Inst Mech Eng H. 2015; 229(5):362–368

[116] Bone MC, Giddins G, Joyce TJ. An analysis of explanted pyrolytic carbon prostheses. J Hand Surg Eur Vol. 2014; 39(6):666–667

[117] Cook SD, Thomas KA, Kester MA. Wear characteristics of the canine acetabulum against different femoral prostheses. J Bone Joint Surg Br. 1989; 71(2):189–197

[118] Kawalec JS, Hetherington VJ, Melillo TC, Corbin N. Evaluation of fibrocartilage regeneration and bone response at full-thickness cartilage defects in articulation with pyrolytic carbon or cobalt-chromium alloy hemiarthroplasties. J Biomed Mater Res. 1998; 41 (4):534–540

[119] Gale LR, Coller R, Hargreaves DJ, Hills BA, Crawford R. The role of SAPL as a boundary lubricant in prosthetic joints. Tribol Int. 2007; 40(4):601–606

[120] Daecke W, Veyel K, Wieloch P, Jung M, Lorenz H, Martini AK. Osseointegration and mechanical stability of pyrocarbon and titanium hand implants in a load-bearing in vivo model for small joint arthroplasty. J Hand Surg Am. 2006; 31(1):90–97

[121] Ross M, James C, Couzens G, Klawitter J. Pyrocarbon small joint arthroplasty of the extremities. In: Revell PA, ed. Joint Replacement Technology. Cambridge, UK: Woodhead Publishing; 2014:628–673

[122] Completo A, Nascimento A, Girão AF, Fonseca F. Biomechanical evaluation of pyrocarbon proximal interphalangeal joint arthroplasty: an in-vitro analysis. Clin Biomech (Bristol, Avon). 2018; 52:72–78

[123] Conolly WB, Rath S. Silastic implant arthroplasty for post-traumatic stiffness of the finger joints. J Hand Surg [Br]. 1991; 16(3):286–292

[124] Ratner BD, Bryant SJ. Biomaterials: where we have been and where we are going. Annu Rev Biomed Eng. 2004; 6:41–75

[125] Agrawal CM, Ray RB. Biodegradable polymeric scaffolds for musculoskeletal tissue engineering. J Biomed Mater Res. 2001; 55(2):141–150

[126] Hutmacher DW, Sittinger M, Risbud MV. Scaffold-based tissue engineering: rationale for computer-aided design and solid free-form fabrication systems. Trends Biotechnol. 2004; 22(7):354–362

[127] Trauner KB. The emerging role of 3D printing in arthroplasty and orthopedics. J Arthroplasty. 2018; 33(8):2352–2354

[128] Zhang BG, Myers DE, Wallace GG, Brandt M, Choong PF. Bioactive coatings for orthopaedic implants-recent trends in development of implant coatings. Int J Mol Sci. 2014; 15(7):11878–11921

[129] Poth N, Seiffart V, Gross G, Menzel H, Dempwolf W. Biodegradable chitosan nanoparticle coatings on titanium for the delivery of BMP-2. Biomolecules. 2015; 5(1):3–19

[130] Motoc MM, Axente E, Popescu C, et al. Active protein and calcium hydroxyapatite bilayers grown by laser techniques for therapeutic applications. J Biomed Mater Res A. 2013; 101(9):2706–2711

[131] Roy M, Fielding GA, Be, yenal H, Bandyopadhyay A, Bose S. Mechanical, in vitro antimicrobial, and biological properties of plasma-sprayed silver-doped hydroxyapatite coating. ACS Appl Mater Interf. 2012; 4(3):1341–1349

3 Proprioception and Neural Feedback in Thumb and Wrist Arthroplasty

Elisabet Hagert and Susanne Rein

Abstract

Proprioception is defined as the conscious and unconscious sensations regulating posture, motion, and joint control. With regard to joint control, proprioception includes the senses of joint position and motion (kinesthesia) as well as feed-forward control. The foundation for a normal joint proprioception includes an intact mechanoreceptor innervation and afferent feedback to the spinal cord and the muscles controlling a joint. In the past decade, ample studies have detailed the mechanoreceptor innervation of the wrist, basal thumb and distal radioulnar joints. In addition, studies on joint reflexes have highlighted the existence of ligamento-muscular reflex arcs to provide both immediate, joint protective, control, as well as slower reflex response for muscle coordination.

In patients with advanced osteoarthritis, however, the innervation pattern in ligamens and synovium is altered, indicating a change in proprioceptive ability and a pattern of pain and inflammation rather than proprioception.

As clinicians, we are of course faced with a challenge when it comes to preserving innervation, but at the same time provide adequate pain relief to our patients. In this chapter, the foundation for hand and wrist proprioception is outlined, with a discussion on the considerations for our patients in need of joint arthroplasty.

Keywords: Joint position sense, kinesthesia, ligament, neuromuscular control, proprioception, sensory nerve endings

> Essential to a great discoverer, in any field of Nature, would seem an intuitive flair for raising the right question. To ask something which the time is not ripe to answer is of small avail. There must be the means for reply and enough collateral knowledge to make the answer worthwhile.
>
> — Sir Charles Scott Sherrington

3.1 Basis of Proprioception for Joint Control

The quote by Sir Charles Scott Sherrington reflects the groundbreaking work that he produced in the early 1900s regarding neuroscience and proprioception; work which led to his Nobel Prize Award in Physiology or Medicine in 1932. His definition of proprioception in 1906 was: "sensations arising in the deep areas of the body, contributing to conscious sensations (*muscle sense*), total posture (*postural equilibrium*), and segmental posture (*joint stability*)."[1] Sherrington went on to further describe these senses as arising from "*receptors in skin, joints and muscles.*"[1] Based on his work more than a hundred years ago, the study of proprioception with regard to joint control has come to fruition in the past two to three decades.[2] As Sherrington said above, there must be "the means for reply and enough collateral knowledge to make the answer worthwhile." What we know today, through global collateral research efforts, is that the proprioception senses may be divided into conscious and unconscious senses (▶ Fig. 3.1), and that these both work in an integrated manner to provide joint control and neuromuscular stability.

3.1.1 Conscious Proprioception Senses

The conscious senses include somatosensory appreciation of touch and motion. For the former, the senses included are primarily tactility, vibration, and pain as arising from receptors in the skin. The latter include kinesthesia (the sense of joint motion), joint position sense, and the sense of muscle force and tension. The origin of the conscious joint proprioception senses is found in skin, muscle, and joint receptors. Skin receptors are primarily of importance in the kinesthesia of finger joints,[3] since the muscles controlling the fingers are located at a distance, in the forearm and hand. Joint receptors are similarly thought to be of importance whenever a muscle traverses more than one major joint,[4] thus limiting the sensitivity of the muscle spindle in detecting motion.

3.1.2 Unconscious Proprioception Senses

The unconscious proprioception senses are the senses related to neuromuscular control of posture, joint stability, and complex-coordinated muscle action, so called feed-forward control.[5,6] Unconscious joint proprioception is primarily influenced by receptors in ligaments and joint capsule, where afferent information from these highly specialized nerve-endings create spinal reflexes for immediate joint control as well as signals to the cerebellum for advanced motor control and planning/execution of joint stability and neuromuscular control.[7,8] To understand the complexity of wrist-and-hand joint proprioception, a

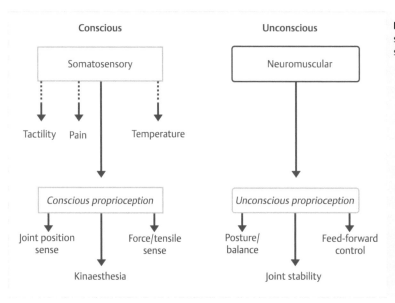

Fig. 3.1 A graphic illustration of the conscious and unconscious proprioceptive senses.

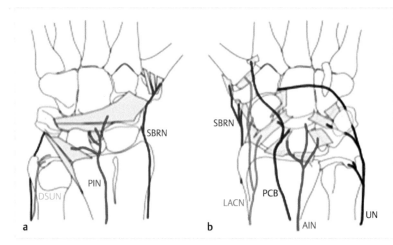

Fig. 3.2 The innervation of the dorsal (**a**) and volar (**b**) wrist, distal radioulnar, and trapeziometacarpal joints: the dorsal sensory branch of the ulnar nerve (DSUN); the posterior interosseous nerve (PIN); the sensory branch of the radial nerve (SBRN); the lateral antebrachial cutaneous nerve (LACN); the palmar cutaneous branch (PCB) of the median nerve; the anterior interosseous nerve (AIN); and the ulnar nerve (UN).

description of sensory nerve endings and their distribution in the wrist and hand will follow.

3.1.3 Sensory Nerve Endings

The innervation of ligaments is characterized by specific sensory nerve endings, which can be classified due to their typical shape (▶ Fig. 3.2) and neurophysiological traits (▶ Table 3.1) according to Freeman and Wyke,[9] modified by Hagert.[10] Sensory nerve endings react to mechanical stimuli, e.g., extremes of ranges of motion, transform them into neural excitations, send this information from the joint via afferent nerves and dorsal root ganglia to the spinal cord, where one part of the information is send to the cerebellum and the cortex, and the other part of the information is used for local or segmental polysynaptic interactions.[6]

According to the classification by Erlanger and Gasser[11] as well as Lloyd[12] and Hunt[13] for afferent and efferent nerve fibers (▶ Table 3.1), the afferents, Ruffini endings, and Pacini corpuscles are myelinated group II and Aβ fibers with nerve conduction velocities of 36 to 72 m/s. Golgi-like endings of the periarticular tissue belong to group II, whereas the originally described Golgi tendon organs of the myotendinous junction are group Ib fibers. The afferents of free nerve endings are either thin myelinated group III and Aδ fibers with a conduction velocity between 4 and 36 m/s or unmyelinated group IV and C fibers with conduction velocities of 0.4 to 2 m/s.[14]

Ruffini Endings

In the late 19th century the Italian histologist Angelo Ruffini[15] described this nerve ending in the skin, which is

Table 3.1 Classification of sensory nerve endings in ligaments

Type	Name	Morphology	Neurophysiological trait	Erlanger/ Gasser	Lloyd/ Hunt	Proprioceptive function	Histological features
I	Ruffini	Dendritic terminal nerve endings, partial or thin encapsulation 50–120 μm	Slowly adapting Low-threshold	A-β	II	Static joint position, kinesthesia changes in velocity/ amplitude	Central axon: PGP9.5, S 100 Capsule: p75 Dendritic nerve endings: S 100, p75, PGP 9.5
II	Pacini	Thick lamellar onion-layered capsule 20–150 μm	Rapidly adapting Low-threshold	A-β	II	Joint acceleration/ deceleration	Central axon: S 100, (PGP 9.5) Capsule: p75
III	Golgi-like	Large spindle-shaped body, thin capsule, small grouped corpuscles within the large corpuscle >150 μm	Rapidly adapting High-threshold	A-β	II	Extreme range of joint motion	Terminal nerve branches: S 100, PGP 9.5 Capsule: p75
IV	Free nerve endings	Often closed to blood vessels, groups, or single fibers	Nonadaptive	A-δ C	III IV	Noxious chemical or mechanical, nocicep-tive or inflammatory stimuli	Axons: S 100, PGP 9.5 Schwann cells: p75
V	Unclassifiable	Variable	Unknown	Unknown	Unknown	Unknown	Variable

Note: The classification of mechanoreceptors in ligaments is based on Freeman and Wyke,[9] modified by Hagert,[10] which characterize the morphology and neurophysiological traits of the various corpuscles. The nerve fiber group classification according to Erlanger and Gasser[11] applies to both, sensory (afferent) and motor (efferent) nerve fibers, whereas the second classification, described by Lloyd[12] and Hunt,[13] applies only to sensory (afferent) nerve fibers.

named after him. Synonyms for this corpuscle are dendritic or spray ending.

Microneurographic recordings from Ruffini endings in cat knee intracapsular ligaments have been shown to be slowly adapting low-threshold receptors that constantly respond during joint movement.[16] Ruffini endings detect static joint position, intra-articular and atmospheric pressure changes, as well as the direction, amplitude, and speed of active and passive joint movement. They respond to axial load and tension, but not to vertical compressive joint forces, highlighting their importance in specifying joint position and rotation. This is required for the regulation of periarticular muscle contracture and neuromuscular joint control.[17]

Pacini Corpuscles

Although Pacini corpuscles are mentioned for the first time by Johannes Gottlieb Lehmann[18] in his doctoral thesis in 1741 and in the same year by the German anatomist and botanist Abraham Vater,[19] this discovery was forgotten for nearly a century.[20] The Italian anatomist Filippo Pacini[21] rediscovered this corpuscle in 1835, which was subsequently named after him. Pacinian corpuscles are fast adapting receptors with a low excitation threshold, which respond to joint accelerations and decelerations.[22]

Golgi-like Endings

The Italian anatomist Camillo Golgi[23] discovered this sensory nerve ending initially as the *"Golgi tendon organ"* in the myotendinous junction in 1878. Named after him, the Golgi-like ending, which is found in ligaments, is a type of spray ending, which originates from the same family as Ruffini endings. Golgi-like endings are slow-adapting receptors, which, in contrast to Ruffini endings, have a high threshold for mechanical stress, making them completely inactive in immobile joints, but important for the detection of extremes of ranges of motion.[24]

Free Nerve Endings

Free nerve endings are nonadaptive high-threshold nociceptors, which respond to different stimuli, e.g., chemical, mechanical, harmful, or inflammatory stimuli. They are mainly located in the interstitium of the densely packed collagen fibers, in the epiligament layer, and in the vicinity of blood vessels.[25,26]

Unclassifiable Corpuscles

Corpuscles, which cannot be classified as Ruffini, Pacini, Golgi-like endings, or free nerve endings, are regarded as unclassifiable corpuscles, type V.[10] The function and

3

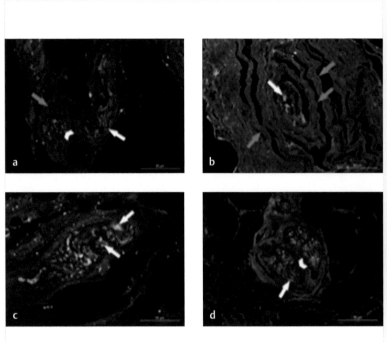

Fig. 3.3 Sensory nerve endings. Simultaneous immunofluorescence imaging of a **(a)** Ruffini ending, **(b)** a Pacini corpuscle, **(c)** a Golgi-like endings, and **(d)** a free nerve ending, stained with protein gene product (PGP) 9.5, S 100 protein, neurotrophin receptor p75, and 4',6 -diamidino-2-phenylindole (DAPI). **(a)** Characteristic dendritic terminal nerve endings are found in Ruffini endings (arrowhead), which are immunoreactive to PGP 9.5, S 100, and p75. The capsule of the Ruffini endings is immunoreactive for p75 (grey arrow). The afferent central axon is clearly visible (white arrow). **(b)** The Pacinian corpuscle has a typical onion-layered capsule, which is immunoreactive for p75 (grey arrows); however, the central axon is immunoreactive for S 100 (white arrow). **(c)** The large Golgi-like ending contains smaller, grouped corpuscles, which are immunoreactive for S 100, p75, and PGP 9.5, within the Golgi-like ending (white arrows). **(d)** Axons of free nerve endings are immunoreactive for PGP 9.5 and S 100 (arrow); their nerve sheaths are immunoreactive for p75 (arrowhead). Original magnification 400 ×.

physiological properties of nonclassifiable corpuscles are currently unknown.

3.2 Innervation Patterns (▶ Fig. 3.3)

3.2.1 Wrist

Articular branches of the radial, ulnar (UN), median, and musculocutaneous nerves are the main contributors to wrist joint innervation.[27] The radial aspect of the radiocarpal joint is innervated by the lateral antebrachial cutaneous nerve (LACN), which is a terminal sensory branch of the musculocutaneous nerve.[28] The central two-thirds of the volar wrist capsule and the volar parts of the scapholunate interosseous ligament (SLIL) are innervated by the anterior interosseous nerve (AIN).[29,30] The palmar cutaneous branch (PCB) of the median nerve innervates the volar midcarpal area.[28] The triangular fibrocartilage complex (TFCC) is mainly innervated by the UN, including branches from the dorsal sensory branch of the UN.[31] The posterior interosseous nerve (PIN) innervates the dorsal wrist capsule, the dorsal aspects of the SLIL, the lunotriquetral interosseous ligament, and the dorsal radiocarpal and intercarpal ligaments.[28,29] Finally, the superficial sensory branch of the radial nerve (SBRN) provides few articular branches to the dorsal and volar radial wrist capsule.[28]

3.2.2 Trapeziometacarpal Joint

Cadaveric dissections of trapeziometacarpal joint (TMJ) have shown that nerve branches to the TMJ arise from the

LACN in 100 % of specimens, the PCB of the median nerve in 70 % of specimens, and the SBRN in 40 % of specimens.[32] Furthermore, the dorsoradial, the dorsocentral, and the posterior oblique ligaments of the TMJ have an abundance of sensory nerve endings.[33] In contrast, little to no innervation have been seen in the anterior oblique ligament. Ruffini endings, which mediate joint position sense, are the predominant mechanoreceptor type with a greater density at the metacarpal insertion of the ligaments.[33] This indicates that joint position sense is an important proprioceptive quality in the highly mobile TMJ.

3.2.3 Distal Radioulnar Joint (DRUJ)

The TFCC is the main stabilizer of the distal radioulnar joint (DRUJ).[34] The seven parts of the TFCC, namely the subsheath of the extensor carpi ulnaris tendon sheath, the ulnocarpal meniscoid, the articular disk, as well as the dorsal and volar radioulnar, ulnolunate, and ulnotriquetral ligaments, are predominantly innervated by free nerve endings.[35]

Since the articular disk and ulnolunate ligament are rarely innervated, both these structures primarily have mechanical functions. Both radioulnar ligaments are richly innervated by all types of sensory nerve endings. Furthermore, the volar radioulnar ligament has the highest number of Ruffini endings, indicating its role in mediating joint position sense. This indicates that both ligaments are important in proprioceptive control of the DRUJ during forearm rotation. The ulnotriquetral ligament, the subsheath of the extensor carpi ulnaris tendon sheath, and the ulnocarpal meniscoid have all types of sensory nerve endings and therefore distinct proprioceptive qualities.[35]

3.3 Innervation Patterns in Osteoarthritis

Proprioception in hand osteoarthritis (OA) has primarily been studied in the TMJ. In an analysis of mechanoreceptor innervation in patients with painful TMJ OA, the innervation patterns were altered as compared to the innervation found in nonarthritic specimens.[36] Where Ruffini corpuscles dominate in the normal joint, the arthritic joint had a marked innervation of unclassifiable corpuscles and free nerve endings, indicating that the nerve endings that normally signal for joint stability and control are diminished and pain receptors dominate.[37] The lack of Ruffini and Pacini corpuscles in TMJ OA may explain why joint position sense has been shown to be impaired in patients with TMJ OA compared to healthy participants.[38]

In a recent publication it was reported that the free nerve endings in tissues around TMJ OA are immunoreactive to markers of the autonomic, sensory, and glutamatergic pathways, which implies that pain in OA is caused by a polymodal neurogenic inflammation.[25] These different nociceptive pathways may explain why anti-inflammatory analgesics or intra-articular corticosteroid injections often help reduce OA-related pain.[39]

3.4 Neural Feedback of the Wrist and Thumb

The intricate joint and mechanoreceptor innervation found in the wrist and TMJ supports the theory that the ligaments of the hand and wrist have an important sensory function in allowing dynamic neuromuscular control of joint stability. In studies on the ligamento-muscular reflexes of the wrist, it has been found that electrical stimulation of the dorsal SLIL elicits immediate, monosynaptic reflexes that serve as joint-protective reflexes.[40] Similarly, electrical stimulation of the dorsoradial ligament of the TMJ elicits joint-protective reflexes that serve to stabilize the TMJ and avoid subluxation of the joint.[41] These reflexes are akin to the anterior cruciate ligament and hamstring ligamento-muscular reflexes around the knee joint[42] that have been shown to have an important role in the proprioception and neuromuscular stability of the knee.[43]

The joint-protective reflexes elicited in the SLIL were found to be entirely eliminated in healthy controls after desensitization of the PIN,[44] suggesting that denervation of a joint will have a major impact on the proprioception of the joint. However a recent publication investigating the effect of complete wrist denervation on wrist proprioception was not able to conclude a difference in proprioception between healthy individuals and patients that

had undergone Wilhelm's denervation procedure, assessed by wrist reflex time, wrist joint position sense, and force sense.[45] The conclusion in this study was that the tests used also stimulated skin receptors and Golgi endings in the musculotendinous unit, both of which are unaffected by wrist denervation.

3.5 Clinical Implications

The indication for thumb or wrist arthroplasty is, in general, to replace a painful/degenerated arthritic joint with an artificial implant that will eliminate/reduce pain while providing a high degree of mobility. The joint to be replaced is likely to have an altered innervation pattern with activated free nerve endings rather than specialized proprioceptors,[36,37] i.e., Ruffini and Pacini corpuscles, meaning reduced proprioception, while the goal of the postoperative rehabilitation is to regain neuromuscular control and proprioceptive function.[46] How should we handle this obvious dilemma; to denervate or reinnervate, that is the question!

3.5.1 The Case for Nerve-Sparing Surgery

A primary goal for arthroplasty surgery must be to cause as little harm as possible and to restore thumb/wrist function. A surgical approach aiming to preserve joint innervation will aid in both postoperative healing of tissues[47,48] and promoting restoration of proprioceptive function through guided rehabilitation.[46] In studies on arthroplasty of the knee it has been found that the arthroplasty itself promoted an improvement in knee proprioception—joint position sense, kinesthesia, and balance—as the arthroplasty surgery both reduced pain and realigned joint capsules and ligaments into more anatomical positions.[49]

Similar findings may be anticipated for wrist and thumb arthroplasties. For instance, a retained innervation appears essential for optimal healing of vascularized joint transfers performed for proximal interphalangeal or metacarpophalangeal joint reconstruction.[50] In arthroplasty where the majority of the ligaments and joint capsule are retained, e.g., an ulnar head replacement, the preserved innervation of the TFCC should assist both healing and postoperative proprioceptive rehabilitation. Nerve-sparing surgical approaches have previously been described in detail for the wrist and DRUJ,[51,52] where the principle is easily understood: approach the joint with care and consideration for the nerve(s) innervating the joint. As in all of medicine, *primum non nocere* (cause no harm).

3.5.2 The Case for Denervation

Given the discussion above on the importance of nerve-sparing approaches, the question remains: is there ever a role for denervation? It is known, for instance, that patients with a history of repetitive or external trauma may suffer painful neuromas in continuity of the PIN.[53] Similar findings are also seen in patients with wrist OA[54] where abnormal enlargement of the PIN may be found and where associated microscopic examination will reveal a fibrotic and neuromatous appearance consistent with a traction neuroma.[54,55] In these cases the PIN is no longer a healthy nerve, capable of reinnervation and proprioceptive functions, but rather a diseased nerve that it appears appropriate to excise as part of a larger wrist salvage procedure or as a solitary procedure for long-term pain relief.[56]

In patients with severe and painful TMJ OA, denervation of the TMJ is found to significantly reduce pain.[32] It is also proposed that denervation of the TMJ affects the innervation of the synovium in the joint, which, in turn, may reduce the neurogenic inflammation, resulting in a relief of pain.[25]

3.6 In Conclusion—to Denervate or Reinnervate?

Let us conclude as we began, with a quote by Sir Charles Scott Sherrington:

This integrative action in virtue of which the nervous system unifies from separate organs an animal possessing solidarity, an individual, is the problem before us.

To exercise caution with a healthy nerve capable of providing reinnervation and proprioception must, in our humble opinion, be the primary goal but with the sober realization that denervation at times is indeed the most likely pain-relieving outcome in a patient with severe joint degeneration and pain. Handle the problem before you.

References

[1] Sherrington CS. The Integrative Action of the Nervous System. New Haven, CT: Yale University Press; 1906

[2] Burke RE. Sir Charles Sherrington's the integrative action of the nervous system: a centenary appreciation. Brain. 2007; 130(Pt 4):887–894

[3] Collins DF, Refshauge KM, Todd G, Gandevia SC. Cutaneous receptors contribute to kinesthesia at the index finger, elbow, and knee. J Neurophysiol. 2005; 94(3):1699–1706

[4] Sturnieks DL, Wright JR, Fitzpatrick RC. Detection of simultaneous movement at two human arm joints. J Physiol. 2007; 585(Pt 3):833–842

[5] Lephart SM, Riemann BL, Fu FH. Introduction to the sensorimotor system. In: Lephart S, Fu FH (Eds). Proprioception and neuromuscular control in joint stability. Champaign, IL: 2000; Human Kinetics, xvii–xiv

[6] Sjölander P, Johansson H, Djupsjöbacka M. Spinal and supraspinal effects of activity in ligament afferents. J Electromyogr Kinesiol. 2002; 12(3):167–176

[7] Paulin MG. The role of the cerebellum in motor control and perception. Brain Behav Evol. 1993; 41(1):39–50

[8] Lephart SM, Fu FH. Proprioception and Neuromuscular Control in Joint Stability. Champaign, IL: Human Kinetics; 2000:1–439

[9] Freeman MA, Wyke B. The innervation of the knee joint:an anatomical and histological study in the cat. J Anat. 1967; 101(Pt 3):505–532

[10] Hagert E. Wrist ligaments: innervation patterns and ligamento-muscular reflexes. 2008; Thesis for doctoral degree (PhD). Karolinska Institutet, Stockholm

[11] Erlanger J, Gasser HS. Electrical Signs of Gassernervous activity. Oxford: Univ Penn Press; 1937

[12] Lloyd DPC. Neuron patterns controlling transmission of ipsilateral hind limb reflexes in cat. J Neurophysiol. 1943; 6:293–315

[13] Hunt CC. Relation of function to diameter in afferent fibers of muscle nerves. J Gen Physiol. 1954; 38(1):117–131

[14] Gilman S. Joint position sense and vibration sense: anatomical organisation and assessment. J Neurol Neurosurg Psychiatry. 2002; 73(5):473–477

[15] Ruffini A. Sur un novel organe nerveux terminal et sur la présence des corpuscles Golgi-Mazzoni dans le conjunctiv sous-cutané de la pulpe des doigts de l'homme. Arch Ital Biol. 1894; 21:249–265

[16] Grigg P, Hoffman AH. Stretch-sensitive afferent neurons in cat knee joint capsule: sensitivity to axial and compression stresses and strains. J Neurophysiol. 1996; 75(5):1871–1877

[17] Grigg P, Hoffman AH. Properties of Ruffini afferents revealed by stress analysis of isolated sections of cat knee capsule. J Neurophysiol. 1982; 47(1):41–54

[18] Lehmann JG. Dissertatio inauguralis medica de consensu partium corporis humani occasione spasmi singularis in manu ejusque digitis ex hernia observati; exposito simul nervorum barchialium et cruralium coalitu peculiari atque papillarum nervearum in digitis dispositio. Wittenberg1741

[19] Vater A. Dissertatio de consensu partium corporis humani occasione spasmi singularis in manu eiusque digitis ex hernia observati exposito simul nervorum brachialium et cruralium coalitu peculiari atque papillarum nervearum in digitis dispositione. In: Haller A, ed. Disputationum anatomicarum selectarum. Göttingen: Vandenhoeck; 1741:953–972

[20] Bentivoglio M, Pacini P. Filippo Pacini: a determined observer. Brain Res Bull. 1995; 38(2):161–165

[21] Pacini F. Sopra un particolare genere di piccoli corpi globosi scoperti nel corpo umano da Filippo Pacini, Alunno interno degli Spedali riuniti di Pistoia. Letter to the Accademia Medico-Fisica di Firenze. 1835

[22] Macefield VG. Physiological characteristics of low-threshold mechanoreceptors in joints, muscle and skin in human subjects. Clin Exp Pharmacol Physiol. 2005; 32(1–2):135–144

[23] Golgi C. Della terminazione dei nervi nei tendini e di un nuovo apparato nervoso terminale muscolo-tendineo. Milano: Atti della Settima Riunione Starordinaria della Societa Italiana di Scienze Naturali in Varese, Tipografia G. Bernardoni; 1878

[24] Skoglund S. Anatomical and physiological studies of knee joint innervation in the cat. Acta Physiol Scand Suppl. 1956; 36(124):1–101

[25] Rein S, Okogbaa J, Hagert E, Manthey S, Ladd A. Histopathological analysis of the synovium in trapeziometacarpal osteoarthritis. J Hand Surg Eur Vol. 2019; 44(10):1079–1088

[26] Rein S, Hagert E, Hanisch U, Lwowski S, Fieguth A, Zwipp H. Immunohistochemical analysis of sensory nerve endings in ankle ligaments: a cadaver study. Cells Tissues Organs. 2013; 197(1):64–76

[27] Ferreres A, Suso S, Foucher G, Ordi J, Llusa M, Ruano D. Wrist denervation:surgical considerations. J Hand Surg [Br]. 1995; 20(6):769–772

[28] Van de Pol GJ, Koudstaal MJ, Schuurman AH, Bleys RL. Innervation of the wrist joint and surgical perspectives of denervation. J Hand Surg Am. 2006; 31(1):28–34

[29] Fukumoto K, Kojima T, Kinoshita Y, Koda M. An anatomic study of the innervation of the wrist joint and Wilhelm's technique for denervation. J Hand Surg Am. 1993; 18(3):484–489

[30] Berger RA. The anatomy of the ligaments of the wrist and distal radioulnar joints. Clin Orthop Relat Res. 2001(383):32–40

[31] Shigemitsu T, Tobe M, Mizutani K, Murakami K, Ishikawa Y, Sato F. Innervation of the triangular fibrocartilage complex of the human

3

wrist: quantitative immunohistochemical study. Anat Sci Int. 2007; 82(3):127–132

[32] Tuffaha SH, Quan A, Hashemi S, et al. Selective thumb carpometacarpal joint denervation for painful arthritis: clinical outcomes and cadaveric study. J Hand Surg Am. 2019; 44(1):64.e1–64.e8

[33] Hagert E, Lee J, Ladd AL. Innervation patterns of thumb trapeziometacarpal joint ligaments. J Hand Surg Am. 2012; 37(4):706–714.e1

[34] Hagert E, Chim H, Moran SL. Anatomy of the distal radioulnar joint and ulnocarpal complex. In: Greenberg JA, ed. Ulnar-sided Wrist Pain: A Master Skills Publication. Chicago, IL: American Society for Surgery of the Hand; 2013:11–21

[35] Rein S, Semisch M, Garcia-Elias M, Lluch A, Zwipp H, Hagert E. Immunohistochemical mapping of sensory nerve endings in the human triangular fibrocartilage complex. Clin Orthop Relat Res. 2015; 473 (10):3245–3253

[36] Mobargha N, Ludwig C, Ladd AL, Hagert E. Ultrastructure and innervation of thumb carpometacarpal ligaments in surgical patients with osteoarthritis. Clin Orthop Relat Res. 2014; 472(4):1146–1154

[37] Ludwig CA, Mobargha N, Okogbaa J, Hagert E, Ladd AL. Altered innervation pattern in ligaments of patients with basal thumb arthritis. J Wrist Surg. 2015; 4(4):284–291

[38] Ouegnin A, Valdes K. Joint position sense impairments in older adults with carpometacarpal osteoarthritis: a descriptive comparative study. J Hand Ther. 2019(Mar):11

[39] Conaghan PG, Peloso PM, Everett SV, et al. Inadequate pain relief and large functional loss among patients with knee osteoarthritis: evidence from a prospective multinational longitudinal study of osteoarthritis real-world therapies. Rheumatology (Oxford). 2015; 54(2):270–277

[40] Hagert E, Persson JK, Werner M, Ljung BO. Evidence of wrist proprioceptive reflexes elicited after stimulation of the scapholunate interosseous ligament. J Hand Surg Am. 2009; 34(4):642–651

[41] Mobargha N, Rein S, Hagert E. Ligamento-muscular reflex patterns following stimulation of a thumb carpometacarpal ligament: an electromyographic study. J Hand Surg Am. 2019; 44(3):248.e1–248.e9

[42] Krogsgaard MR, Dyhre-Poulsen P, Fischer-Rasmussen T. Cruciate ligament reflexes. J Electromyogr Kinesiol. 2002; 12(3):177–182

[43] Fridén T, Roberts D, Ageberg E, Waldén M, Zätterström R. Review of knee proprioception and the relation to extremity function after an anterior cruciate ligament rupture. J Orthop Sports Phys Ther. 2001; 31(10):567–576

[44] Hagert E, Persson JK. Desensitizing the posterior interosseous nerve alters wrist proprioceptive reflexes. J Hand Surg Am. 2010; 35(7):1059–1066

[45] Rein S, Winter J, Kremer T, Siemers F, Range U, Euchner N. Evaluation of proprioception in denervated and healthy wrist joints. J Hand Surg Eur Vol. 2020; 5(4):408–413

[46] Hagert E. Proprioception of the wrist joint: a review of current concepts and possible implications on the rehabilitation of the wrist. J Hand Ther. 2010; 23(1):2–17

[47] Mammoto T, Seerattan RA, Paulson KD, Leonard CA, Bray RC, Salo PT. Nerve growth factor improves ligament healing. J Orthop Res. 2008; 26(7):957–964

[48] Salo P. The role of joint innervation in the pathogenesis of arthritis. Can J Surg. 1999; 42(2):91–100

[49] Swanik CB, Lephart SM, Rubash HE. Proprioception, kinesthesia, and balance after total knee arthroplasty with cruciate-retaining and posterior stabilized prostheses. J Bone Joint Surg Am. 2004; 86(2):328–334

[50] Ju J, Li L, Hou R. Transplantation of a free vascularized joint flap from the second toe for the acute reconstruction of defects in the thumb and other fingers. Indian J Orthop. 2019; 53(2):357–365

[51] Hagert E, Ferreres A, Garcia-Elias M. Nerve-sparing dorsal and volar approaches to the radiocarpal joint. J Hand Surg Am. 2010; 35(7):1070–1074

[52] Garcia-Elias M, Hagert E. Surgical approaches to the distal radioulnar joint. Hand Clin. 2010; 26(4):477–483

[53] Carr D, Davis P. Distal posterior interosseous nerve syndrome. J Hand Surg Am. 1985; 10(6 Pt 1):873–878

[54] Dellon AL. Partial dorsal wrist denervation: resection of the distal posterior interosseous nerve. J Hand Surg Am. 1985; 10(4):527–533

[55] Lluch A. Treatment of radial neuromata and dysesthesia. Tech Hand Up Extrem Surg. 2001; 5(3):188–195

[56] Peltz TS, Yapp LZ, Elherik FK, Breusch SJ. Patient satisfaction and outcomes of partial wrist denervation in inflammatory arthritis. Clin Rheumatol. 2019; 38(11):2995–3003

3

4 Outcome Measurement in Hand and Wrist Arthroplasty

Miriam Marks

Abstract

This chapter summarizes the most suitable patient-reported outcome measures (PROMs) for assessing patients with hand and wrist arthroplasties, explains the measurement properties ideally required for a PROM and provides guidance on choosing the appropriate outcome measure for various aims and settings. Furthermore, the challenges of incorporating PROMs into daily clinical practice are described and some tips are given for the interpretation of outcome scores.

Keywords: Patient-reported outcome measure, measurement properties, reliability, validity, responsiveness, Michigan Hand Outcomes Questionnaire, Patient-Rated Wrist Evaluation, core set, minimal important change, patient acceptable symptom state

4.1 Introduction

Without measuring treatment outcome, we can neither improve our hand surgical interventions nor demonstrate their effectiveness. Outcome measures help to not only quantify patient benefit but also identify problems and limitations of a particular intervention.

Besides the objective clinical measures such as range of motion, strength, or the evaluation of radiographs, subjective patient-reported outcome measures (PROMs) have become indispensable. The systematic use of information from PROMs leads to better communication and decision making between doctors and patients, and improves patient satisfaction with care.[1]

Standardized and validated PROMs are essential to monitor the disease process, to evaluate its outcome as well as the associated socioeconomic consequences. In the modern world with its increasing focus on containment of healthcare costs, measureable outcome data can form the basis for negotiations with health authorities.

4.2 Frequently Used PROMs Suitable for Patients Undergoing Hand Arthroplasty

A wide variety of outcome measures are available for assessing patients with hand disorders. A literature review analyzing studies including patients with osteoarthritis (OA) of the thumb carpometacarpal (CMC) joint, for example, revealed that there were 21 different questionnaires in use.[2] Similar findings have been reported for Dupuytren studies, whereby only 14% used validated PROMs.[3] The diversity in reporting outcomes makes it difficult to compare results among studies, e.g., in meta-analyses. ▶ Table 4.1 highlights the most common and validated PROMs suitable for patients with hand or wrist arthroplasty.

4.2.1 Michigan Hand Outcomes Questionnaire (MHQ)[8]/Brief MHQ[16]

The MHQ is a 37-item questionnaire, which is divided into six subscales: hand function, activities of daily living (ADL), pain, work performance, aesthetics, and satisfaction with hand function. It takes about 15 minutes to complete and yield results for each hand separately. The total score ranges from 0 to 100, with a higher score indicating better hand performance. The MHQ has been translated and cross-culturally adapted into several languages. Overall, it shows good measurement properties for many hand disorders.[9]

In order to reduce responder burden, the brief Michigan Hand Outcomes Questionnaire (briefMHQ) was developed as a shorter version of the original tool with only 12 items.[16] Similar to the original MHQ, the brief version has excellent measurement properties for various hand disorders.[16] However, it is neither possible to derive subscales scores nor distinguish between the right and left hand using the brief version. The brief MHQ also yields a summary score between 0 and 100 with higher scores indicating better overall hand function.

More information and questionnaire templates (freely available) can be found here: http://mhq.lab.medicine.umich.edu/

4.2.2 Patient-Rated Wrist Evaluation (PRWE)[4,5]

The PRWE is a 15-item scale specifically designed for patients with wrist disorders. The 15 items are divided into the two subscales of pain and function. The items are scored on a 0 to 10 numeric rating scale. Both subscales can be calculated independently and a total score combining these constructs can also be calculated. In contrast to the MHQ, the total PRWE score of 100 is associated with higher levels of pain and disability.

Recently, a decision-tree version has been developed[19] allowing a faster completion of the questionnaire. Based on the answer given to a question, the computer selects the most appropriate subsequent question. At the end, the patient only has to answer six questions instead of 15 yet still giving a score highly similar to that of the original version.

PRWHE[20] was introduced later by replacing the term "wrist" by "wrist/hand" allowing for a broader assessment

Table 4.1 Most common and validated patient-reported outcome measures (PROMs) specific for patients undergoing arthroplasty at the hand/wrist

Name	Target population	No. of items	Domains	Pros/Cons
PRWE[4,5,6,7]	Wrist conditions (e. g., distal radius fractures)	15 items	Two subscales: pain and function	Pros: Good measurement properties, subscales can be scored individually Cons: Potential item redundancy
MHQ[8,9,10,11,12,13,14,15]	All hand conditions	37 items	Six subscales: overall hand function, activities of daily living, pain, work performance, aesthetics, satisfaction	Pros: Good measurement properties, scores both hands separately, subscales can be scored individually Cons: Quite long
Brief MHQ[13,16,17,18]	All hand conditions	12 items	Six domains: overall hand function, activities of daily living, pain, work performance, aesthetics, satisfaction	Pros: Good measurement properties, short Cons: Subscales cannot be scored individually

Abbreviations: MHQ, Michigan Hand Outcomes Questionnaire; PRWE, Patient-Rated Wrist Evaluation.

of hand conditions. The PRWHE has two additional questions considering hand aesthetics. Both questionnaires are commonly used in hand studies and their measurement properties are known to be sound for various hand conditions.[6]

More information and questionnaire templates (freely available) can be found at the following link: https://srs-mcmaster.ca/research/musculoskeletal-outcome-measures

4.2.3 Disability of the Arm, Shoulder, and Hand Questionnaire (DASH)[21]/ *Quick*DASH[22]

The DASH is an upper extremity-specific 30-item questionnaire; the *Quick*DASH is the shortened form with 11 items. They are the most commonly used questionnaires in hand surgery. Several studies attest to their sound measurement properties.[23,24,25,26,27] But the DASH and *Quick*DASH intended to measure function of the entire upper extremity and not just the hand. The questionnaires contain items relevant to shoulder-and-elbow function that significantly influence the total score. Therefore, it is recommended to use a hand-specific questionnaire for the primary evaluation of hand surgical procedures. The DASH might still have its place, for example, in assessing more widespread conditions such as rheumatoid arthritis, where the whole upper extremity is involved and the effect of a single intervention on global function requires evaluation.

More information and questionnaire templates (freely available) can be found here: http://www.dash.iwh.on.ca

4.2.4 Patient-Reported Outcomes Measurement Information System (PROMIS)[28]

The PROMIS tool consists of an item bank related to physical, mental, and social health. The items can be administered either as a fixed short form or computer adaptive test (CAT). The CAT uses an algorithm based on the item-response theory that selects successive questions based on the answer to the previous item. There are many tools available for different health conditions. For patients with hand conditions, the PROMIS UE is most relevant. The CAT version includes 46 items and the short form consists of seven items all answered on a 5-point Likert scale. The results generate a final T-score with a standardized normative value of the mean (± standard deviation) equivalent to 50 (± 10).

The main benefit of the PROMIS lies in its speed of completion. It is reliable and highly correlated to the DASH/*Quick*DASH.[29,30] However, like the DASH, the tool includes items influenced by shoulder function. Responsiveness of the PROMIS UE is considerably lower than that of the MHQ or carpal tunnel questionnaire.[31]

More information and questionnaire templates (freely available for individual research) can be found at the following link: http://www.healthmeasures.net/explore-measurement-systems/promis

4.2.5 Patient-Specific Functional Scale (PSFS)[32]

The PSFS is an individual outcome measure allowing patients to rate their individual health problems. The patient indicates at least three specific activities that they are unable to do or have difficulty with and rates them on a scale ranging from 0 to 10, where 10 indicates being unable to perform the activity and 0 means the patient is able to perform the activity at the same level as prior to their injury or disorder, i.e., normally for them.

The advantage of this scale is that health issues not considered by traditional questionnaires can be assessed. For example, the PSFS might be useful for patients with unique functional demands such as athletes who would score highly in traditional outcome measures, but still experience problems specific to their discipline. On the other hand, the PSFS may also be used to assess patients with greater activity restrictions who are not able to perform the tasks given in traditional questionnaires.

The disadvantage is that the PSFS cannot be compared so easily across patients and especially studies. Although the score has been shown to be reliable, there is only a weak correlation with the DASH. Therefore, it is suggested that the PSFS is used as a complementary tool in conjunction with traditional outcome measures.[33,34]

4.2.6 Single Assessment Numeric Evaluation (SANE) Score[35]

The SANE is a global, single-question PROM. Patients indicate their answer on a scale ranging from 0 to 100 based on the question: *How would you rate your* [e.g., hand] *today as a percentage of normal? (100% = normal).* Originally developed for patients with shoulder conditions, the SANE has also been used to assess the outcomes of knee surgery. It correlates moderately to well with other shoulder- and knee-specific scores.[36] Although it is a very quick and easy evaluation of the patient's subjective condition, it cannot replace existing comprehensive questionnaires. By using only one global question, the domains affecting the answer cannot be distinguished. The clinician is unable to conclude if the score is based on pain, function, appearance, or another related factor. Therefore, the SANE is recommended only as a supplementary evaluation.[36]

4.2.7 Quality-of-Life Measures

Quantifying quality of life can be used as a secondary outcome measure and is essential for economic evaluations. In such studies, estimating the quality-adjusted life years (QALYs) is required. The most popular questionnaires from which QALYs can be derived include the EuroQol EQ-5D[37] and the Short Form-36 (SF-36)[38] or its brief version, the SF-12.[39]

Two versions of the EQ-5D are available, the first of which includes three response options per question (EQ-5D-3L), while the second and more sensitive version consists of five response options (EQ-5D-5L). Each version addresses the five dimensions of mobility, self-care, normal activity, pain/discomfort, and anxiety/depression. Its measurement properties have been investigated widely for different musculoskeletal disorders.[40] The final score ranges from –0.285 to 1.0 (English value set)[41] with higher scores indicating better health status. It is freely available for noncommercial research.

The SF-36 and SF-12 include 36 and 12 questions, respectively, which generate two component summary measures of physical and mental health. The scores range from 0 to 100 with higher scores representing better health, the norm value being a mean of 50 (± 10). These health surveys show sound measurement properties in patients with various musculoskeletal disorders, e.g., OA and rheumatoid arthritis patients,[42] distal radius fractures,[43] as well as those with carpal tunnel syndrome.[44] License fees apply for the Short Form questionnaires.

More information can be found at the following link for the EQ-5D: https://euroqol.org

And the following link can be checked for the short form questionnaires: https://www.optum.com/solutions/life-sciences/answer-research/patient-insights/sf-health-surveys.html

4.2.8 Further Validated Hand-Specific PROMs

Apart from the PROMs suitable for patients undergoing hand arthroplasty described above, other PROMs are freely available for specific hand conditions.

The UnitéRhumatologique des Affections de la Main (URAM) scale is a 9-item questionnaire specifically designed for patients with Dupuytren's disease.[45] The Boston Carpal Tunnel Questionnaire (BCTQ) or Levine scale[46] covers the domains relevant for patients with carpal tunnel syndrome. Both PROMs have sound measurement properties and are recommended for the assessment of these specific populations.

4.3 Core Sets

Outcome measures should cover all domains of interest to comprehensively assess the health status of a patient. For example, the dimensions of objective data (clinical measures, radiological criteria), functional outcome (hand- and extremity-specific), and patient-rated subjective data (quality of life, function, and pain) together with socioeconomic data and comorbidities are of interest. This implies the use of many different outcome measure tools, which may contribute to a large administrative burden for both the healthcare provider and patient. If available, core sets assessing clinical and patient-reported outcomes as well as complications are recommended, such as the already established core sets for assessing patients with distal radius fractures[47] or hand OA.[48]

4.4 Measurement Properties

Colloquially, a "validated" outcome measure indicates that a tool has sound measurement or psychometric properties of reliability, validity, responsiveness, and interpretability. The COnsensus-based Standards for the selection of health Measurement Instruments (COSMIN) group has established the following categories and definitions[49,50,51,52]:

4.4.1 Reliability

Reliability is defined as the degree to which the measurement is free from measurement error and is usually established by test–retest reliability (intraclass correlation coefficient, ICC), internal consistency (Cronbach's alpha), and measurement error (standard error of measurement, SEM). An ICC of greater than or equal to 0.7 is considered acceptable, with values of 0.8 or higher considered optimal. Cronbach's alpha values lying between 0.7 and 0.9 indicate good internal consistency; higher values may demonstrate redundancy among the questionnaire items.

4.4.2 Validity

Validity can be subdivided into three separate components of content, construct, and criterion validity:

Content validity is the degree to which the content of an instrument is an adequate reflection of the construct to be measured. For example, an instrument aiming at assessing obesity should include information on both weight and height and not solely on the weight of a person.

Construct validity measures the degree to which the scores of an instrument are consistent with hypotheses. These hypotheses may include correlations with other tools measuring the same construct or differences between relevant groups. A hypothesis for a pain questionnaire might be that it is highly correlated (i.e., correlation coefficient > 0.7) with the pain visual analog scale.

Criterion validity is often confused with construct validity by testing correlations to similar outcome measures. It correctly refers to the degree to which an instrument adequately reflects a "gold standard." There are no existing gold standard PROMs, except for the long-version form of any short-version questionnaire; for example, the MHQ is the gold standard for the brief MHQ and the DASH for the QuickDASH.

4.4.3 Responsiveness

Responsiveness is defined as the ability of an instrument to detect change over time. In a similar manner to validity testing, responsiveness has to be assessed using a construct approach with the formulation of a priori hypotheses. These hypotheses may include assumptions about the expected effect, which can be analyzed by calculating effect sizes (ES) or the standardized response mean (SRM). Values of 0.2 and 0.5 indicate a small and a medium effect, respectively, whereas values greater than or equal to 0.8 indicate a large effect.[53] Such a hypothesis might be that the instrument under investigation yields an ES of > 0.8 or that the ES is higher than that of the comparative instrument.

4.4.4 Interpretability

The interpretability of a questionnaire is defined as the degree to which qualitative meaning can be ascribed to its quantitative scores. It includes the minimal important change (MIC), minimal important difference (MID), or floor/ceiling effects (see below).

A detailed summary of the criteria for sound measurement properties is outlined by Prinsen et al.[54]

4.5 Choosing an Appropriate Outcome Measure

The selection of an appropriate outcome measure is challenging because the tool must not only focus on

Table 4.2 Roadmap for selecting an appropriate outcome measure

Steps	Questions to ask
Step 1	Does it measure what I want to measure? Have a look at the items. Do they reflect the construct you want to assess? If you want to examine hand function, the tool to choose will most likely be different from that used to assess pain.
Step 2	Is it suitable for my population? Some tools are disease specific. The URAM scale, for example, is specifically designed for patients with Dupuytren's disease and is therefore unsuitable for assessing patients with wrist OA.
Step 3	Are the measurement properties sound? Check if the tool has been tested for reliability, validity, and responsiveness in your target population. Especially, responsiveness frequently differs between tools and indications.
Step 4	Frequently used and documented in the literature? To compare results of different studies, e.g. in a meta-analysis analogous outcome measures should be used. Avoid less commonly used tools.
Step 5	Is it feasible? How much time does it take to complete? Do you need special scoring software? How can you incorporate it in your daily practice? Is it licensed?
Step 6	Select outcome measure

Based on Marks M. Which patient-reported outcomes shall we use in hand surgery? J Hand Surg Eur Vol. 2020; 45: 5–11.

the specific domain to be measured (e. g., pain), but needs to be suitable for the target population. Using an outcome measure designed for patients with Dupuytren's disease is inappropriate for patients with distal radius fractures. Furthermore, the measurement properties of the instrument have to be suitable for the aim and target population and it is important that the instrument has been frequently applied and documented in the literature to allow for adequate comparisons to be made with one's own results. Last but not least, the feasibility of the outcome measure needs to be evaluated for its regular use and integration into daily practice with low administrative burden. Patients should be able to complete the questionnaire quickly and without difficulties. A roadmap for the selection of a suitable outcome measure is outlined in ▶ Table 4.2, and a decision tree to find the appropriate PROM for patients with hand or wrist arthroplasties is shown in ▶ Fig. 4.1.

4.6 Collecting and Processing Outcome Measures

Having chosen an appropriate outcome measure, the next challenge awaits: the integration into daily business and the processing of resultant data. It is often forgotten that the standardized measurement of an outcome requires time and money. Prior to data collection, it is important to define what is going to be done with the data. It is our duty to patients to analyze all data provided by them. The collection of data without analysis is only a burden to the patient so is unethical. Therefore, it should be defined at the outset if the data is going to be used internally for patient monitoring or quality assurance. Is it intended for routine documentation in a registry or for a clinical trial?

Data collection requires a multidisciplinary team comprising a clinician, a study nurse, a data manager, and IT staff who are familiar with good clinical practice (GCP) guidelines. If the data are part of a clinical trial, a statistician, monitor, and medical writer may also be necessary.

A professional database that conforms to international laws and regulations as well as protects patients' data has to be developed a priori. The use of Excel for research purposes is outdated, since data can be easily manipulated or misplaced. The development and maintenance of such a database, e.g., REDCap (www.project-redcap.org)[55] or secuTrial (www.secutrial.com), requires the expertise of a research associate and IT staff.

It is preferable to distribute the questionnaires to patients electronically. If patients are unable to complete electronic questionnaires, a study nurse is required to hand out paper forms for completion as well as for transferring the patient information to the database increasing the administrative burden and the potential for transcription errors.

4.7 Interpretation of Outcomes

Traditionally, study outcomes were interpreted based on p-values. If a p-value is below the "magic" threshold of 0.05, the treatment was considered as significantly effective. However, as highlighted by the American Statistical Association, the p-value does not measure the magnitude of an effect.[56] It is influenced by the sample size, whereby a small difference in a large study population will most likely reveal a significant p-value, although the effect is small.

Therefore, the interpretation of study results based on what is important to the patient has become increasingly popular.[57,58] There are several underlying concepts looking at the patient's perspective of a successful treatment.

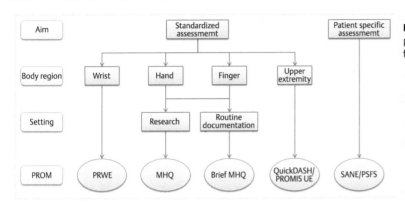

Fig. 4.1 Decision tree for finding a suitable patient-reported outcome measure (PROM) for patients with hand/wrist arthroplasty.

4.7.1 Minimal Important Difference (MID) and Minimal Important Change (MIC)

The MID is the smallest difference between patients or groups that is considered important.[51,59,60]

The MIC is the smallest change in score which patients perceive as important.[51,59] Changes exceeding this value can be considered relevant for the patient. There are several studies in hand surgery investigating the MIC and MID for several hand conditions and two reviews summarizing available data.[58,61]

Apart from the MID and MIC, the related term of Minimal Clinically Important Difference (MCID) has also been defined.[62] However, it is suggested to adhere to the established terminology promoted by the COSMIN group,[51,59] whereby the MID considers differences between groups or patients and the MIC defines the "within group or patient" differences. For example, in a randomized controlled trial (RCT) investigating two different surgeries in patients with thumb CMC OA, it is important to look at the differences in outcome scores. If the difference at follow-up is higher than a defined MID value, which is 12 points for the brief MHQ,[63] a clinically relevant difference between the two interventions can be assumed.

In an observational study, the MIC helps in the interpretation of a treatment effect between baseline and follow-up. If the change in the brief MHQ, for example, is higher than the defined MIC of 16 points,[63] it can be concluded that the intervention resulted in a subjective relevant improvement for the patient.

4.7.2 Patient Acceptable Symptom State (PASS)

PASS is the value beyond which patients consider themselves well.[64] For patients with hand conditions, there are two studies investigating the PASS in patients with thumb CMC joint OA[63] and after proximal interphalangeal joint arthroplasty.[17]

The MID/MIC and PASS are useful tools to interpret the outcome of individual patients during clinical routine, to appraise study results, and to calculate sample sizes for a study. During clinical practice the surgeon can judge if a treatment has had a subjectively important effect for the patient and if the patient is satisfied despite potential residual symptoms. For the interpretation of study results, knowledge of the MIC and PASS is crucial to look beyond the p-values, which do not consider the magnitude of a treatment effect and depend heavily on the sample size.[17]

4.8 Conclusion

Selecting an appropriate outcome measure is challenging and enough time should be spent on this process. Measurement properties and feasibility have to be considered. For the assessment of personal or unit practice, I recommend using the brief MHQ as it is quick to administer and is suitable for almost all patients with hand conditions. For a research study, the instrument has to match the research question. Oftentimes, more than one tool is required to answer the primary and secondary research questions. The original MHQ might be a good basis for the assessment of various hand conditions in clinical studies. However, other tools might be more suitable, depending on the exact research question.

References

[1] Nelson EC, Eftimovska E, Lind C, Hager A, Wasson JH, Lindblad S. Patient reported outcome measures in practice. BMJ. 2015; 350:g7818

[2] Marks M, Schoones JW, Kolling C, Herren DB, Goldhahn J, VlietVlieland TPM. Outcome measures and their measurement properties for trapeziometacarpal osteoarthritis: a systematic literature review. J Hand Surg Eur Vol. 2013; 38(8):822–838

[3] Ball C, Pratt AL, Nanchahal J. Optimal functional outcome measures for assessing treatment for Dupuytren's disease: a systematic review and recommendations for future practice. BMC MusculoskeletDisord. 2013; 14(1):131

[4] MacDermid JC. Development of a scale for patient rating of wrist pain and disability. J Hand Ther. 1996; 9(2):178–183

[5] MacDermid JC. The PRWE/PRWHE update. J Hand Ther. 2019; 32(2):292–294

[6] Mehta SP, MacDermid JC, Richardson J, MacIntyre NJ, Grewal R. A systematic review of the measurement properties of the patient-rated wrist evaluation. J Orthop Sports PhysTher. 2015; 45(4):289–298

[7] Mulders MAM, Kleipool SC, Dingemans SA, et al. Normative data for the Patient-Rated Wrist Evaluation questionnaire. J Hand Ther. 2018; 31(3):287–294

[8] Chung KC, Pillsbury MS, Walters MR, Hayward RA. Reliability and validity testing of the Michigan Hand Outcomes Questionnaire. J Hand Surg Am. 1998; 23(4):575–587

[9] Shauver MJ, Chung KC. The Michigan hand outcomes questionnaire after 15 years of field trial. PlastReconstrSurg. 2013; 131(5):779e–787e

[10] Marks M, Audigé L, Herren DB, Schindele S, Nelissen RG, VlietVlieland TP. Measurement properties of the German Michigan Hand Outcomes Questionnaire in patients with trapeziometacarpal osteoarthritis. Arthritis Care Res (Hoboken). 2014; 66(2):245–252

[11] Kroon FPB, Boersma A, Boonen A, et al. Performance of the Michigan Hand Outcomes Questionnaire in hand osteoarthritis. Osteoarthritis Cartilage. 2018; 26(12):1627–1635

[12] Chung BT, Morris SF. Reliability and internal validity of the michigan hand questionnaire. Ann PlastSurg. 2014; 73(4):385–389

[13] Busuioc SA, Karim M, Efanov JI, et al. The Michigan Hand Questionnaire and Brief Michigan Hand Questionnaire were successfully translated to Canadian French. J Hand Ther. 2018; 31(4):564–567

[14] Waljee JF, Chung KC, Kim HM, et al. Validity and responsiveness of the Michigan Hand Questionnaire in patients with rheumatoid arthritis: a multicenter, international study. Arthritis Care Res (Hoboken). 2010; 62(11):1569–1577

[15] Nolte MT, Shauver MJ, Chung KC. Normative values of the Michigan Hand Outcomes Questionnaire for patients with and without hand conditions. PlastReconstrSurg. 2017; 140(3):425e–433e

[16] Waljee JF, Kim HM, Burns PB, Chung KC. Development of a brief, 12-item version of the Michigan Hand Questionnaire. PlastReconstrSurg. 2011; 128(1):208–220

[17] Marks M, Hensler S, Wehrli M, Schindele S, Herren DB. Minimal important change and patient acceptable symptom state for patients after proximal interphalangeal joint arthroplasty. J Hand Surg Eur Vol. 2019; 44(2):175–180

[18] Wehrli M, Hensler S, Schindele S, Herren DB, Marks M. Measurement properties of the Brief Michigan Hand Outcomes Questionnaire in patients with Dupuytrencontracture. J Hand Surg Am. 2016; 41(9):896–902

[19] van der Oest MJW, Porsius JT, MacDermid JC, Slijper HP, Selles RW. Item reduction of the patient-rated wrist evaluation using decision tree modelling. DisabilRehabil. 2019; •••:1–8

[20] MacDermid JC, Tottenham V. Responsiveness of the disability of the arm, shoulder, and hand (DASH) and patient-rated wrist/hand evaluation (PRWHE) in evaluating change after hand therapy. J Hand Ther. 2004; 17(1):18–23

[21] Hudak PL, Amadio PC, Bombardier C, The Upper Extremity Collaborative Group (UECG). Development of an upper extremity outcome measure: the DASH (disabilities of the arm, shoulder and hand) [corrected]. Am J Ind Med. 1996; 29(6):602–608

[22] Beaton DE, Wright JG, Katz JN, Upper Extremity Collaborative Group. Development of the QuickDASH: comparison of three item-reduction approaches. J Bone Joint Surg Am. 2005; 87(5):1038–1046

[23] Rodrigues J, Zhang W, Scammell B, et al. Validity of the Disabilities of the Arm, Shoulder and Hand patient-reported outcome measure (DASH) and the Quickdash when used in Dupuytren's disease. J Hand Surg Eur Vol. 2016; 41(6):589–599

[24] Forget NJ, Jerosch-Herold C, Shepstone L, Higgins J. Psychometric evaluation of the Disabilities of the Arm, Shoulder and Hand (DASH) with Dupuytren's contracture: validity evidence using Rasch modeling. BMC MusculoskeletDisord. 2014; 15:361

[25] Kennedy CA, Beaton DE, Smith P, et al. Measurement properties of the QuickDASH (disabilities of the arm, shoulder and hand) outcome measure and cross-cultural adaptations of the QuickDASH: a systematic review. Qual Life Res. 2013; 22(9):2509–2547

[26] Gummesson C, Ward MM, Atroshi I. The shortened disabilities of the arm, shoulder and hand questionnaire (QuickDASH): validity and reliability based on responses within the full-length DASH. BMC MusculoskeletDisord. 2006; 7(1):44

[27] Kleinlugtenbelt YV, Krol RG, Bhandari M, Goslings JC, Poolman RW, Scholtes VAB. Are the patient-rated wrist evaluation (PRWE) and the disabilities of the arm, shoulder and hand (DASH) questionnaire used in distal radial fractures truly valid and reliable? Bone Joint Res. 2018; 7(1):36–45

[28] Cella D, Riley W, Stone A, et al. PROMIS Cooperative Group. The Patient-Reported Outcomes Measurement Information System (PROMIS) developed and tested its first wave of adult self-reported health outcome item banks: 2005–2008. J Clin Epidemiol. 2010; 63(11):1179–1194

[29] Brodke DJ, Saltzman CL, Brodke DS. PROMIS for orthopaedic outcomes measurement. J Am AcadOrthopSurg. 2016; 24(11):744–749

[30] Fidai MS, Saltzman BM, Meta F, et al. Patient-reported outcomes measurement information system and legacy patient-reported outcome measures in the field of orthopaedics: a systematic review. Arthroscopy. 2018; 34(2):605–614

[31] Mahmood B, Chongshu C, Qiu X, Messing S, Hammert WC. Comparison of the Michigan Hand Outcomes Questionnaire, Boston Carpal Tunnel Questionnaire, and PROMIS Instruments in carpal tunnel syndrome. J Hand Surg Am. 2019; 44(5):366–373

[32] Stratford P, Gill C, Westaway M, Binkley J. Assessing disability and change on individual patients: a report of a patient specific measure. Physiother Can. 1995; 47(4):258–263

[33] Rosengren J, Brodin N. Validity and reliability of the Swedish version of the Patient Specific Functional Scale in patients treated surgically for carpometacarpal joint osteoarthritis. J Hand Ther. 2013; 26(1):53–60, quiz 61

[34] Wright HH, O'Brien V, Valdes K, et al. Relationship of the Patient-Specific Functional Scale to commonly used clinical measures in hand osteoarthritis. J Hand Ther. 2017; 30(4):538–545

[35] Williams GN, Gangel TJ, Arciero RA, Uhorchak JM, Taylor DC. Comparison of the Single Assessment Numeric Evaluation method and two shoulder rating scales:outcomes measures after shoulder surgery. Am J Sports Med. 1999; 27(2):214–221

[36] Furtado R, MacDermid J. Clinimetrics: single assessment numeric evaluation. J Physiother. 2019; 65(2):111

[37] EuroQol Group. EuroQol: a new facility for the measurement of health-related quality of life. Health Policy. 1990; 16(3):199–208

[38] Ware JE, Kosinski M, Dewey JE, Gandek B. SF-36 Health Survey: Manual and Interpretation Guide. Lincoln, RI: Quality Metric Inc.; 2000

[39] Ware JEJr, Kosinski M, Gandek B, et al. User's Manual for the SF-12v2 Health Survey. 2nd ed. Lincoln, RI: QualityMetric Incorporated; 2010

[40] Grobet C, Marks M, Tecklenburg L, Audigé L. Application and measurement properties of EQ-5D to measure quality of life in patients with upper extremity orthopaedic disorders: a systematic literature review. Arch Orthop Trauma Surg. 2018; 138(7):953–961

[41] Devlin NJ, Shah KK, Feng Y, Mulhern B, van Hout B. Valuing health-related quality of life: an EQ-5D-5L value set for England. Health Econ. 2018; 27(1):7–22

[42] Gandhi SK, Salmon JW, Zhao SZ, Lambert BL, Gore PR, Conrad K. Psychometric evaluation of the 12-item short-form health survey (SF-12) in osteoarthritis and rheumatoid arthritis clinical trials. Clin Ther. 2001; 23(7):1080–1098

[43] MacDermid JC, Richards RS, Donner A, Bellamy N, Roth JH. Responsiveness of the short form-36, disability of the arm, shoulder, and hand questionnaire, patient-rated wrist evaluation, and physical impairment measurements in evaluating recovery after a distal radius fracture. J Hand Surg Am. 2000; 25(2):330–340

[44] Keith MW, Masear V, Amadio PC, et al. Treatment of carpal tunnel syndrome. J Am AcadOrthopSurg. 2009; 17(6):397–405

[45] Beaudreuil J, Allard A, Zerkak D, et al. URAM Study Group. UnitéRhumatologique des Affections de la Main (URAM) scale: development and validation of a tool to assess Dupuytren's disease-specific disability. Arthritis Care Res (Hoboken). 2011; 63(10):1448–1455

[46] Levine DW, Simmons BP, Koris MJ, et al. A self-administered questionnaire for the assessment of severity of symptoms and functional status in carpal tunnel syndrome. J Bone Joint Surg Am. 1993; 75(11):1585–1592

4

[47] Goldhahn J, Beaton D, Ladd A, Macdermid J, Hoang-Kim A, Distal Radius Working Group of the International Society for Fracture Repair (ISFR), International Osteoporosis Foundation (IOF). Recommendation for measuring clinical outcome in distal radius fractures: a core set of domains for standardized reporting in clinical practice and research. Arch Orthop Trauma Surg. 2014; 134(2):197–205

[48] Kloppenburg M, Bøyesen P, Smeets W, et al. Report from the OMERACT Hand Osteoarthritis Special Interest Group: advances and future research priorities. J Rheumatol. 2014; 41(4):810–818

[49] De Vet HCW, Terwee CB, Mokkink LB, Knol DL. Measurement in Medicine. Cambridge: Cambridge University Press; 2011

[50] Terwee CB, Bot SD, de Boer MR, et al. Quality criteria were proposed for measurement properties of health status questionnaires. J Clin Epidemiol. 2007; 60(1):34–42

[51] Mokkink LB, Terwee CB, Knol DL, et al. The COSMIN checklist for evaluating the methodological quality of studies on measurement properties: a clarification of its content. BMC Med Res Methodol. 2010; 10:22

[52] Mokkink LB, Terwee CB, Patrick DL, et al. The COSMIN study reached international consensus on taxonomy, terminology, and definitions of measurement properties for health-related patient-reported outcomes. J Clin Epidemiol. 2010; 63(7):737–745

[53] Cohen J. A power primer. Psychol Bull. 1992; 112(1):155–159

[54] Prinsen CA, Vohra S, Rose MR, et al. How to select outcome measurement instruments for outcomes included in a "Core Outcome Set": a practical guideline. Trials. 2016; 17(1):449

[55] Harris PA, Taylor R, Thielke R, Payne J, Gonzalez N, Conde JG. Research electronic data capture (REDCap): a metadata-driven methodology and workflow process for providing translational research informatics support. J Biomed Inform. 2009; 42(2):377–381

[56] Wasserstein RL, Lazar NA. The ASA's statement on p-values: context, process, and purpose. Am Stat. 2016; 70(2):129–133

[57] Harris JD, Brand JC, Cote MP, Faucett SC, Dhawan A. Research pearls: the significance of statistics and perils of pooling. Part 1: clinical versus statistical significance. Arthroscopy. 2017; 33(6):1102–1112

[58] Marks M, Rodrigues JN. Correct reporting and interpretation of clinical data. J Hand Surg Eur Vol. 2017; 42(9):977–979

[59] de Vet HC, Beckerman H, Terwee CB, Terluin B, Bouter LM. Definition of clinical differences. J Rheumatol. 2006; 33(2):434–, author reply 435

[60] Rodrigues JN. Different terminologies that help the interpretation of outcomes. J Hand Surg Eur Vol. 2020; 45(1):97–99

[61] Rodrigues JN, Mabvuure NT, Nikkhah D, Shariff Z, Davis TR. Minimal important changes and differences in elective hand surgery. J Hand Surg Eur Vol. 2015; 40(9):900–912

[62] Engel L, Beaton DE, Touma Z. Minimal clinically important difference: a review of outcome measure score interpretation. Rheum Dis Clin North Am. 2018; 44(2):177–188

[63] Marks M, Grobet C, Audigé L, Herren DB. Clinical thresholds of symptoms for deciding on surgery for trapeziometacarpal osteoarthritis. J Hand Surg Eur Vol. 2019; 44(9):937–945

[64] Tubach F, Ravaud P, Baron G, et al. Evaluation of clinically relevant states in patient reported outcomes in knee and hip osteoarthritis: the patient acceptable symptom state. Ann Rheum Dis. 2005; 64(1):34–37

4

5 The Norwegian Arthroplasty Register

Ynvar Krukhaug

Abstract

The Norwegian Arthroplasty Register (NAR) is a nationwide register that receives information on primary and revision joint replacements performed in Norway.

From 1994 to 2018, 300 primary total wrist replacements were performed. The survival of the total wrist arthroplasties in the NAR is similar to other studies of wrist arthroplasties, but not as good as most total knee and hip arthroplasties. The annual number of total wrist replacements changed over time. The number of arthroplasties for inflammatory arthritis reduced (p < 0.001), but operations for osteoarthritis increased (p < 0.001).

From 1994 to 2011, 515 primary thumb CMC joint arthroplasties were registered in 432 patients. The overall 5-year and 10-year survivals were 91% and 90%, respectively. There were no statistically significant differences between the implant brands (p = 0.60). The annual number of arthroplasties performed due to IA decreased (p = 0.003), whereas the number for OA increased (p < 0.001) during the period.

From 1994 to 2018, 3786 primary MCP joint arthroplasties were registered. During the period, 768 prostheses were revised. The annual number of primary prosthesis has decreased over the last 20 years.

From 1994 through 2018, 105 primary PIP arthroplasties were registered. Sixteen (13%) have been revised. The annual number of primary prosthesis in PIP has remained constant over the last 20 years.

Keywords: register, documentation, outcome, arthroplasty, wrist replacement, proximal interphalangeal joint, metacarpophalangeal joint, thumb carpometacarpal joint

5.1 Introduction

The Norwegian Arthroplasty Register (NAR) is a nationwide register that receives information on primary and revision joint replacements performed in Norway.

The NAR started to collect data on total hip replacements in 1987. In 1994, this register was extended to include all artificial joints.[1] Individual reports are received from all seven hospitals that perform total wrist replacements in the country (population: 5.3 million at January 1, 2019).

The completeness of registration in the NAR was recently evaluated by comparing it to the mandatory reporting of administrative data to the Norwegian Patient Register (NPR); it was found to be 97% for hip replacements, 97% for knee replacements, 94% for all primary ankle replacements, and 86% for wrist replacements (The annual report from NAR, http://nrlweb.ihelse.net/eng/Rapporter/Report2018_english.pdf).

One explanation for the under-reporting could be that relative to the hip and knee, few wrist replacements are performed, and for this reason reporting to the Arthroplasty Register is not so well established among wrist surgeons.

The magnitude of under-reporting is unclear, however, as the NBD code group (except for NBD 8) of the NOMESCO 2006 coding system, which is used by the hospitals in their reports to the NPR, does not require it to be specified whether the prosthesis has been inserted in the radiocarpal joint or in other joints in the carpus. Also, the code NBD 99 applies to any prosthesis operation in the wrist or hand. Thus, the NPR data on wrist implants most probably also include data from implants in joints other than the radiocarpal joint.[2] We have no reason to believe that there is any systematic under-reporting to the NAR.

5.2 Wrist Replacements

From 1994 to 2018, 300 primary total wrist replacements were performed (▶ Table 5.1). Three types of wrist prostheses were used: "Biax," "Motec Wrist," and "ReMotion Wrist."

The diagnoses were grouped into "inflammatory arthritis" (IA) ($n = 130$) comprising rheumatoid arthritis and psoriatic arthritis, and into "noninflammatory arthritis" (NIA) ($n = 170$) comprising primary osteoarthritis (OA), postfracture disorders, ligament injuries, and joint destruction after infection.

5.2.1 Method

The NAR has registered wrist replacements since 1994. From 1994 to 2018, 300 patients had 300 primary wrist replacements (90 Biax prostheses of which 80 were cementless, 154 cementless Motec, and 56 ReMotion arthroplasties). Prostheses survival was analyzed using Cox regression analyses. The three implant designs were compared and time trends were analyzed.

5.2.2 Results

The annual number of total wrist replacements changed over time. The number of arthroplasties for IA reduced ($p < 0.001$), but operations for NIA increased ($p < 0.001$). These findings are consistent with a general trend for arthroplasty of other joints.[3,4,5,6,7]

The survival of the total wrist arthroplasties in the NAR is similar to other studies of wrist arthroplasties, but not

Table 5.1 Demography

Type of prosthesis	Number of primary prostheses	Percentage of women	Mean age [range] years	Cause: non-inflammatory arthritis (numbers)	Cause: inflammatory arthritis (numbers)	Number of hospitals	Mean number of operations per hospital [range]	Number of revisions (%)	Median follow-up (y)
Biax	90	89%	57 [28–77]	6	84	5	18 [1–46]	21	15.2
ReMotion	56	43%	59 [20–79]	53	3	4	14 [3–27]	7	4.3
Motec	154	47%	55[17–79]	111	43	5	31 [4–94]	33	9.0
Total	300	59%	56 [17–85]	170	130	9	21 [1–94]	61	9.0

Table 5.2 Reasons for revision (more than one reason could be given)

Brand	Biax	ReMotion	Motec	Total
Proximal component loosening	3	1	2	6
Distal component loosening	9	3	14	26
Dislocation	2	–	–	2
Instability	4	–	–	3
Axis problems	7	1	4	12
Deep infection	1	2	5	8
Pain	8	–	13	21
Wear of liner	3	–	–	3
Total number of revisions	21	7	33	61

as good as most total knee and hip arthroplasties (▶ Table 5.1 and ▶ Table 5.2, and ▶ Fig. 5.1).

5.3 CMC IA Replacements

The NAR has registered thumb carpometacarpal (CMC) joint arthroplasties since 1994.

From 1994 to 2011, 515 primary thumb CMC joint arthroplasties were registered in 432 patients. Thirty-six cases were excluded from the analysis; 12 because they had been operated on with rarer implants (Custom made in 5 and Avanta in 7), 16 due to missing information about implant brand, and 8 due to missing (5) or rare (3) diagnoses.

Four different brands of CMC implants were included in the analysis: "Silastic Trapezium" (Swanson Silastic), "Swanson Titanium Basal" (Swanson Titanium), "Elektra," and "Motec."

The patient diagnoses were stratified in two groups: "inflammatory arthritis" (IA) (108) and "osteoarthritis" (OA) (371). In the IA group 99 cases had rheumatoid arthritis, 8 had psoriatic arthritis, and 1 had lupus.

5.3.1 Results

The rate of thumb CMC joint arthroplasties did not change during the study period ($p = 0.55$) (▶ Fig. 5.2). The number of arthroplasties performed due to IA decreased ($p = 0.003$), whereas the number for OA increased ($p < 0.001$).[6]

Type of Prosthesis

The Swanson Silastic and Titanium implants were used in both diagnostic groups.

The Motec and the Elektra implants were only used in patients with OA (▶ Table 5.3). The median follow-up time was longer for the Swanson Silastic (7.9 years) and the Swanson Titanium (11.7 years) than for the Elektra (2.0 years) and Motec (1.9 years) implants ($p < 0.001$). The median follow-up for all prostheses as a group was 7.4 years.

Revision and Survival

Forty-two (8.8%) of the 479 CMC implants were revised (▶ Table 5.3). The mean time until the first revision was 7.0 (95 CI: 6.6–7.5) years. When interposition implants (Swanson Silastic and Swanson Titanium) were compared to the total prostheses (Elektra and Motec), no statistical significant difference was found in terms of prosthesis survival ($p = 0.70$; ▶ Table 5.4). Similarly there were no differences when the analysis was limited to patients with OA ($p = 0.55$).

The overall 5-year and 10-year survivals were 91% (95 CI: 88–93) and 90% (95 CI: 87–93), respectively. There were no statistically significant differences between the implant brands ($p = 0.60$; ▶ Table 5.4 and ▶ Fig. 5.2). The implant with the highest number of registered cases and longest follow-up time (Swanson Silastic) had 5- and 10-year survivals of 90% and 89%, respectively.

Dislocation ($n = 20$) and pain ($n = 23$) were the most frequent reasons for revision (▶ Table 5.5). Among the 42 patients who underwent revision, the implants were removed in 19 cases. In the remaining cases, the whole implant or parts of the implant were exchanged.

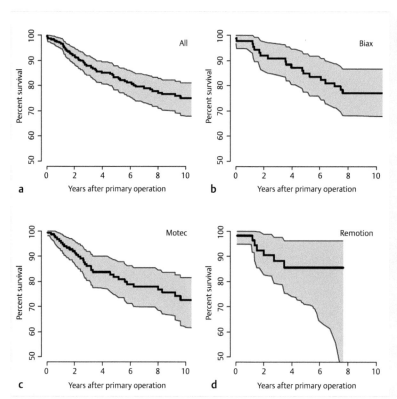

Fig. 5.1 Survival (Kaplan–Meier) with confidence interval (95% CI) in red. All implants (a), Biax (b), Motec (c), ReMotion (d).

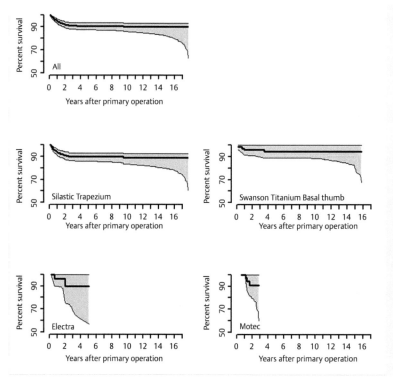

Fig. 5.2 Kaplan–Meier survival curves.

Table 5.3 Demography

Prosthesis	Number of primary prostheses	Percentage of women	Mean age [range] years	Osteoarthritis (OA)	Inflammatory arthritis (IA)	Number of hospitals	Mean number of operations per hospital [range]	Number of revisions	Median follow-up (y)
Silastic Trapezium	326	89%	64 [21–86]	239	97	14	23 [2–185]	33	7.9
Swanson Titanium Basal	71	82%	63 [38–82]	60	11	4	18 [1–52]	4	11.7
Elektra	29	72%	62 [50–72]	29	0	1	29 [29–29]	2	2.0
Motec	53	60%	63 [51–85]	53	0	3	18 [4–38]	3	1.9
Total	479	84%	64 [21–86]	371	108	16	30 [1–202]	42	7.4

Table 5.4 Five- and 10-year survival and hazard rate ratios (RR) from an unadjusted Cox-regression model on thumb carpometacarpal (CMC) joint arthroplasties reported to the Norwegian Arthroplasty Register 1994–2011

Prosthesis brand (number of implants)	5-year survival (95% CI)	10-year survival (95% CI)	RR (95% CI)	p-value
Swanson Silastic (326)	90% (86–93)	89% (85–93)	1[a]	0.60
Swanson Titanium (71)	94% (89–100)	94% (89–100)	0.50 (0.18–1.42)	0.20
Elektra (29)	90% (75–100)	–	0.80 (0.19–3.35)	0.76
Motec (53)	91% (81–100)[b]	–	0.73 (0.22–2.38)	0.60
All prostheses (479)	91% (88–93)	90% (87–93)		

[a]The Swanson Silastic was used as the reference prostheses against which the others were compared.
[b]The number represents 3-year survival because of insufficient follow-up.

Table 5.5 Reasons for revisions (more than one reason for each case is possible)

Reason for revision operation	Swanson Silastic	Swanson Titanium	Elektra	Motec	Total
Loosening	1	1	1	3	6
Dislocation	18	1	1		20
Instability	5		1		6
Pain	19	3		1	23
Total number of revisions	33	4	2	3	42

Risk Factors for Revision

The gender of the patient (hazard rate ratio [RR] females vs. males 1.0 [95% CI 0.4–2.5]), age (RR for each 10 years increase 1.0 [95% CI 0.7–1.3]), and diagnostic group (RR IA vs. OA 0.6 [95% CI 0.3–1.4]) did not influence the risk of revision.

Thumb CMC joint arthroplasties were performed in 16 hospitals in Norway during the study period. The number of arthroplasties performed in each hospital during the observation period ranged from 1 to 70 prostheses. The revision rate in hospitals performing more than 30 (5 hospitals) operations was not statistically different to the revision rate in hospitals that had performed fewer than 30 operations.

5

5.4 Finger Joint Replacement

The NAR has registered replacements in the metacarpophalangeal (MCP) and proximal interphalangeal (PIP) joints since 1994.

5.4.1 MCP Joint Replacement

From 1994 to 2018, 3,786 primary MCP joint arthroplasties were registered.

The annual number of primary prosthesis has decreased over the last 20 years, but the number of revisions has remained relatively constant (▶ Fig. 5.3). All prostheses are uncemented. The prosthesis brands used are listed in ▶ Table 5.6.

During the period, 768 prostheses were revised. The reasons for revisions are shown in ▶ Table 5.7.

5.4.2 PIP Joint Replacement

From 1994 through 2018, 105 primary PIP arthroplasties were registered.

The annual number of primary prosthesis in PIP has remained constant over the last 20 years. Sixteen (13%) have been revised.

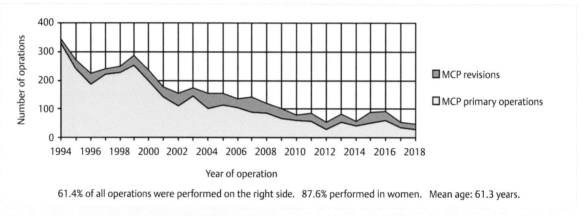

61.4% of all operations were performed on the right side.   87.6% performed in women.   Mean age: 61.3 years.

Fig. 5.3 Annual number of metacarpophalangeal (MCP) operations.

Table 5.6 Metacarpophalangeal (MCP) joint prostheses used in primary operations

Prostheses	1994–09	2010	2011	2012	2013	2014	2015	2016	2017	2018	Total
Silastic HP 100	1814	53	49	27	25		5	1	5		1979
Avanta	554	1					1		4		560
Silastic HP 100 II	2	5	6		28	41	45	56	26	26	235
NeuFlex	196										198
Ascension MCP	26	1	2			1		2		2	34
MCS	6										6
SR Avanta								2			2
Moje	1										1
Total	**2601**	**60**	**57**	**27**	**53**	**42**	**51**	**61**	**35**	**26**	**3015**

Table 5.7 Metacarpophalangeal (MCP) joint prostheses—reasons for revisions

Year	Loose proximal comp.	Loose distal comp.	Dislocation	Instability	Malalignment	Deep infection	Fracture (near implant)	Pain	Defect polyethylene	Fractured/defect component	Other	Missing
2018			4	7	1		6	5		8	4	
2017			1	3			9	4			10	
2016			5	5	8	1	2	10	9	5	9	
2015	6	2		6		1		15	9	8	10	
2014		1		4				2	4		5	
2013				4	13			13		10	1	
2012			1	2	4			10	4	13	1	
2011					6	2		13		12	8	
2010	1	1	2				2	3		10	3	
2009	1	2	3	2	2	4		6	3	22	5	
2008		1	2	4	15	4		13	5	10	5	
2007		3	11	8	2	1		16		39		4
2006			4	10	4	1		7	4	11		1
2005			5	6	6			12	5	24	4	2
2004	2	5		8	8			12		30	5	4
2003		1	1		9			8	1	17	2	
2002		3		12	7			15		27	4	
2001		3	3	4	7			11	3	9	10	
2000		2	1	2	1	4	8	4		20	5	1
1999		1	4	3	6		4	7		14	8	
1998		1	1	3	5		1	2		11	1	
1997		1	3	4	4	1		8		11	1	
1996				8				13		22	7	2
1995	4				4		7	12		13	5	
1994					1		1	1		2	4	6
Total	14	27	51	105	113	19	40	222	47	348	117	20

Note: Revision reasons are not mutually exclusive. More than one reason for revision is possible.

References

[1] Havelin LI. The Norwegian Joint Registry. Bull Hosp Jt Dis. 1999;58(3):139–147

[2] Espehaug B, Furnes O, Havelin LI, Engesaeter LB, Vollset SE, Kindseth O. Registration completeness in the Norwegian Arthroplasty Register. Acta Orthop. 2006;77(1):49–56

[3] da Silva E, Doran MF, Crowson CS, O'Fallon WM, Matteson EL. Declining use of orthopedic surgery in patients with rheumatoid arthritis? Results of a long-term, population-based assessment. Arthritis Rheum. 2003;49(2):216–220

[4] Pedersen AB, Johnsen SP, Overgaard S, Søballe K, Sørensen HT, Lucht U. Total hip arthroplasty in Denmark: incidence of primary operations and revisions during 1996–2002 and estimated future demands. Acta Orthop. 2005;76(2):182–189

[5] Weiss RJ, Stark A, Wick MC, Ehlin A, Palmblad K, Wretenberg P. Orthopaedic surgery of the lower limbs in 49,802 rheumatoid arthritis patients: results from the Swedish National Inpatient Registry during 1987 to 2001. Multicenter Study Ann Rheum Dis. 2006;65(3):335–341

[6] Fevang BTS, Lie SA, Havelin LI, Engesaeter LB, Furnes O. Reduction in orthopedic surgery among patients with chronic inflammatory joint disease in Norway, 1994-2004. Arthritis Rheum. 2007;57(3):529–532

[7] Krukhaug Y, Lie SA, Havelin LI, Furnes O, Hove LM. Results of 189 wrist replacements. A report from the Norwegian Arthroplasty Register. Acta Orthop. 2011;82(4):405–409

6 The History of Arthroplasty in the Hand and Wrist

Michael Brodbeck

Abstract

The human dream of replacing a destroyed joint is as old as Greek mythology. Before the 19th century, amputation of an infected limb was the surgical treatment of choice to save the human body from septicemia and death. In 1536, the first attempt to excise a joint while maintaining the distal part of the limb so as to restore motion at the level of the former joint was recorded and is accredited to Ambroise Paré, a barber who served in the French military. In 1890, Themistocles Gluck performed and recorded the very first total wrist arthroplasty. In 1962, Alfred B. Swanson introduced the concept of flexible implants for the reconstruction of small joints of the extremities and performed the first ever biocompatibility studies of silicone in bone, which revolutionized the surgical treatment of the arthritic hand. The finger joint silicone implant remains the golden standard of care more than 50 years later. The history of joint replacement in the hand was followed by various developments in material, design, tribology and bone anchorage over the decades. This chapter gives a brief historical overview of some concepts and implants in hand arthroplasty.

Keywords: history, arthroplasty, prosthesis, replacement, implant, wrist, metacarpophalangeal joint, interphalangeal joint, distal radioulnar joint, trapeziometacarpal joint

6.1 The Very Early History

6.1.1 The Era of Zeus and His Fellow Gods

The human dream of replacing a destroyed joint is as old as Greek mythology and depicted through the legend of "The Ivory Shoulder": Tantalus, king at Mount Sipylus in Anatolia, cut his son Pelops into pieces, made his flesh into a stew, and served it to the gods on Olympus to test their omniscience. The gods perceived the deception and left the meal untouched. Only Demeter, deep in grief after the abduction of her daughter Persephone, absentmindedly accepted the offering and ate the left shoulder. Zeus, the father of the gods, commanded Hermes, who could freely move between the worlds of mortal and divine and was the conductor of souls into the afterlife, to put the remaining pieces of Pelops in a cauldron. As one of the Three Fates who spin the thread of life, Clotho assisted Hermes in bringing Pelops back to life. Demeter replaced the missing shoulder with a chunk of ivory,[1] a material used in the modern age by Themistocles Gluck for the first total wrist implant in 1890.

6.1.2 Amputation—Upper Paleolithic to the Middle Ages

Before the 19th century, amputation of an infected limb was the surgical treatment of choice to save the human body from septicemia and death. It is one of the oldest surgical procedures. In the caves of Gargas in southwestern France, several negative imprints from the Upper Paleolithic period—about 22,000 to 25,000 years BP—show mutilated hands with a loss of some or all fingers. Almost all possible combinations occur, including part or total loss of a thumb. From the knowledge of more modern practices among various tribes, one can assume that these French paintings represent a form of mutilation carried out for ritual or religious purposes. Yet other more natural events including trauma, frostbite, leprosy, and Raynaud's phenomenon can contribute to such imprints of hands and amputated fingers that have also been found on other continents of the world.[2]

During the Islamic Golden Age, the most common reason for amputation was punishment for crimes. Consequently, some patients refused amputation for medical reasons because it would identify them as criminals. The first artificial hand replacement dates from the Egyptian and Roman times; an Egyptian cosmetic hand was found on a mummy dating from 200 BC, and the Roman general Marcus Sergius (167 BC) lost his right hand and used an artificial metal one with which he continued to fight in battle.[2]

6.2 Milestones in the Modern History of Wrist Arthroplasty

6.2.1 Resection Arthroplasty

In 1536, the first attempt to excise a joint while maintaining the distal part of the limb so as to restore motion at the level of the former joint was recorded. This intervention is accredited to a barber who served in the French military, Ambroise Paré. Known as the founder of French surgery, he resected an elbow joint of a patient with a destructive infection.[3]

Two centuries later, a German surgeon, Johann Ulrich Beyer, serving in the Prussian army documented the first wrist resection for the musketeer, Adam Kilian, who sustained a severe crush trauma caused by a howitzer. Despite fulminant infection and severe blood loss, "complete recovery" was achieved four months later; the final outcome was a natural-looking, nonfunctional hand.[4]

At the end of the 18th century, Victor Moreau and his son, two surgeons from Bar-le-Duc in France, reported their experiences with joint resections to the "Académie

Royale de Chirurgie" and published a book describing their technique. However, they did not receive credit for their contribution to wrist arthroplasty.[5]

A common dream of surgeons from the earlier days was to make a stiff joint movable and painless by means of an arthroplasty technique. John Rhea Barton is often credited with having performed the first resection arthroplasty in Lancaster, Pennsylvania in 1826. His observations that pseudarthrosis of long bones were often painless inspired him to create an artificial pseudarthrosis in the proximal femur, which may provide a limited degree of controlled hip movement. In seven minutes and without the benefit of modern anesthesia, he performed a subtrochanteric osteotomy just above the level of the lesser trochanter. The wound was left open to develop the expected postoperative infection and early mobilization was enforced.[6]

After introducing the foundations of modern surgery in the 19th century—namely, anesthesia and Lister's concept of aseptic surgery in 1888—an explosive development in surgery took place in Europe and the United States.[6] Surgeons including Kocher, Lister, von Langenbeck, and Ollier all followed Barton's concept of early mobilization after joint resection. Von Langenbeck recommended the technique of subperiosteal dissection to ensure that some degree of bone restoration might occur.[7]

6.2.2 Interposition Arthroplasty

Interposing material between the resected joint was a logical progression from the simple resection procedures. It is accredited to John Murray Carnochan of New York, who described the interposition of a small block of wood after resecting the mandibular neck to mobilize an ankylosed jaw in 1840. Twenty years later, Aristide Verneuil, a French surgeon, used soft parts for interposition, initially using muscle followed by adipose tissue and fascia.[6] Adipose tissue interposition was soon discarded because of its rapid absorption. By the end of the 19th century, a plethora of materials was tested and used: skin, glass, pig's bladder, celluloid, rubber, magnesium, and gold foil. In 1894, Péan, recognizing the reactivity of human tissues, used platinum plates as interpositional material in human joints including the wrist. Murphy widely advocated the use of fascia lata for interposition arthroplasties of the hip and knee from 1902; he performed his first wrist interposition arthroplasty after 1910. This method found widespread use in Europe at the beginning of the 20th century.[3]

6.2.3 The First Total Knee and Wrist Replacement—Themistocles Gluck (1853–1942)

Themistocles Gluck was born in Jassy, Romania in 1853, the son of a famous German doctor who was the

attending physician to the royal family. In 1873, Gluck began his preclinical medical studies in Leipzig and continued in Berlin, where Virchow and von Langenbeck were among his teachers. He was von Langenbeck's last assistant; he received the title of university professor in 1883. Upon von Langenbeck's retirement, Gluck did not receive a position to continue his university career and so worked as an industrial physician in Berlin until 1890, when he was appointed as head of surgery at the Kaiser- und Kaiserin-Friedrich-Kinderkrankenhaus in Berlin.

His early work concentrated on using guide rails for tissue regeneration following nerve and tendon replacement. He was interested in the field of tissue transplantation. After experimenting with autologous transplantation and heterologous transplants in animals, he began to work with foreign materials. He successfully bridged tendon, muscle, and bone defects by interposing silk and catgut suture bundles, and named the resulting fibrous tissue formation "autoplastic." During his services as a doctor in the two Balkan Wars of 1877 and 1885, Gluck used nickel-coated steel plates and screws for internal fracture fixation. After performing animal experiments with inserts of aluminum, wood, glass, celluloid, and steel, he decided that ivory was the most suitable material for implantation because it would be incorporated into bone with minimal inflammatory response. He began using ivory intramedullary pegs and intramedullary nails for fracture fixation. Gluck rapidly developed models for the total replacement of shoulder, elbow, hand, and knee joints. More than 65 years before Sir John Charnley, he already used bone cement and experimented with a variety of substances including copper amalgam, plaster of Paris, and putty materials (i.e., resin with pumice stone or gypsum), which hardened rapidly after mixing.

On 20 May 1890, Gluck performed his first ivory total knee replacement, which was followed by a total wrist replacement three weeks later on 9 June 1890 (▶ Fig. 6.1). Overall, he completed four total arthroplasties (three knees and one wrist) in septic joints affected by tuberculosis. Although the short-term results were strikingly successful, all ultimately failed due to chronic infection.

Gluck intended to present his implant arthroplasties to the International Medical Congress in 1890. For this purpose, he prepared a skeleton with several implants at the hip, shoulder, elbow, wrist, and knee, which became well-known as the "skeleton of Paris." A former superior, von Bergmann, refused Gluck's participation at the congress and in preventing his lecture wrote: "As the leader of German surgery I cannot allow that you discredit German science in front of a platform of international surgical specialists. My pupils and I will fight you with all means."[3] Finally, only the "skeleton of Paris" was exhibited and Gluck stopped his work on joint replacement.

In his later years, Gluck was honored for his work. In 1921, he reported on the good long-term outcome of his

6

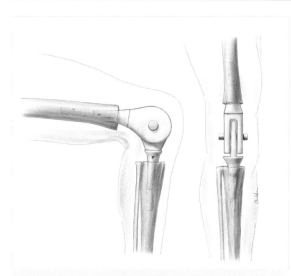

Fig. 6.1 Gluck's first ivory knee prosthesis. Drill holes in the shaft were made as slots for horizontal ivory peg fixation. (This image is provided courtesy of Dr. Samuel Christen, St. Gallen, Switzerland.)

6

implants at the 45th German Society for Surgery annual meeting. If his first implants had not been used to treat tuberculous joints, the humiliation of 1891 might not have occurred. However, his rationale was that these joints were completely destroyed by tuberculosis and there was nothing to lose by his experimental surgery. In 1922, he was made an "extraordinary professor" and in 1930, at the age of 77, was invited to join the honor roll of the German Surgical Society. Themistocles Gluck died in Berlin aged nearly 90 on 25 April 1942.[8]

6.2.4 The Concept of Flexible Implant Arthroplasty—Alfred B. Swanson (1923–2016)

Alfred Bertil Swanson, the son of Swedish parents, was born in 1923 in Wisconsin, USA. He graduated from the University of Illinois medical school in 1947 and subsequently underwent orthopaedic training at Illinois, Northwestern, and Indiana universities. Starting his career at the time of the thalidomide disaster and the great polio epidemic, Swanson was interested in treating children with polio, cerebral palsy, congenital limb differences, and arthritic deformities of the hand. He became Professor of Surgery at Michigan State University and served three terms between 1963 and 1978 as Chief of Staff at the Mary Free Rehabilitation Hospital. As a member of numerous national and international societies, he presented lectures and surgical demonstrations worldwide. He authored more than 300 publications, many of them together with his wife, Geneviève de Groot Swanson. He was President of the American Society for Surgery of the Hand (1979–1980), and Secretary General (1976–1983), President

(1983–1989), and Historian (1990–2003) of the International Federation of Societies for Surgery of the Hand (IFSSH). Swanson died at the age of 93 in 2016.

By applying silicone as an internal pad for below-knee amputations, Swanson discovered that this material would be suitable for joint arthroplasty.[9] In 1962, he introduced the concept of flexible implants for the reconstruction of small joints of the extremities and performed the first ever biocompatibility studies of silicone in bone. The Swanson one-piece implant comprises an intramedullary stem on either side bridged by a hinge. The inherent flexibility of the silicone elastomer allows flexion and extension at the hinge of the implant and provides a dampening effect on the bone. The implant is stiff enough to maintain joint alignment after bony resection and soft tissue balancing. Silicone implants have been machine tested for more than 130 million cycles without evidence of breakdown.[9] Swanson described two processes that occur with implantation and theoretically enhance implant performance. The first process is "encapsulation" or development of a fibrous joint capsule surrounding the implant, which enhances joint stability. The second process is the "piston effect" or the gliding motion of the stems within the medullary canals during joint flexion and extension. Theoretically, the piston effect increases the lifespan of the implant because forces are dispersed over a broad area of the implant. Gliding also allows a greater range of motion (ROM).[10] The original Swanson implant was made from a heat-vulcanized, medical-grade silicone elastomer stock. Swanson's silicone elastomer implant fulfilled most of his criteria for an ideal joint replacement: maintenance of joint space, preservation of stable joint motion, simple and efficient design, simple and durable fixation, resistance to stress and deterioration, biologically and mechanically acceptable to host, ease of manufacturing and sterilization, and facilitating rehabilitation.[9]

Swanson's concepts of a nonrigid prosthesis and the development of silicone elastomer, titanium, and other implants for small joint reconstruction revolutionized the surgical treatment of the arthritic hand, upper extremity, and forefoot. His work has benefited millions of arthritis sufferers worldwide and the finger joint silicone implant remains the golden standard of care more than 50 years later.

6.3 Early Design Developments in Wrist Arthroplasty

Due to its predictable functional outcome, the achievement of pain relief and its cost effectiveness, total hip replacement has been referred to as "the operation of the 20th century."[11] Nonetheless, replacements of other joints (excluding knee replacements) have been less predictable. The history of wrist replacement began with Swanson's concept of silicone arthroplasty followed by various developments in material, design, tribology, and bone anchorage over the decades. With the diversity of contemporary wrist arthroplasties to date, there is no single optimal standard; it also remains unclear whether the concept of arthroplasty is superior to total wrist arthrodesis for a large majority of patients.

6.3.1 First Generation: Elastomer Flexible Hinge Design

The Swanson implant was the first commonly used wrist prosthesis developed in 1967. It is a double-stemmed, flexible hinge silicone prosthesis, which acts as a spacer between the hand and forearm and allows some motion (▶ Fig. 6.2). Following the concepts of "encapsulation" and the "piston effect," the implant was not intended for bone fixation, but to allow motion between the implant and bone, and over time, fibrous tissue would form around the wrist joint. A proximal row carpectomy including the distal edge of the capitate and removal of the distal radius and ulnar head was performed to create space for the barrel-shaped midsection of the implant. The core of the implant was reinforced with Dacron (polyethylene terephthalate [PET]) to provide axial stability and resistance to rotational force. In 1974, the original silicone rubber was

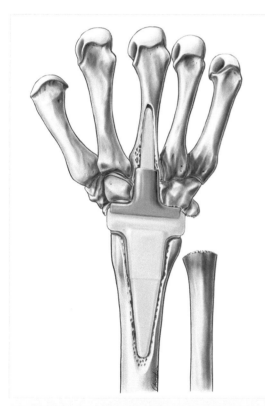

Fig. 6.2 Swanson's silicone flexible-hinged wrist implant. In a subsequent version, titanium grommets were applied to protect the silicone from rubbing against sharp bone. (This image is provided courtesy of Dr. Samuel Christen, St. Gallen, Switzerland.)

changed to a high-performance silicone elastomer that is more biocompatible and resistant to wear and fatigue. There have been several updates of the initial design to address breakage and wear, which include the application of titanium grommets in 1982 to protect the elastomer from rubbing against sharp bone. Swanson reported good pain relief, an acceptable ROM (34-degree flexion, 26-degree extension, 10-degree radial, and 18-degree ulnar deviation), a significant improvement in grip strength, and a relatively low complication rate in 181 wrists with a mean follow-up of 4 (range 0.5–10) years; 25 wrists were revised and 3 wrists were converted to arthrodesis.[12] These results have been difficult to reproduce by other working groups, and high complication rates for fracture, destructive silicone synovitis, persistent pain, and extensor tendon imbalance have been reported.[13] Prosthetic fracture occurs in up to 50% of patients, usually at the junction of the distal stem and barrel, although the incidence has decreased with the addition of metal grommets.[14] The reported incidence of silicone synovitis is 30%.[15]

6.3.2 Second Generation: Multicomponent Implants

In the 1970s, a second generation of hard-bearing multicomponent implants was introduced. There is no consensus on the definition of this implant type, although they generally consist of a radial component and a carpal component that is fixed to one or more metacarpal bones. Most of these implants are no longer available on the market because of unsatisfactory long-term results and the associated adverse events of loosening, soft tissue imbalance and dislocation.

Ball-and-Socket Designs

Meuli/MWP III

H. C. Meuli from Berne, Switzerland introduced his original prosthesis in 1972, an unconstrained reversed ball-and-socket implant. The proximal and distal metal components had two pliable prongs for cement fixation in the radius and metacarpal bones, respectively. The initial head on the proximal component was made of polyester, which resulted in marked tissue reactions in some of the first patients. It was abandoned in favor of high-molecular-weight polyethylene (HMWPE). Additionally, the center of rotation was too far radial, which resulted in significant ulnar deviation. The prosthetic design was modified in 1978 with a slightly volar and ulnar offset to the axis.[16] To adjust for problems with stability and imbalance, the Meuli 3rd generation implant (MWP III) was released in 1986 ▶ Fig. 6.3. The prosthesis was made from a titanium alloy with a corundum, rough-blasted surface for implantation using either cement or a press-fit technique. The nitride-coated ball was fixed to the proximal component and articulated with a relatively deep

6

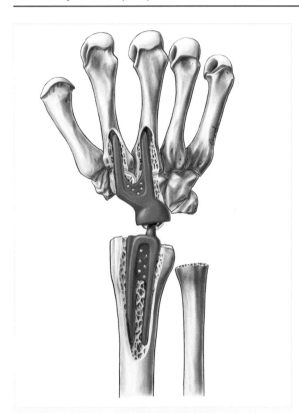

Fig. 6.3 The Meuli reversed ball-and-socket implant has undergone three generations of development. (This image is provided courtesy of Dr. Samuel Christen, St. Gallen, Switzerland.)

ultra-HMWPE (UHMWPE) socket distally. The anchoring prongs of the carpal component were angled 15 degree dorsal to the median axis. Meuli published satisfactory clinical results of 38 MWP III implants with a mean follow-up of 5.5 (range 3–9.5) years, but a revision rate of 30%.[17] The working group of Cooney revised 53 of 140 Meuli wrist implants as a result of dislocation, implant loosening, soft tissue deformity, median nerve compression, tendon rupture, and hematomas.[18]

Elos/Gibbon/Motec

A. Reigstad and colleagues developed the Elos prosthesis, a modular ball-and-socket wrist implant in the late 1990s.[19] Despite the ball-and-socket design and long metacarpal stem, the Motec implant should, in fact, be considered as an implant of the third generation, and will be discussed in further detail later in Chapter 26.

Constrained Designs

Figgie/Trispherical

H. E. Figgie III and colleagues developed the only fully constrained wrist prosthesis in 1977. The trispherical implant has metacarpal and radial components articulating with a HMWPE bearing and an axle restraint. The axle prevents dislocation, but does not absorb the load produced under normal activities of daily living.[20] Long-term results have been documented in 34 patients with rheumatoid arthritis (RA) at a mean follow-up of 9 (range 5–11) years.[21] Twenty-eight wrists were rated as good to excellent. The mean arc of flexion and extension improved from 35 to 50 degree. There were no deep infections or dislocations. Two wrists both required the removal of the implant and conversion to an arthrodesis, one for loosening and the other due to persistent pain. Postoperative tendon attrition occurred in six wrists, all of which had preoperative tendon ruptures necessitating tendon transfer. Radiographs showed radiolucency in seven wrists including seven around the metacarpal stem and one around the radial stem.[21] Lorei et al reported a 9% (8 implants) revision rate at a mean of 8.7 (range 3–18) years for 87 trispherical total wrist implants[22]; the primary complications were loosening, attritional rupture of extensor tendons and late sepsis. Five patients underwent implant removal and arthrodesis, two revision arthroplasty, and the last a resection arthroplasty.

Volz/Arizona Medical Center

R. G. Volz was inspired by the success of Charnley's low friction concept in hip arthroplasty using metal articulating with polyethylene and bone fixation with methyl methacrylate cement. In 1973, he designed a semiconstrained cemented wrist implant at the Arizona Medical Center based on these concepts (▶ Fig. 6.4). The implant had a hemispherical design with radii of two different dimensions to achieve motion in two planes without rotation, whilst providing 90-degree flexion/extension and 50-degree radial/ulnar deviation. The depth of the metal on polyethylene interface was designed to provide sufficient stability, especially to distraction forces. Proximal and distal component cementation further enhanced prosthesis stability.[23] Wrist imbalance was the main cause of poorer results with the double-prong metacarpal component, which was later modified to a single-prong counterpart. Long-term review at a mean of 8.6 (range 3.5–12.5) years in patients mostly with RA demonstrated pain relief in 83 to 86% with a flexion/extension arc of 49 degree and a radial/ulnar deviation arc of 25 degree. Metacarpal loosening was noted in 22%, a loss in carpal height in 24% and radial loosening in 6%.[24] Bone resorption under the collar of the radial component occurred in 79%.[25]

Convex–Concave Ellipsoidal Component Designs

Biaxial

The Biaxial implant was developed by and used at the Mayo Clinic since the early 1980s. It has a cobalt-chrome (CoCr) alloy metacarpal component with an ellipsoidal-

6

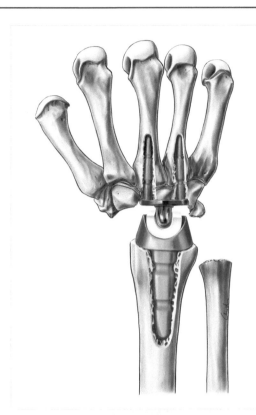

Fig. 6.4 Volz designed a semiconstrained implant. The original metacarpal component had two prongs, which was later modified to a single prong. (This image is provided courtesy of Dr. Samuel Christen, St. Gallen, Switzerland.)

shaped head articulating against a UHMWPE bearing surface attached to the metal radial component. The long stem of the metacarpal component is inserted into the middle finger metacarpal, and a small stud that fits into the trapezoid bone provides additional stability and fixation. Cement is used to fix the metacarpal and radial stems into position, but press-fit fixation is possible. The proximal surfaces of the implant also have a porous coating for enhanced stress distribution at the cement fixation interface.[26]

Cobb and Beckenbaugh performed a retrospective review of 46 patients with RA treated with the Biaxial implant with a mean follow-up of 6.5 (range 5–9.9) years. The authors reported significant improvements in pain, ROM (extension and radial deviation), and grip strength. While the Biaxial total wrist prosthesis had an overall 5-year survival of 83 % (67 % without cement), there was radiographic loosening in 22 % with subsequent revision in eight cases.[26] A systematic literature review showed that 22 (8 %) of 278 Biaxial implants in seven patient series were reported to have dislocated.[27] A retrospective review of 32 Biaxial total wrist implants found a survival rate of 81 % after 7 years.[28] Thirty-one complications were noted and 22 wrists showed signs of radiographic

loosening. Overall, ROM improved with the exception of pronation, and both the mean pain and DASH scores improved.

Guépar/Horus

The Guépar was developed by Y. Alnot in Paris, France in 1979. The radial component is made entirely of UHMWPE and is cemented into the radius. The carpal component has a metal plate that is fixed by two screws into the index and middle finger metacarpals. An egg-shaped CoCr alloy–bearing surface is then fitted over the plate and secured with a small screw. The distal radius and ulna are resected and a straight cutting plane is prepared at the level of the proximal capitate.[29]

In a retrospective follow-up of 72 wrists with a mean follow-up of 4 (range 1–10) years, 11 wrists underwent revision due to loosening of the small screw and proximal components. Osteolysis and bone resorption was noted under the carpal plate, which increased with time.[29] A redesigned version of the implant is marketed as the Horus total wrist prosthesis since 2009.

Universal

The Universal wrist implant, developed by J. Menon, is an unconstrained arthroplasty with titanium radial and carpal components. The concave articular surface of the radial component has a 20-degree inclination with a Y-shaped stem surrounded by a titanium mesh for bone ingrowth. The component can be inserted with or without bone cement. With this particular implant, almost 95 % of the capitate is preserved along with part of the scaphoid and triquetrum. Primary fixation of the carpal plate is in the capitate and not in the medullary canal of the middle finger metacarpal. The carpal component is ovoid with three holes in the carpal plate for screw fixation into the carpal/metacarpal bones. A convex toroid-shaped HMWPE inlay slides over the carpal plate and is locked in place by a locking pin. The surgical technique involves an intercarpal arthrodesis at the level of the distal carpal resection through the proximal pole of the capitate, including the distal scaphoid, resection of the ulnar head, and an inclined resection of the distal radius.[30] The initial results for 37 wrists after a mean follow-up of 6.7 years (range 48–120 mo) were good pain relief in 88 % and an increase in the flexion/extension arc from 73 to 96 degrees. But there was a complication rate of 28 % which included dislocations, radial component loosening, and deep infection.[30] In a second, revised design, the distal component was altered to have a centrally placed peg with indentations and screws on each side (▶ Fig. 6.5). The radial-sided distal screw was made longer in order to allow for improved purchase in the index finger metacarpal. Cement was used on the proximal side and for the distal peg. Prospective results of 19 revised Universal implants in 15 patients with RA showed a high rate of

6

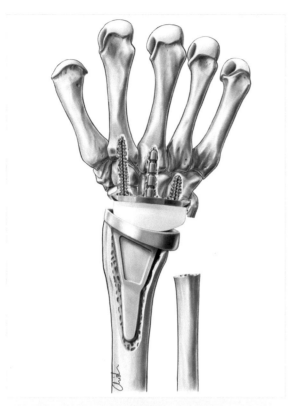

Fig. 6.5 Several concave–convex ellipsoidal component wrist arthroplasty designs were developed in the 1980s and early 1990s including the Universal implant. These early implants share relative extensive bone resection and fixation in the metacarpal bones by bridging the carpometacarpal (CMC). (This image is provided courtesy of Dr. Samuel Christen, St. Gallen, Switzerland.)

failure with 50% revision rate at the latest follow-up at average 7.3 (range 5.0–10.8) years. Nine prostheses (45%) had undergone revision surgery because of carpal component loosening.[31]

Destot

The Destot prosthesis was designed in 1991 in France and Belgium to specifically treat posttraumatic osteoarthritis (OA). With a sandblasted and porous-coated steel proximal and distal component, UHMWPE radial cup, proximal steel carpal ball, condylar UHMWPE cylinder, and distal steel component, the distal component is designed to stay next to the triquetrum after resection of the scaphoid and lunate, while preserving the distal radioulnar joint (DRUJ).

Levadoux and Legré published their experiences treating 28 stage 2 or 3 scapholunate advanced collapse (SLAC) and scaphoid nonunion advanced collapse (SNAC) wrists in 25 patients with a mean follow-up of 47 (range 12–72) months.[32] A high rate of revisions and distal component loosening were observed. The revisions included

three wrists revised due to pain or infection. The 4-year survival rate was 85%. The mean ROM increased for flexion/extension from 26/20 to 48/41 degree, for radial/ulnar deviation from 7/25 to 15/22 degree, and for pronation/supination from 60/45 to 90/77 degree. The mean grip strength increased from 20 to 32 kgf.[32]

Anatomic Physiologic (APH)

The APH wrist prosthesis was designed and introduced by S. Radmer and colleagues in Berlin, Germany.[33] The implant, developed for patients with RA, is a two-component hydroxyapatite-coated CoCr alloy prosthesis with titanium-coated stems for cement-free implantation. The articular surface of the radial component and the mobile-bearing surface of the carpal component have a radioulnar inclination of 10 degree. The distal component is anchored in the middle finger metacarpal and distal carpal bones.[33] Although short-term outcome was good, the results gradually deteriorated. At a mean follow-up of 52 (range 24–73) months, 39 of 40 patients required revision surgery mainly because of loosening with subsequent dislocation.[34] Severe titanium wear staining the soft tissues was noted at every revision.

6.4 Contemporary Designs in Wrist Arthroplasty

In the literature, there is a lack of consensus on the definition of implant generation. Currently available arthroplasties are inconsistently referred to as third- or fourth-generation implants. In this overview, the third-generation implants encompass all currently available multicomponent implants. The majority of third-generation implants as well as those made of pyrocarbon, which can also be referred to as fourth-generation prostheses, will be discussed in further detail later in this book.

6.4.1 Third Generation: Minimal Bone Resection

The third generation of wrist arthroplasties was designed with the goal of minimizing bone resection, sparing the DRUJ, avoiding fixation in the metacarpal bones, restoring the "anatomical" centers of wrist rotation and improving soft tissue balance and stability. An exception is the Motec design, which differs because its fixation with a large screw in the radius and middle finger metacarpal uses a ball-and-socket joint; this implant has been referred to as a second-generation implant.[35] A recently published systematic review of total wrist arthroplasty and wrist arthrodesis shows significantly lower overall complication rates for the newer generation implants compared to their older counterparts that are defined as second-generation implants in this overview. Survival rates of 78% at 15 years (Universal

6

2), 95 % at 8 years (Maestro), 90 % at 9 years (ReMotion), and 86 % at 10 years (Motec) have been reported.[35] Those current available implants will be discussed in further detail in a subsequent chapter of this book.

6.5 Arthroplasty of the Distal Radioulnar Joint (DRUJ)

6.5.1 Resection/Interposition Arthroplasty

For the arthritic DRUJ, several nonprosthetic procedures have been described in the past, which are still common solutions in the armamentarium of many hand surgeons. The Darrach's procedure involves the resection of the ulnar head.[36] The first description of ulnar head resection was documented in the French literature in 1855 by J. F. Malgaine; this method was used for irreducible open dislocations to prevent infection with subsequent loss of the whole hand. For acute injuries, E. M. Moore was the first to mention this procedure in the American literature in 1880, and C. Lauenstein made his contribution to the German literature in 1887.[37] Segmental resection of the ulna shaft without arthrodesis of the DRUJ was first performed by the French surgeons R. Le Fort and P. Colo-lian in 1918, but is often cited as the Lauenstein procedure.[37] Segmental resection of the distal ulna shaft with radioulnar arthrodesis known as the Sauve–Kapandji procedure was described by L. Sauvé and M. Kapandji in 1936[38] and modified by I. A. Kapandji in 1986.[39] Longitudinal hemi-resection of the distal ulna was described in the 1980s by W. H. Bowers with interposition of either the dorsal capsule or an "anchovy" made of tendon/muscle,[40] and by H. K. Watson who performed a "matched" distal ulna resection leaving the ulnar shaft-styloid axis along with the triangular fibrocartilage (TFC) complex and the distal ulnar ligamentous attachments intact.[41]

Although modifications of these "salvage procedures" have evolved, complications related to instability of the distal forearm remain the most common problem leading to pain often related to ulnoradial impingement, and weakness of grip and torsional forearm strength.[42] Optimal load transfer from the wrist to the elbow requires a functioning DRUJ. About 20 % of the total load passes into the ulnar through the normal DRUJ.[43] The greatest forces of up to 34 % occur through the ulna in supination. If the ulnar head is excised, only 1.8 to 2.7 % of the total load is transmitted to the ulna at the wrist.[44]

6.5.2 Ulna Head Replacement

Partial DRUJ arthroplasty was developed in the 1970s by replacing the ulnar head with a silastic implant.[45] Due to the extremely high bone resorption rates of up to 100 %, and high (40–63 %) rates of prosthesis migration or breakage, these implants are no longer used.[46,47] In recognizing the shortcomings of silicone rubber implants, a group of European and US hand surgeons, under the leadership of T. J. Herbert, designed a modular ulnar head replacement that was released onto the market in 1995. This system comprises a ceramic ulnar head fitting onto a metallic stem for insertion into the ulna.[48] The head is capable of rotating on the stem as the radius dynamically rotates around the ulna. Soon after the release of the Herbert ulnar head prosthesis, similar implants became available from several other manufacturers. The predominantly used implants are the Avanta U-Head or Integra First Choice ulna head replacement. The outcomes of these implants are described in more detail in Chapters 31 to 33.

6.5.3 Partial Ulna Head Replacement

The Eclypse implant, developed by M. Garcia-Elias, is a pyrocarbon spacer used for DRUJ hemiarthroplasty. It replaces the articular portion of the ulnar head while preserving the insertion of the TFC at the level of the fovea, the ulnocarpal ligaments, and the extensor carpi ulnaris sheath.[49] This implant is described in more detail in Chapter 34.

6.5.4 Total DRUJ Replacement

As an alternative to the "salvage procedures" of the destroyed DRUJ described earlier, L. R. Scheker designed a total DRUJ replacement. The Aptis total DRUJ replacement prosthesis consists of a semiconstrained and modular implant designed to replace the function of the ulnar head, the sigmoid notch of the radius, and the TFC ligaments. The ulnar components include a press-fit endomedullary CoCr alloy stem with a titanium plasma-sprayed surface for osteointegration, and a UHMWPE ball. The ulnar head is attached to the radial plate intraoperatively to ensure that the adequate level of implant constraint is maintained.[50] This implant is described in more detail in Chapter 35.

6.6 Arthroplasty of Metacarpophalangeal and Proximal Interphalangeal Joints

6.6.1 Resection/Interposition Arthroplasty

Stiffness of metacarpophalangeal (MCP) and proximal interphalangeal (PIP) joints after trauma was the stimulus for developing partial or complete resection arthroplasties in an effort to regain some motion.

In 1946, S. B. Fowler described a technique for the MCP joint in which the metacarpal head was shaped in a transverse pointed end by resecting dorsal and volar half

6

wedges.[51] A thin line of bone was left to articulate with the center of the proximal phalanx base. The former sliding joint was changed to a hinge joint, which allowed only limited flexion. In severe volar-dislocated rheumatoid MCP joint deformities, Fowler recommended an additional tenodesis of the extensor tendon to the proximal phalanx base so as to prevent recurrence of volar dislocation.[51] In 1956, D. C. Riordan modified the technique by excising only the volar wedge from the metacarpal head and immobilizing the joint with a Kirschner wire to allow the collateral ligaments to heal to their new insertion on the dorsal cortex of the metacarpal.[51]

Inspired by the positive outcome of the Vitallium (CoCrMo alloy) cup arthroplasty of the hip,[52] M. S. Burman and R. H. Abrahamson attempted an interposition arthroplasty of the MCP and PIP joints in 1943 with Vitallium and Lucite (methyl methacrylate) caps which lead to lateral joint instability.[53] In the 1964 fourth edition of Bunnell's Surgery of the Hand, an interposition arthroplasty technique is described using fascia lata.[54]

K. Vainio and colleagues introduced an interposition arthroplasty of the MCP joint in RA patients in 1968. They resected the metacarpal head and interposed the distal stump of the transected extensor tendon into the joint, sewing it down to the volar plate and additionally transposed the radial interosseous muscles.[55]

In the late 1960s, A. Tupper described a resection arthroplasty of the MCP joint, interposing the proximally detached volar plate and suturing it to the dorsal edge of the resected metacarpal.[56]

There is general agreement that the long-term follow-up of RA patients who receive any type of resection arthroplasty eventually reveals absorption and shortening of the metacarpal bone accompanied by progressive instability, recurrence of volar subluxation, ulnar drift, and finger shortening.[51]

The earliest report on resection arthroplasty of the PIP joint without interposing any material was published in 1954 by Carroll and Taber who presented 30 cases of deformed and ankylosed PIP joints with a follow-up ranging from 6 months to 7 years.[57] They resected the distal part of the proximal phalanx through a mid-lateral approach. A Kirschner wire was passed through the middle phalanx to maintain joint distraction for 6 weeks.

For the PIP joint, volar plate arthroplasty was not immediately applicable during this early time because the volar plate was responsible for joint stability to prevent dorsal subluxation during hyperextension. In 1967, R. G. Eaton adapted the volar plate interposition arthroplasty for post-traumatic PIP joint destruction. The volar plate was detached from the middle phalanx and sutured into a trough in the base of the middle phalanx to reconstruct the volar articular surface. The aim of this reconstruction was to restore a smooth gliding surface to the base of the middle phalanx.[58] Satisfactory function and pain-free motion were reported after a mean follow-up of 11.5 years.[59]

6.6.2 Transplant Arthroplasty

As early as 1910, the German surgeon H. Wolff reported the successful autologous transplantation of an entire proximal phalanx of the second toe, with its periosteum and both joints, in a case of tuberculosis affecting the proximal phalanx of a female ring finger.[60] Three years later, W. Goebel used the same procedure for a case of enchondroma.[60] Oeleker performed a cadaver joint transplantation in the case of an ankylosed PIP joint sustained after a gunshot wound.[10] In 1948, W. C. Graham and D. C. Riordan replaced several metacarpal heads with fourth metatarsal heads and published satisfactory 1-year postoperative ROM without any radiological signs of degenerative changes.[61] In 1954, Graham replaced an entire thumb MCP joint in a 3-year-old boy with a fourth metatarsophalangeal joint.[10] Transplant arthroplasty using the vascularized toe transfer technique will be discussed in further detail later in Chapter 10.

6.6.3 Hinged Implant Arthroplasty

E. B. Brannon and G. Klein developed a metal, hinged prosthesis for posttraumatic damaged joints of the finger in selected cases, which would serve as an alternative to amputation or arthrodesis. In 1959, they published their results in 14 patients with a follow-up of approximately 3 years. The original device made of steel, is now a titanium implant consisting of both uncemented proximal and distal stems articulating with a hinge that is locked by a screw (▶ Fig. 6.6). Significant bone resorption around the stems, longitudinal rotation, and subsidence led to revision with fixation of the stems to the adjacent bone by staples.[62] As a result, A. E. Flatt developed another hinged, metal prosthesis with two-pronged stems for rheumatoid MCP and PIP joints.[63]

Although several types of hinged MCP and PIP implants have been developed, they all share common problems. Lateral as well as subluxation forces are transmitted through the implant shaft and place stress on the bone–stem interface. Bone resorption with subsequent loosening or fracture around the intramedullary shaft, fibrosis around the hinge mechanism, fracturing of prongs, screw failure, wear within the conventional hinge mechanism with subsequent deposit of metallic debris, and breakdown of the overlying skin have been documented.[63,64,65,66]

6.6.4 One-Piece Polymer Arthroplasty

After the unsatisfactory results of metal-hinged implants, the use of plastics was favored. Several polymer one-piece prostheses were then developed in the late 1960s. Polypropylene and silicone are relatively cheap, inert, durable, and simple to mold.[64] The former allowed the design of a thin hinge to complement flexion while good

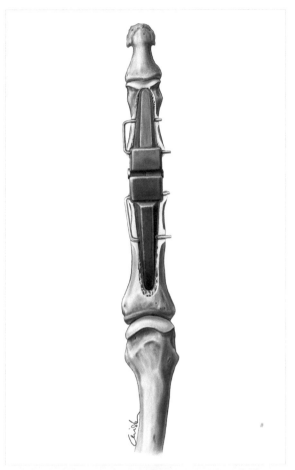

Fig. 6.6 Brannon and Klein developed a metal-hinged implant for cement-free metacarpophalangeal (MCP) and proximal interphalangeal (PIP) arthroplasties in posttraumatic damaged joints. (This image is provided courtesy of Dr. Samuel Christen, St. Gallen, Switzerland.)

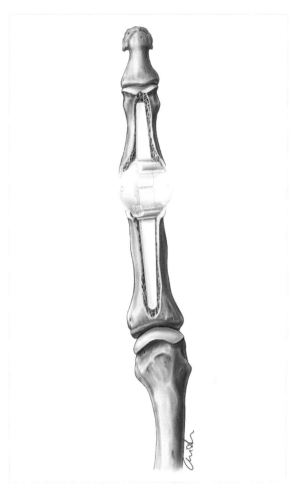

Fig. 6.7 Nicolle and Calnan designed an encapsulated thin-hinged implant with a polypropylene body and silicone capsule. (This image is provided courtesy of Dr. Samuel Christen, St. Gallen, Switzerland.)

lateral stability was retained. Under axial compression, however, buckling of the hinge and subsequent subluxation occurred. F. V. Nicolle and J. S. Calnan developed a thin-hinged polyethylene implant with an encapsulating silicone polymer balloon to prevent direct contact between soft tissues and the hinge[64] (▶ Fig. 6.7). J. J. Niebauer and colleagues designed a laminated silicone-Dacron, thin-hinge device with stems covered by a Dacron mesh to provide fibrous fixation.[67,68]

Swanson began the development of various novel MCP and PIP implants in 1962. The basic design of these devices comprised a single silicone unit with tapered proximal and distal stems and a dorsal offset hinge region.[9] The broad stem-hub junction resisted buckling, but the tensile stress in the convex aspect of the hinge under a bending moment increased disproportionately as the square of thickness and inversely with length. Over time this led to fracture in or near the hinge element and the development of cold flow deformities or structural changes.[65] Later

improvements involved alterations of the silicone polymer composition to provide greater strength and the inclusion of protective metal grommets at the stem-hub junction to prevent erosion at the bone ends.[69] The Swanson-designed silicone implant has, nonetheless, remained the joint replacement of choice for several decades.

6.6.5 Metalloplastic Arthroplasty

Metalloplastic designs proliferated after the success of total hip arthroplasties that used metal and polyethylene articular components. These hybrid material designs used several different concepts to establish a workable articulation and stable intramedullary fixation. Most relied on a captive metal element rotating within a UHMWPE bearing, whereas others were designed to be implanted at the MCP and PIP joints. The greater the constraint, the greater the stresses that were transmitted through the prosthesis to the stem–bone interface. Breakage, erosion, contracture,

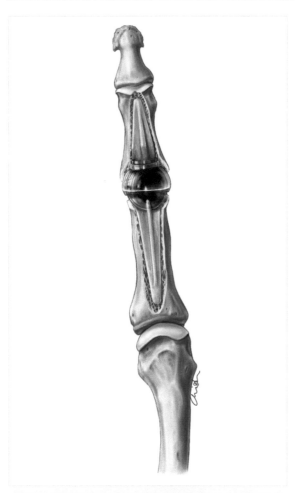

Fig. 6.8 The Nicolle implant is one example from a wide variety of constrained metalloplastic arthroplasty designs available for treating metacarpophalangeal (MCP) and proximal interphalangeal (PIP) joints in the past. (This image is provided courtesy of Dr. Samuel Christen, St. Gallen, Switzerland.)

and other adverse events have plagued many of these initiatives[65]($\triangleright$ Fig. 6.8).

6.6.6 Surface Replacement Arthroplasty

In 1979, R. L. Linscheid and J. H. Dobyns developed the first anatomical surface replacement arthroplasty (SRA) for the PIP joint at the Mayo Clinic.[70] SRA aims to recreate the center of rotation of the native joint, which allows for a combination of rolling and sliding at the terminal ends of motion. Implant stability is achieved through preservation of the collateral ligaments and volar plate, implant–bone interface integration, and inherent implant design. The initial Mayo SRA was an internally constrained prosthesis. Progressive erosion of the cortical bone and consecutive migration of the implant led to unsatisfactory results.[70] To overcome these problems, the original design

was adapted to incorporate a proximal bicondylar CoCr alloy component articulated with a distal, pure UHMWPE double-concave component designed for cementation. They reported particularly good results in the treatment of degenerative arthritis and somewhat better results with a dorsal approach. The complication rate was almost 30 % and included events of instability, ulnar deviation, swan-neck deformity, flexion contracture, tenodesis, and joint subluxation.[70] The prosthesis design was modified in 2000 to incorporate a titanium-stemmed distal component to support press-fit cementless fixation.[71] Based on this specific concept, several implants have come onto the market over the past two decades. Some of the latest PIP joint SRAs will be discussed in further detail in Chapters 9 and 12 to 15.

6.6.7 Pyrocarbon Implant Arthroplasty

R. D. Beckenbaugh developed the first pyrocarbon implant for the MCP joint. As a cementless two-component implant, this device is fixed to the bone by press-fit into the medullary canal and was applied for the first time in 1979.[72] The concept was adapted for the PIP joint with initially promising results. However, since the introduction of the PIP pyrocarbon implant, numerous studies have published variable long-term results.[73] Pyrocarbon arthroplasty of the MCP and PIP joints will be discussed in more detail later in Chapter 12.

6.7 Arthroplasty of the Trapeziometacarpal (TMC) Joint

6.7.1 Interposition Arthroplasty

Soft Tissue

The most common surgical treatment of TMC arthritis is trapeziectomy with soft tissue interposition with or without ligament reconstruction.[74,75,76,77] Overall, good pain relief is achieved, but opinions are varied with regard to whether proximal migration of the first metacarpal bone results in decreased pinch strength.[78,79,80,81] Long-term studies, in fact, show that patients have a weak lateral pinch after tendon interposition arthroplasties. Therefore, this treatment is mainly reserved for older, less-demanding patients who do not engage in occupations requiring manual labor or heavy machinery.[78,80,81]

Silicone

The first TMC arthroplasty consisting of trapeziectomy and replacement with a silicone implant was performed in 1965 by Swanson. It resulted in a good ROM and grip strength.[82] Since this time, silicone arthroplasty of the TMC joint has been extensively used and studied by many surgeons. Patient-related outcome measures (PROMs) such as pain relief and function have generally been comparable with alternative surgical treatments such as trapeziectomy and its variants. However, radiographic changes showing periprosthetic lysis, subsidence of the thumb metacarpal, long-term implant failure because of fracture, and resultant silicone giant cell synovitis with bone resorption are major adverse events associated with this implant.[83,84,85,86,87,88]

Artelon

The Artelon TMC spacer is a T-shaped, biodegradable polycaprolactone-based polyurethane urea material proposed for use in isolated cases of TMC arthritis. The device has two modes of action: first, it stabilizes the carpometacarpal (CMC) joint by augmenting the joint capsule, and second, it resurfaces the distal part of the trapezium. The device aimed to provide a scaffold for tissue ingrowth and prevent impingement between the bones of the CMC joint. The wings of the implant are typically fixed with two screws. In vitro degradation studies revealed that complete hydrolysis of Artelon takes approximately 6 years.[89] In the pilot study by Nilsson and colleagues, this implant showed superior results for key and tripod pinch function compared to trapeziectomy and ligament reconstruction and tendon interposition (LRTI) arthroplasty.[89] However, a randomized controlled, multicenter follow-up study showed that pain and postoperative swelling were more common in Artelon-treated patients compared to those treated with trapeziectomy and LRTI arthroplasty, which was accompanied by a lack of increase in key and tripod pinch.[90] Several patients treated with Artelon underwent subsequent implant removal. Biopsies of the removed soft tissues and synovium in revision cases revealed a granulomatous foreign body giant cell reaction to the implant.[91,92,93]

Pyrocarbon

Pyrocarbon interposition arthroplasty for the arthritic TMC joint has been described by P. Bellemère and colleagues in 2011.[94] Depending on the configuration, implants can be used after total or partial trapeziectomy or inserted into the TMC joint space.[73] These implants—known under the names of Pyrocardan, PyroDisk, and PI2—will be discussed in further detail later in Chapters 19 and 20.

6.7.2 Hemiarthroplasty of the TMC Joint

Titanium

In an effort to address the silicone wear problem, Swanson selected unalloyed titanium as an alternative material for spacer implants, and performed a TMC joint hemiarthroplasty with this metal component in 1984. Swanson published excellent clinical results after a mean follow-up of 5 years with radiographic bone remodeling around the base of the implant within the first 6 months after surgery that remained stable.[95] Nevertheless, radiological loosening with implant settling and abnormal wear of the trapezoid bone were seen frequently and led to failure rates of up to 20%.[96,97] The mismatch in the stiffness of titanium, which has a 1000 times higher Young's modulus of elasticity than cortical bone, may be responsible for the high localized stresses leading to implant loosening.[97]

Pyrocarbon

The first-generation pyrocarbon TMC hemiarthroplasty implant—the PyroHemiSphere prosthesis—was initially designed for use in the MCP joint and represents the proximal component of this implant.[98] The NuGrip is the second generation of this implant specifically designed for the TMC joint and will be discussed in further detail in Chapter 19.

6.7.3 Total TMC Arthroplasty

Ball-and-Socket Design

The earliest total TMC joint replacement involved a cemented ball-and-socket implant with a UHMWPE cup inserted into the trapezium and a CoCr alloy stem in the metacarpal designed by J. Y. de la Caffinière and Aucouturier in 1971.[99] Early investigations showed overall good clinical results, although there were several cases of asymptomatic radiographic loosening of the trapezium component.[100,101,102] A long-term follow-up of 8.5 (range 2–16) years revealed an implant survival rate of only 72% and an overall loosening rate of 44%.[103]

Several implants have been developed in the past decade with the aim of overcoming the most frequent complications of early dislocation and component loosening in the long term. Most of the currently available total TMC arthroplasty devices have a ball-and-socket design. The outcomes of these implants are described in more detail in Chapter 18.

Dual mobility might be an effective concept to reduce dislocation and still provide a good ROM. Mechanically, there are two concentric articulations: a small one represented by the neck moving against a cup and a greater one represented by the cup moving against the trapezium implant.[104] Developments in implant fixation technique, optimizing the long metacarpal lever arm and different surface coating for durable osteointegration might be effective in reducing component loosening. Several of the most recent implants such as the MAÏA, Ivory, Moovis, or Touch prostheses will be discussed in further detail in Chapter 21.

6

Acknowledgment

We thank Dr. Samuel Christen (Kantonsspital St. Gallen) for drawing the pictures and Dr. Melissa Wilhelmi (Schulthess Klinik) for manuscript editing.

References

[1] PacheCO. Pelops. In: Pache CO, ed. Baby and Child Heroes in Ancient Greece. Urbana, IL: University of Illinois Press;2004:84–94

[2] Friedmann LW. Amputations and prostheses in primitive cultures. Bull Prosthet Res. 1972; 10–17:105–138

[3] Ritt MJ, Stuart PR, Naggar L, Beckenbaugh RD. The early history of arthroplasty of the wrist:from amputation to total wrist implant. J Hand Surg [Br]. 1994; 19(6):778–782

[4] BeyerJU. Zwanzigste Wahrnehmung. In: Bilguer JU, ed. Chirurgische Wahrnehmungen welche meistens während dem von 1756 bis 1763 gedauerten Krieg über in denen Königlich Preussischen Feldlazarethen von verschiedenen Wundärzten aufgezeichnet. Berlin: Wever; 1763:443–444

[5] Chauvin F, Schiele P, Chauvin E, Fischer Cossu-Ferra V, Fischer LP. Les docteurs Moreau de Bar-le-Duc: Victor Moreau (1746-1799) et Pierre-Félix Moreau (1778-1846). Les premières resections ostéo-articulaires. Hist Sci Med. 2002; 36(3):250–251

[6] Thompson FR. An essay on the development of arthroplasty of the hip. Clin Orthop Relat Res. 1966; 44(44):73–82

[7] Rosenfeld JF, Nicholson JJ. History and design considerations for arthroplasty around the wrist. Hand Clin. 2013; 29(1):1–13

[8] Eynon-Lewis NJ, Ferry D, Pearse MF. Themistocles Gluck: an unrecognised genius. BMJ. 1992; 305(6868):1534–1536

[9] Swanson AB. Finger joint replacement by silicone rubber implants and the concept of implant fixation by encapsulation. Ann Rheum Dis. 1969; 28 Suppl 5:47–55

[10] Berger RA. A brief history of finger arthroplasty. Iowa Orthop J. 1989; 9:77–82

[11] Learmonth ID, Young C, Rorabeck C. The operation of the century: total hip replacement. Lancet. 2007; 370(9597):1508–1519

[12] Swanson AB, de Groot Swanson G, Maupin BK. Flexible implant arthroplasty of the radiocarpal joint:surgical technique and long-term study. Clin Orthop Relat Res. 1984(187):94–106

[13] Reigstad O. Wrist arthroplasty: bone fixation, clinical development and mid to long term results. Acta Orthop Suppl. 2014; 85(354): 1–53

[14] Capone RA, Jr. The titanium grommet in flexible implant arthroplasty of the radiocarpal joint: a long-term review of 44 cases. Plast Reconstr Surg. 1995; 96(3):667–672

[15] Lawler EA, Paksima N. Total wrist arthroplasty. Bull NYU Hosp Jt Dis. 2006; 64(3–4):98–105

[16] Meuli HC. Meuli total wrist arthroplasty. Clin Orthop Relat Res. 1984 (187):107–111

[17] Meuli HC. Total wrist arthroplasty:experience with a noncemented wrist prosthesis. Clin Orthop Relat Res. 1997(342):77–83

[18] Cooney WP, III, Beckenbaugh RD, Linscheid RL. Total wrist arthroplasty:problems with implant failures. Clin Orthop Relat Res. 1984 (187):121–128

[19] Reigstad A, Reigstad O, Grimsgaard C, Røkkum M. New concept for total wrist replacement. J Plast Surg Hand Surg. 2011; 45(3):148–156

[20] Figgie HE, III, Ranawat CS, Inglis AE, Straub LR, Mow C. Preliminary results of total wrist arthroplasty in rheumatoid arthritis using the trispherical total wrist arthroplasty. J Arthroplasty. 1988; 3(1):9–15

[21] Figgie MP, Ranawat CS, Inglis AE, Sobel M, Figgie HE, III. Trispherical total wrist arthroplasty in rheumatoid arthritis. J Hand Surg Am. 1990; 15(2):217–223

[22] Lorei MP, Figgie MP, Ranawat CS, Inglis AE. Failed total wrist arthroplasty:analysis of failures and results of operative management. Clin Orthop Relat Res. 1997(342):84–93

[23] Volz RG. The development of a total wrist arthroplasty. Clin Orthop Relat Res. 1976(116):209–214

[24] Bosco JA, III, Bynum DK, Bowers WH. Long-term outcome of Volz total wrist arthroplasties. J Arthroplasty. 1994; 9(1):25–31

[25] Dennis DA, Ferlic DC, Clayton ML. Volz total wrist arthroplasty in rheumatoid arthritis: a long-term review. J Hand Surg Am. 1986; 11(4):483–490

[26] Cobb TK, Beckenbaugh RD. Biaxial total-wrist arthroplasty. J Hand Surg Am. 1996; 21(6):1011–1021

[27] Boeckstyns ME. Wrist arthroplasty: a systematic review. Dan Med J. 2014; 61(5):A4834

[28] Harlingen Dv, Heesterbeek PJ, J de Vos M. High rate of complications and radiographic loosening of the biaxial total wrist arthroplasty in rheumatoid arthritis: 32 wrists followed for 6 (5–8) years. Acta Orthop. 2011; 82(6):721–726

[29] Fourastier J, Le Breton L, Alnot Y, Langlais F, Condamine JL, Pidhorz L. La prothèse totale radio-carpienne Guépar dans la chirurgie du poignet rhumatoïde. A propos de 72 cas revus. Rev Chir Orthop Repar Appar Mot. 1996; 82(2):108–115

[30] Menon J. Universal total wrist implant: experience with a carpal component fixed with three screws. J Arthroplasty. 1998; 13 (5):515–523

[31] Ward CM, Kuhl T, Adams BD. Five to ten-year outcomes of the Universal total wrist arthroplasty in patients with rheumatoid arthritis. J Bone Joint Surg Am. 2011; 93(10):914–919

[32] Levadoux M, Legré R. Total wrist arthroplasty with Destot prostheses in patients with posttraumatic arthritis. J Hand Surg Am. 2003; 28(3):405–413

[33] Radmer S, Andresen R, Sparmann M. Wrist arthroplasty with a new generation of prostheses in patients with rheumatoid arthritis. J Hand Surg Am. 1999; 24(5):935–943

[34] Radmer S, Andresen R, Sparmann M. Total wrist arthroplasty in patients with rheumatoid arthritis. J Hand Surg Am. 2003; 28 (5):789–794

[35] Berber O, Garagnani L, Gidwani S. Systematic review of total wrist arthroplasty and arthrodesis in wrist arthritis. J Wrist Surg. 2018; 7(5):424–440

[36] Darrach W. Partial excision of lower shaft of ulna for deformity following Colles's fracture. Ann Surg. 1913; 57:764–765

[37] Buck-Gramcko D. On the priorities of publication of some operative procedures on the distal end of the ulna. J Hand Surg [Br]. 1990; 15(4):416–420

[38] Sauvé L, Kapandji M. Nouvelle technique de traitement chirurgical des luxations récidivantes isolées de l'extrémité inferieure du cubitus. J Chir (Paris). 1936; 47:589–594

[39] Kapandji IA. The Kapandji-Sauvé operation:its techniques and indications in non rheumatoid diseases. Ann Chir Main. 1986; 5(3): 181–193

[40] Bowers WH. Distal radioulnar joint arthroplasty: the hemiresection-interposition technique. J Hand Surg Am. 1985; 10(2):169–178

[41] Watson HK, Ryu JY, Burgess RC. Matched distal ulnar resection. J Hand Surg Am. 1986; 11(6):812–817

[42] Sauerbier M, Hahn ME, Berglund LJ, An KN, Berger RA. Biomechanical evaluation of the dynamic radioulnar convergence after ulnar head resection, two soft tissue stabilization methods of the distal ulna and ulnar head prosthesis implantation. Arch Orthop Trauma Surg. 2011; 131(1):15–26

[43] Werner FW, Palmer AK, Fortino MD, Short WH. Force transmission through the distal ulna: effect of ulnar variance, lunate fossa angulation, and radial and palmar tilt of the distal radius. J Hand Surg Am. 1992; 17(3):423–428

[44] Shaaban H, Giakas G, Bolton M, Williams R, Scheker LR, Lees VC. The distal radioulnar joint as a load-bearing mechanism: a biomechanical study. J Hand Surg Am. 2004; 29(1):85–95

6

[45] Swanson AB. Implant arthroplasty for disabilities of the distal radio-ulnar joint:use of a silicone rubber capping implant following resection of the ulnar head. Orthop Clin North Am. 1973; 4(2):373–382

[46] Sagerman SD, Seiler JG, Fleming LL, Lockerman E. Silicone rubber distal ulnar replacement arthroplasty. J Hand Surg [Br]. 1992; 17(6):689–693

[47] Stanley D, Herbert TJ. The Swanson ulnar head prosthesis for post-traumatic disorders of the distal radio-ulnar joint. J Hand Surg [Br]. 1992; 17(6):682–688

[48] van Schoonhoven J, Fernandez DL, Bowers WH, Herbert TJ. Salvage of failed resection arthroplasties of the distal radioulnar joint using a new ulnar head prosthesis. J Hand Surg Am. 2000; 25(3):438–446

[49] Garcia-Elias M. Eclypse: partial ulnar head replacement for the isolated distal radio-ulnar joint arthrosis. Tech Hand Up Extrem Surg. 2007; 11(1):121–128

[50] Scheker LR. Implant arthroplasty for the distal radioulnar joint. J Hand Surg Am. 2008; 33(9):1639–1644

[51] Riordan DC, Fowler SB. Arthroplasty of the metacarpophalangeal joints: review of resection-type arthroplasty. J Hand Surg Am. 1989; 14 2 Pt 2:368–371

[52] Hernigou P. Smith-Petersen and early development of hip arthroplasty. Int Orthop. 2014; 38(1):193–198

[53] Steinberg DR, Steinberg ME. The early history of arthroplasty in the United States. Clin Orthop Relat Res. 2000(374):55–89

[54] BunnellS, ed. Surgery of the Hand. 4th ed. Philadelphia: JB Lippincott; 1964

[55] Hellum C, Vainio K. Arthroplasty of the metacarpophalangeal joints in rheumatoid arthritis with transposition of the interosseus muscles. Scand J Plast Reconstr Surg. 1968; 2(2):139–143

[56] Tupper JW. The metacarpophalangeal volar plate arthroplasty. J Hand Surg Am. 1989; 14(2 Pt 2):371–375

[57] Carroll RE, Taber TH. Digital arthroplasty of the proximal interphlangeal joint. J Bone Joint Surg Am. 1954; 36-A(5):912–920

[58] Eaton RG, Malerich MM. Volar plate arthroplasty of the proximal interphalangeal joint: a review of ten years' experience. J Hand Surg Am. 1980; 5(3):260–268

[59] Dionysian E, Eaton RG. The long-term outcome of volar plate arthroplasty of the proximal interphalangeal joint. J Hand Surg Am. 2000; 25(3):429–437

[60] Gohla T, Metz Ch, Lanz U. Non-vascularized free toe phalanx transplantation in the treatment of symbrachydactyly and constriction ring syndrome. J Hand Surg [Br]. 2005; 30(5):446–451

[61] Graham WC, Riordan DC. Reconstruction of a metacarpophalangeal joint with a metatarsal transplant. J Bone Joint Surg Am. 1948; 30A(4):848–853

[62] Brannon EW, Klein G. Experiences with a finger-joint prosthesis. J Bone Joint Surg Am. 1959; 41-A(1):87–102

[63] Flatt AE, Ellison MR. Restoration of rheumatoid finger joint function. 3. A follow-up note after fourteen years of experience with a metallic-hinge prosthesis. J Bone Joint Surg Am. 1972; 54(6):1317–1322

[64] Nicolle FV, Calnan JS. A new design of finger joint prosthesis for the rheumatoid hand. Hand. 1972; 4(2):135–146

[65] Linscheid RL. Implant arthroplasty of the hand: retrospective and prospective considerations. J Hand Surg Am. 2000; 25(5):796–816

[66] Yamamoto M, Chung KC. Implant arthroplasty: selection of exposure and implant. Hand Clin. 2018; 34(2):195–205

[67] Niebauer JJ, Shaw JL, Doren WW. Silicone-dacron hinge prosthesis: design, evaluation, and application. Ann Rheum Dis. 1969; 28(5):56–58

[68] Niebauer JJ, Landry RM. Dacron-: silicone prosthesis for the metacarpophalangeal and interphalangeal joints. Hand. 1971; 3(1):55–61

[69] Swanson AB, Maupin BK, Gajjar NV, Swanson GD. Flexible implant arthroplasty in the proximal interphalangeal joint of the hand. J Hand Surg Am. 1985; 10(6 Pt 1):796–805

[70] Linscheid RL, Dobyns JH. Total joint arthroplasty:the hand. Mayo Clin Proc. 1979; 54(8):516–526

[71] Johnstone BR, Fitzgerald M, Smith KR, Currie LJ. Cemented versus uncemented surface replacement arthroplasty of the proximal interphalangeal joint with a mean 5-year follow-up. J Hand Surg Am. 2008; 33(5):726–732

[72] Beckenbaugh RD. Preliminary experience with a noncemented nonconstrained total joint arthroplasty for the metacarpophalangeal joints. Orthopedics. 1983; 6(8):962–965

[73] Bellemère P. Pyrocarbon implants for the hand and wrist. Hand Surg Rehabil. 2018; 37(3):129–154

[74] Burton RI, Pellegrini VD, Jr. Surgical management of basal joint arthritis of the thumb. Part II. Ligament reconstruction with tendon interposition arthroplasty. J Hand Surg Am. 1986; 11(3):324–332

[75] Froimson AI. Tendon interposition arthroplasty of carpometacarpal joint of the thumb. Hand Clin. 1987; 3(4):489–505

[76] Weilby A. Tendon interposition arthroplasty of the first carpo-metacarpal joint. J Hand Surg [Br]. 1988; 13(4):421–425

[77] Sigfusson R, Lundborg G. Abductor pollicis longus tendon arthroplasty for treatment of arthrosis in the first carpometacarpal joint. Scand J Plast Reconstr Surg Hand Surg. 1991; 25(1):73–77

[78] Dell PC, Brushart TM, Smith RJ. Treatment of trapeziometacarpal arthritis: results of resection arthroplasty. J Hand Surg Am. 1978; 3(3):243–249

[79] Iyer KM. The results of excision of the trapezium. Hand. 1981; 13(3):246–250

[80] Gibbons CER, Gosal HS, Choudri AH, Magnussen PA. Trapeziectomy for basal thumb joint osteoarthritis: 3- to 19-year follow-up. Int Orthop. 1999; 23(4):216–218

[81] Downing ND, Davis TRC. Trapezial space height after trapeziectomy: mechanism of formation and benefits. J Hand Surg Am. 2001; 26(5):862–868

[82] Swanson AB, deGoot Swanson G, Watermeier JJ. Trapezium implant arthroplasty:long-term evaluation of 150 cases. J Hand Surg Am. 1981; 6(2):125–141

[83] Pellegrini VD, Jr, Burton RI. Surgical management of basal joint arthritis of the thumb. Part I. Long-term results of silicone implant arthroplasty. J Hand Surg Am. 1986; 11(3):309–324

[84] Minamikawa Y, Peimer CA, Ogawa R, Howard C, Sherwin FS. In vivo experimental analysis of silicone implants on bone and soft tissue. J Hand Surg Am. 1994; 19(4):575–583

[85] Lanzetta M, Foucher G. A comparison of different surgical techniques in treating degenerative arthrosis of the carpometacarpal joint of the thumb:a retrospective study of 98 cases. J Hand Surg [Br]. 1995; 20(1):105–110

[86] Lehmann O, Herren DB, Simmen BR. Comparison of tendon suspension-interposition and silicon spacers in the treatment of degenerative osteoarthritis of the base of the thumb. Ann Chir Main Memb Super. 1998; 17(1):25–30

[87] Bezwada HP, Webber JB. Questions regarding the Swanson silicone trapezium implant. J Bone Joint Surg Am. 2002; 84(5):872–, author reply 872–873

[88] Minami A, Iwasaki N, Kutsumi K, Suenaga N, Yasuda K. A long-term follow-up of silicone-rubber interposition arthroplasty for osteoarthritis of the thumb carpometacarpal joint. Hand Surg. 2005; 10(1):77–82

[89] Nilsson A, Liljensten E, Bergström C, Sollerman C. Results from a degradable TMC joint Spacer (Artelon) compared with tendon arthroplasty. J Hand Surg Am. 2005; 30(2):380–389

[90] Nilsson A, Wiig M, Alnehill H, et al. The Artelon CMC spacer compared with tendon interposition arthroplasty. Acta Orthop. 2010; 81(2):237–244

[91] Choung EW, Tan V. Foreign-body reaction to the Artelon CMC joint spacer: case report. J Hand Surg Am. 2008; 33(9):1617–1620

[92] Giuffrida AY, Gyuricza C, Perino G, Weiland AJ. Foreign body reaction to artelon spacer: case report. J Hand Surg Am. 2009; 34(8):1388–1392

[93] Robinson PM, Muir LT. Foreign body reaction associated with Artelon: report of three cases. J Hand Surg Am. 2011; 36(1):116–120

[94] Bellemère P, Gaisne E, Loubersac T, Ardouin L, Collon S, Maes C. Pyrocardan implant: free pyrocarbon interposition for resurfacing trapeziometacarpal joint. Chir Main. 2011; 30:S28–S35

6

[95] Swanson AB, de Groot Swanson G, DeHeer DH, et al. Carpal bone titanium implant arthroplasty: 10 years experience. Clin Orthop Relat Res. 1997(342):46–58

[96] Phaltankar PM, Magnussen PA. Hemiarthroplasty for trapeziometacarpal arthritis - a useful alternative? J Hand Surg [Br]. 2003; 28(1): 80–85

[97] Naidu SH, Kulkarni N, Saunders M. Titanium basal joint arthroplasty: a finite element analysis and clinical study. J Hand Surg Am. 2006; 31(5):760–765

[98] Vitale MA, Hsu CC, Rizzo M, Moran SL. Pyrolytic carbon arthroplasty versus suspensionplasty for trapezial-metacarpal arthritis. J Wrist Surg. 2017; 6(2):134–143

[99] de la Caffinière JY, Aucouturier P. Trapezio-metacarpal arthroplasty by total prosthesis. Hand. 1979; 11(1):41–46

[100] Søndergaard L, Konradsen L, Rechnagel K. Long-term follow-up of the cemented Caffinière prosthesis for trapezio-metacarpal arthroplasty. J Hand Surg [Br]. 1991; 16(4):428–430

[101] Nicholas RM, Calderwood JW. De la Caffinière arthroplasty for basal thumb joint osteoarthritis. J Bone Joint Surg Br. 1992; 74(2):309–312

[102] Chakrabarti AJ, Robinson AH, Gallagher P. De la Caffinière thumb carpometacarpal replacements: 93 cases at 6 to 16 years follow-up. J Hand Surg [Br]. 1997; 22(6):695–698

[103] van Cappelle HG, Elzenga P, van Horn JR. Long-term results and loosening analysis of de la Caffinière replacements of the trapeziometacarpal joint. J Hand Surg Am. 1999; 24(3):476–482

[104] Dreant N, Poumellec MA. Total thumb carpometacarpal joint arthroplasty: a retrospective functional study of 28 MOOVIS prostheses. Hand (N Y). 2019; 14(1):59–65

6

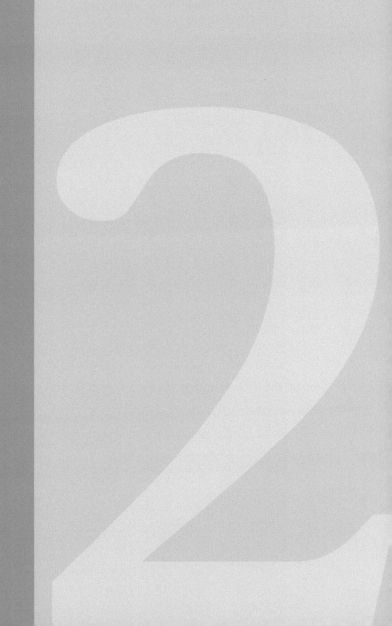

Section 2

Arthroplasty of Finger Joints

Section 2A

MCP Arthroplasty

7 Failure Analysis of Silicone Implants in Metacarpophalangeal and Proximal Interphalangeal Joints

Grey Giddins and Tom Joyce

Abstract

Silicone implant arthroplasty of the metacarpophalangeal and proximal interphalangeal joints has dominated joint replacement in the fingers for decades. Despite their generally positive clinical results, issues remain with Silicone rubber (silastic) implants, the most important being fracture. Although there are reported fracture rates of up to 65% at 15 years, by the time of failure a fibrous pseudojoint has formed, so that replacement of the implant is not always necessary.

The three main designs are the Swanson, the Sutter, and the NeuFlex. For Swanson and Sutter MCP joint prostheses, fracture generally occurs at the junction of the distal stem and the body of the implant. For the NeuFlex, it can break there, but most commonly fractures across the hinge. For Sutter MCP joint prostheses in particular, it has been shown that fracture is initiated on the dorsal aspect of the implant and travels in a palmar direction, likely due to the dominance of subluxing forces in rheumatoid metacarpophalangeal joints. While it has been claimed for many years that hard bearing two-piece implants more akin to the anatomy of finger joints will supersede the nonanatomical single-piece silicone designs, this has not been achieved clinically, despite many clever designs being proposed. It may be that improvements to current silicone designs will be an important next step for finger joint replacement.

Keywords: metacarpophalangeal, proximal interphalangeal, prosthesis, silicone, Swanson, Sutter, NeuFlex, fracture, failure, implant

7.1 Introduction

Single-piece silicone implants are the commonest metacarpophalangeal (MCP) and proximal interphalangeal (PIP) joint replacements[1]; MCP joints tend to be replaced far more often than the PIP joints[1] and there is more data on their outcomes. While a number of different designs of silicone implant have been proposed, all share a central hinge section intended to keep the ends of the finger bones separated and two stems which fit into holes reamed in the bones on each side of the joint (▶ Fig. 7.1). The most commonly implanted design is the Swanson prosthesis.[2] This implant has been supplied with titanium grommets which slip over the stems and are intended to protect the relatively soft silicone material from damage by bone although are not typically inserted. The second main design is the Sutter which is also known as the Avanta.[3] More recently, the NeuFlex design from De Puy

has been available, with pre-flexed stems,[4] in contrast to the colinear stems of the Swanson and Sutter implants (▶ Fig. 7.1).

Despite the successes of single-piece silicone implants, a key concern is implant fracture.[2,3,4,5] It has been reported that approximately two-thirds of silicone finger implants fracture after 14 to 17 years in the body.[6,7] It is also known that fracture rates increase with duration in vivo; radiographic fracture rates of 7% at 5 years, 42% at 10 years, and 65% at 15 years have been reported.[8] Nevertheless, once these implants fracture, a fibrous pseudojoint is formed, providing some stability so that a revision operation may not be necessary.[9] Boe et al[8] reported on 325 silicone MCP joint implants. Of these 325 implants, 22 were revised; the majority of these (14/22) were fractured. Of 214 MCP joint implants with radiographic follow-up greater than 2 years, 80 (37%) were fractured. The authors stated that implant fracture was significantly associated with increasing age, female gender, increased body mass index, osteoarthritis, posttraumatic arthritis, and diabetes mellitus.[8] Although less information is

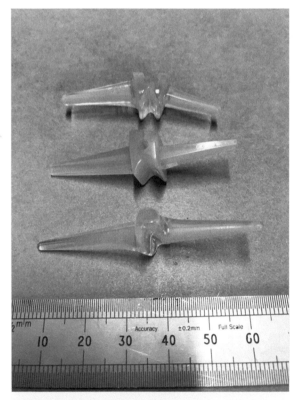

Fig. 7.1 Silicone metacarpophalangeal (MCP) implants, from top to bottom, NeuFlex, Sutter, and Swanson.

available for silicone PIP joint implants, there are common features with silicone MCP joint implants. For Swanson PIP joint implants, a high incidence of in vivo fracture was noted but as for the MCP joints these do not necessarily lead to revision.[10] At a mean follow-up of 10 years, 21 of 38 (55%) Swanson PIP joint implants had fractured. Four implants from this cohort were removed, three for implant fracture. This high rate of in vivo fracture is similar to that seen in the MCP joint implants and this commonality should be recognized. For NeuFlex PIP joint implants, at a mean follow-up of 39 months, a 10% fracture rate was reported.[11] Herren et al stated that 44% of silicone PIP implant revision operations were associated with implant breakage.[12] The authors also reviewed 70 published papers and stated that the most common reason for revision (in 40% of cases) was implant breakage. They did not define what type of silicone implant they used. Fracture rates are summarized in ▶ Table 7.1.

7.2 Failure Mechanisms

For Swanson and Sutter MCP joint prostheses, fracture generally occurs at the junction of the distal stem and the body of the implant,[3,13] but can occur at the proximal stem and body. In contrast a recent study has shown that the NeuFlex implants appear to fracture primarily across the hinge,[4] but can occur at the stem-body junction or both (▶ Fig. 7.2).

It was presumed previously that once an implant fracture occurred the stresses were dissipated and further fracture would not occur but this recent study[4] challenges that idea. The mechanism for this is not understood. If the prevalence of fractures could be reduced it would be expected that silicone finger implants would function better for longer and thus provide greater patient benefit. Before cases of fracture can be reduced, the origins of fracture need to be understood. An analysis of 12 explanted Sutter MCP joint silicone implants[14] determined that the fracture started on the dorsal aspect of the distal stem and travelled in a palmar direction. This fracture initiation point may have been caused by bone impingement from the cortical bone of the proximal phalanx, due to the subluxing forces which dominate in rheumatoid MCP joints or simply the direction of the forces (typically into ulnar deviation and flexion) causing the greatest tearing moment at the dorsoradial corner of the

Table 7.1 Fracture rates of silicone implants in metacarpophalangeal (MCP) and proximal interphalangeal (PIP) joints

Reference	Implant	Follow-up	Fracture rate	Joint
Joyce et al[3]	Sutter	42 mo	27% (11 of 41 implants)	MCP
Joyce and Giddins[4]	NeuFlex	59 mo	77% (23 of 30 explants)	MCP
Trail et al[6]	Swanson	17 y	66% (of 1336 implants)	MCP
Goldfarb and Stern[7]	Swanson	14 y	67% (99 of 148 implants)	MCP
Goldfarb and Stern[7]	Sutter	14 y	52% (31 of 60 implants)	MCP
Boe et al[8]	Not stated	>2 y	37% (80 of 214 implants)	MCP
Bales et al[10]	Swanson	10 y	55% (21 of 38 implants)	PIP
Bouacida et al[11]	NeuFlex	39 mo	10% (3 of 28 implants)	PIP
Herren et al[12]	Not stated	8.3 y	44% (of 27 patients)	PIP

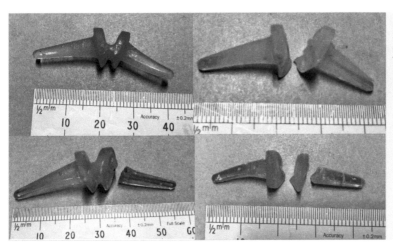

Fig. 7.2 Different positions of fracture seen with NeuFlex metacarpophalangeal (MCP) joint explants. Top left, no fracture; top right, fracture at hinge; bottom left, fracture at distal stem; bottom right, fracture at hinge and at distal stem.

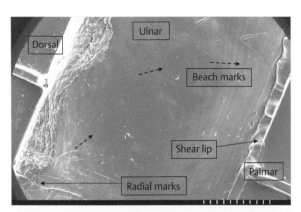

Fig. 7.3 Scanning Electron Microscope image of the fracture face of an explanted silicone metacarpophalangeal (MCP) implant, showing crack initiation (radial marks), crack progression (black dashed arrows overlaying beach marks), and final area of fracture (shear lip).

proximal stem insertion into the implant body. In contrast, there was relatively little damage on the palmar aspect of the stems of the implants. In addition, classic features of fatigue fractures were seen on the explants.[14] These features included "radial marks" which indicated the origin of fracture on the dorsal aspect of the distal stem, toward the radial side (▶ Fig. 7.3). Next, "beach marks" showed fatigue crack propagation in an arc from radial to ulnar and from dorsal to palmar (▶ Fig. 7.3). Lastly, a "shear lip" on the palmar aspect indicated the final area of fracture of the silicone implant (▶ Fig. 7.3). Fatigue fractures are the typical failure mode with silicone finger implants.

Possible causes of crack initiation include poor surgical handling damaging the implant at operation and damage from sharp bone edges. Poor handling rarely leads to overt implant tears but there may be microscopic damage later leading to failure. Sharp bone edges can clearly damage the implant surfaces. Because of these worries grommets were introduced but did not seem to affect failure rates and are largely not used.[6] Eccentric loading appears to be the commonest cause of crack progression as shown in ▶ Fig. 7.3. These forces will eventually tear the dorsoulnar corner of the insertion of the distal stem into the body (or the hinge for NeuFlex implants). The tears then propagate in response to the continuing deforming forces. Plastic deformation occurs with prolonged ulnar deviation as shown in intact explants and in simulated jigs.[15]

7.3 Material Properties

Silicone refers to a family of materials. Each manufacturer of finger implants uses its own medical-grade silicone, for example, "Flexspan," "Silflex II," and "Anasil" but aside from these names, relatively few of the material properties are divulged.[16] It is known that the silicone used in the Swanson implant has changed over

time, in an effort to reduce the fracture rate.[7] Based on findings from failure analysis, the key material properties required, after biocompatibility, are crack growth resistance, to counter crack propagation, and abrasion resistance, to counter crack initiation. It should also be recognized that sample thickness has an effect on crack propagation, with the crack growth rate higher for thinner samples.[17] In other words, under the same loading conditions, a larger/thicker sample will survive longer than a thinner sample. As an alternative biomaterial, polyurethane is said to have greater crack growth resistance than silicone[18] and it has higher tear and abrasion resistance than silicone.[17] Interestingly, a comparative clinical trial of 21 silicone (Swanson) and 23 polyurethane (Swanson-shape) MCP joint implants were reported on 4.5 years (range 3–5) postoperatively.[19] There was one implant fracture in each group leading the authors to conclude that polyurethane gave no worse clinical results than silicone.[19] It is possible that this was too short a time and too small a cohort to see any significant difference between the materials. Potentially, alternative materials could be usefully reinvestigated.

7.4 Improving Silicone Implants

In future, silicone implants may be replaced by hard-bearing implants for MCP or PIP joint destruction; this statement is likely to have been written many times in the last 30 years. Nonetheless this "prediction" has largely blocked research into silicone implants as they are felt likely to be replaced soon. As this "soon" appears still to be some time away, optimization of silicone implants may help patients sooner. The aims of any changes should be to prevent fracture initiation and/or crack propagation. Much of this line of enquiry will be related to materials used to construct the implants. Unfortunately, it is unlikely that there will be commercial or research funding to tackle this issue. Implant shape changes may help to increase longevity of the implants; this could be instituted more easily. Reducing the postoperative ranges of motion particularly in MCP joint arthroplasties may allow adequate function but greater longevity; this is not currently established.

7.5 Conclusion

Silicone finger implants have provided a simple and reasonably reliable implant for decades particularly for lower demand patients. Even higher demand patients may gain good long-term pain relief, even if they never achieve good strength and stability. As yet, silicone finger implants have not been superseded. For this reason, they continue to have a role in contemporary hand surgical practice. It may be that newer designs of silicone implants will improve their outcomes, perhaps in conjunction with changes in rehabilitation.

7

References

[1] Norwegian_Arthroplasty_Register. Nasjonalt Register for Leddproteser. 2018; http://nrlweb.ihelse.net/eng/Rapporter/Report2018_english.pdf. Accessed April 14, 2019

[2] Joyce TJ, Unsworth A. A literature review of "failures" of the Swanson finger prosthesis in the metacarpophalangeal joint. Hand Surg. 2002; 7(1):139–146

[3] Joyce TJ, Milner RH, Unsworth A. A comparison of ex vivo and in vitro Sutter metacarpophalangeal prostheses. J Hand Surg [Br]. 2003; 28(1): 86–91

[4] Joyce TJ, Giddins G. Sites of fractures in explanted NeuFlex® silicone metacarpophalangeal joint prostheses. J Hand Surg Eur Vol. 2018; 43(10):1083–1087

[5] Weiss A-PC, Moore DC, Infantolino C, Crisco JJ, Akelman E, McGovern RD. Metacarpophalangeal joint mechanics after 3 different silicone arthroplasties. J Hand Surg Am. 2004; 29(5):796–803

[6] Trail IA, Martin JA, Nuttall D, Stanley JK. Seventeen-year survivorship analysis of silastic metacarpophalangeal joint replacement. J Bone Joint Surg Br. 2004; 86(7):1002–1006

[7] Goldfarb CA, Stern PJ. Metacarpophalangeal joint arthroplasty in rheumatoid arthritis: a long-term assessment. J Bone Joint Surg Am. 2003; 85(10):1869–1878

[8] Boe C, Wagner E, Rizzo M. Long-term outcomes of silicone metacarpophalangeal arthroplasty: a longitudinal analysis of 325 cases. J Hand Surg Eur Vol. 2018; 43(10):1076–1082

[9] Swanson AB. Flexible implant arthroplasty for arthritic finger joints: rationale, technique, and results of treatment. J Bone Joint Surg Am. 1972; 54(3):435–455

[10] Bales JG, Wall LB, Stern PJ. Long-term results of Swanson silicone arthroplasty for proximal interphalangeal joint osteoarthritis. J Hand Surg Am. 2014; 39(3):455–461

[11] Bouacida S, Lazerges C, Coulet B, Chammas M. Proximal interphalangeal joint arthroplasty with Neuflex® implants: relevance of the volar approach and early rehabilitation. Chir Main. 2014; 33(5):350–355

[12] Herren DB, Keuchel T, Marks M, Schindele S. Revision arthroplasty for failed silicone proximal interphalangeal joint arthroplasty: indications and 8-year results. J Hand Surg Am. 2014; 39(3):462–466

[13] Joyce TJ, Unsworth A. The design of a finger wear simulator and preliminary results. Proc Inst Mech Eng H. 2000; 214(5):519–526

[14] Joyce TJ. Analysis of the mechanism of fracture of silicone metacarpophalangeal prostheses. J Hand Surg Eur Vol. 2009; 34(1):18–24 (British and European Volume)

[15] Drayton P, Morgan BW, Davies MC, Giddins GEB, Miles AW. A biomechanical study of the effects of simulated ulnar deviation on silicone finger joint implant failure. J Hand Surg Eur Vol. 2016; 41(9):944–947

[16] Joyce TJ. Currently available metacarpophalangeal prostheses: their designs and prospective considerations. Expert Rev Med Devices. 2004; 1(2):193–204

[17] Alnaimat FA, Shepherd DET, Dearn KD. Crack growth in medicalgrade silicone and polyurethane ether elastomers. Polym Test. 2017; 62:225–234

[18] Hutchinson DT, Savory KM, Bachus KN. Crack-growth properties of various elastomers with potential application in small joint prostheses. J Biomed Mater Res. 1997; 37(1):94–99

[19] Sollerman CJ, Geijer M. Polyurethane versus silicone for endoprosthetic replacement of the metacarpophalangeal joints in rheumatoid arthritis. Scand J Plast Reconstr Surg Hand Surg. 1996; 30(2):145–150

7

8 Silicone Interposition Arthroplasty for MCP and PIP joints

Sarah E. Sasor and Kevin C. Chung

Abstract

The metacarpophalangeal (MCP) and proximal interphalangeal (PIP) joints can be deformed and disabled by arthritis. Treatment is challenging, owing to bony destruction and tendon imbalances. Reconstruction of a stable, mobile, pain-free joint is crucial to restore hand function. Silicone arthroplasty is indicated in patients with severe pain, deformity, or loss of function. Patients can expect 30 to 40 degrees of motion in the MCP joint and 60 degrees of motion in the PIP joint after arthroplasty. This chapter describes indications, techniques, and outcomes for MCP and PIP joint silicone arthroplasty.

Keywords: silicone arthroplasty, implant arthroplasty, interposition arthroplasty, small joint replacement, finger joint replacement, proximal interphalangeal joint, metacarpophalangeal joint, rheumatoid arthritis, scleroderma, silicone implant

8.1 Introduction

Dr. Alfred Swanson introduced a hinged, silicone implant for finger joint replacement in Grand Rapids, Michigan, USA in 1962.[1,2] The implant was designed to relieve pain, provide reasonable motion, and reduce joint deformity. He published his first series of 222 proximal phalangeal joint arthroplasties in 1973 which showed promising short-term results.[1] Although surgical indications and techniques have evolved over the past 60 years, the implant design and general principles of small joint silicone arthroplasty remain largely unchanged.

8.2 Characteristics of Silicone Implants

Silicone is biologically inert and has many properties that are ideal for small joint reconstruction. It is heat stable and has excellent flexion and force dampening characteristics. Unlike rigid implants, silicone implants are softer than bone and do not stimulate bony resorption. They act as dynamic spacers after joint resection by providing internal stability and maintaining finger alignment.

Fixation of silicone implants is not needed. Implants are supported by the surrounding ligamentous structures and become encapsulated by fibrous tissue shortly after insertion.[3] Early motion is essential to promote the development of a functionally adapted capsule. The implant glides within the capsule to permit greater range of motion as the implant finds the best position with respect to the axis of rotation of the joint. Motion is often maintained in the setting of implant fracture – the joint continues to function as a simple, resection arthroplasty. Once the implant has served its purpose as a spacer, the stable capsuloligamentous structures support the joint.[4]

8.3 MCP Joint Arthroplasty

8.3.1 Indications

Metacarpophalangeal joint (MCPJ) arthritis is commonly rheumatic or inflammatory but can also occur after trauma or with age-related degeneration. The index and middle finger MCPJs are typically affected first.[5,6] Silicone arthroplasty is considered in patients with severe pain, deformity, or loss of function. Arthroplasty is favored in rheumatoid patients when ulnar drift and volar subluxation cannot be passively reduced.

8.3.2 Contraindications

Silicone MCPJ arthroplasty is contraindicated in patients with poor wound healing capacity, inadequate soft tissue, infection, excessive bony erosion, or fatty replacement of the bone with inability to support an implant.

8.3.3 Preoperative Evaluation

In rheumatoid patients, wrist deformity and distal radio-ulnar joint (DRUJ) instability must be addressed before the MCPJs. Radial deviation of the wrist leads to progressive ulnar drift at the MCPJs, and DRUJ instability can result in attritional rupture of the extensor tendons. Examination of the MCPJs often reveals ulnar subluxation of the extensor tendon into the valley between the metacarpal heads (► Fig. 8.1). If the MCPJ deformity is passively correctable, soft tissue reconstruction is possible—synovectomy and extensor tendon centralization with cross-intrinsic transfer of the ulnar lateral band. Arthroplasty is indicated when the deformity is severe (> 15 degrees of ulnar drift or > 20 degrees of extensor lag) or cannot be passively corrected.

In scleroderma patients, boutonniere deformities are common. Sclerosis of the joint capsule, collateral ligaments, and flexor tendon sheath and attenuation of the central slip lead to volar displacement of the lateral bands and flexion contracture at the proximal interphalangeal joint (PIPJ). Patients compensate by hyperextending the MCPJ (► Fig. 8.2).

Standard, three-view radiographs of the affected joint are required. Bone quality is assessed for its ability to accept an implant. Articular damage, loss of joint space, joint incongruity, and bony alignment are evaluated (► Fig. 8.3). Radiographs of the wrist are also obtained if any pathology is suspected.

8

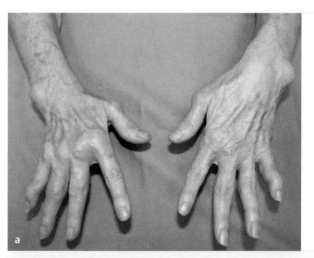
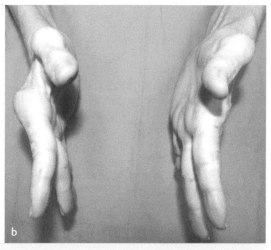

Fig. 8.1 (a, b) Preoperative evaluation of a 59-year-old female with rheumatoid arthritis. Ulnar drift and volar subluxation of the fingers at the metacarpophalangeal joints (MCPJs).

8

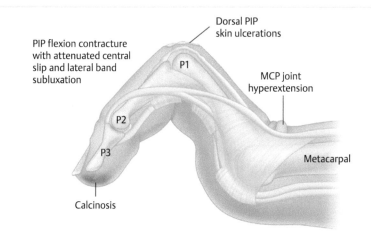

PIP flexion contracture with attenuated central slip and lateral band subluxation

Dorsal PIP skin ulcerations

P1

MCP joint hyperextension

P2

P3

Metacarpal

Calcinosis

Fig. 8.2 Boutonniere deformity in scleroderma. (Reproduced with permission from Kamnerdnakta S., Kelley B. P., Chung K. C. Silicone Metacarpophalangeal Arthroplasty (SMPA). In: Operative Techniques: Hand and Wrist Surgery. (Ed: Chung K. C.). Elsevier; 2018.)

8.3.4 Surgical Anatomy

The MCPJ is an asymmetric condylar joint—the ovoid articular surface of the metacarpal fits into an elliptical cavity at the base of the proximal phalanx. The metacarpal head is sloped volarly and ulnarly. Motion is permitted in two planes: flexion-extension and radioulnar deviation.

The volar plate, collateral ligaments, and extensor mechanism stabilize the joint. The sagittal bands center the extensor tendon over the joint and prevent bowstringing during hyperextension. The intrinsic muscles insert onto the lateral bands which pass volar to the axis of rotation of the MCPJ and produce flexion, adduction, and adduction forces (▶ Fig. 8.4).

The MCPJ is commonly affected in rheumatoid arthritis. Attenuation of the radial collateral ligament from synovitis results in volar subluxation of the proximal phalanx and ulnar drift of the fingers. Chronic joint subluxation contributes to intrinsic muscle contracture which may require release and cross-intrinsic transfer at the time of arthroplasty. Alternatively, in lieu of ulnar lateral band releases, the metacarpal head can be aggressively resected to decrease the tension on the lateral bands.

8.3.5 Approach

The dorsal approach provides expeditious access to the MCPJ. A longitudinal or lazy-S incision centered at the joint is used for access to a single MCPJ. Multiple arthroplasties are performed through a single, extended transverse incision (▶ Fig. 8.5) or multiple longitudinal incisions. Care is taken to preserve the dorsal veins to reduce postoperative swelling.

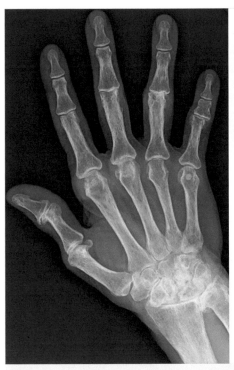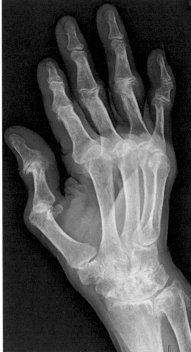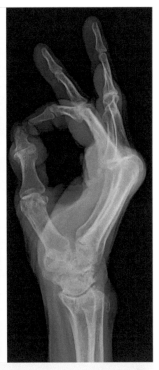

Fig. 8.3 Standard 3-view radiographs show volar and ulnar subluxation of the proximal phalanges on the metacarpal heads.

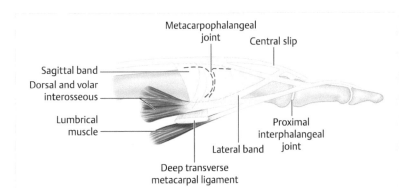

Fig. 8.4 Anatomy of metacarpophalangeal joint. (Reproduced with permission from Kamnerdnakta S., Kelley B. P., Chung K. C. Silicone Metacarpophalangeal Arthroplasty (SMPA). In: Operative Techniques: Hand and Wrist Surgery. (Ed: Chung K. C.). Elsevier; 2018.)

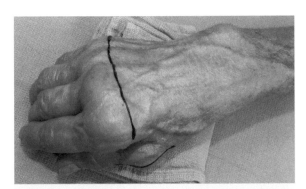

Fig. 8.5 Transverse incision for dorsal approach to the metacarpophalangeal joints (MCPJs).

8.3.6 Authors' Preferred Technique

The skin is incised and the subcutaneous tissue is elevated off the extensor mechanism. The radial sagittal band is incised and the extensor tendon is retracted. The joint capsule is incised longitudinally and synovectomy is performed. The collateral ligaments are released at their proximal attachment on the metacarpal head. A sagittal saw is used to remove the articular surface of the metacarpal head (▶ Fig. 8.6). The MCPJ should then easily reduce into normal alignment. If the joint remains tight or the finger ulnarly deviated, ulnar intrinsic release is performed. If soft tissue tightness persists, consider release of the volar plate or resection of additional metacarpal bone.

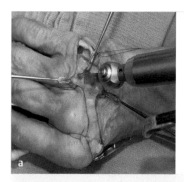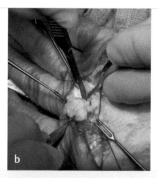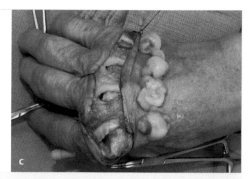

Fig. 8.6 (a–c) Resection of the metacarpal heads with an oscillating saw.

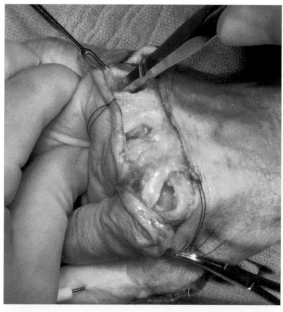

Fig. 8.7 Broaching the medullary canal of the proximal phalanx.

An awl is used to open the medullary canals of the proximal phalanx and metacarpal. The medullary canals of the proximal phalanx are prepared first for index, middle, and small finger MCPJ arthroplasty. For the ring finger, the order is reversed due to the narrow canal of the fourth metacarpal; the metacarpal is broached first and the implant size determined before preparing the proximal phalanx to avoid over reaming.

On the proximal phalanx, the starting point of the awl is at the junction of the dorsal and middle third of the articular surface. The awl is inserted with a gentle twisting motion. The smallest distal broach is then inserted straight into the medullary canal of the proximal phalanx in the path created by the awl (▶ Fig. 8.7). Orientation of the broach must be maintained during insertion and withdrawal—typically, the numbered side of the broach is placed parallel with the dorsal cortex. If the broach is twisted, it may asymmetrically enlarge the medullary cavity and create a poor fit with the implant stem. The

broach should be inserted to its full depth to create enough space for the implant stem. Take care to insert the broaches along the central axis of the phalanx—breaking the dorsal or volar cortex can destabilize the implant. Broaches are increased in size until the desired implant size is reached.

The same process is repeated for the metacarpal. With the articular surface removed, the awl inserts easily into the medullary canal. Broaches are sequentially inserted to their full depth until the implant size is reached. The largest implant that the medullary canal will accept is selected for a snug fit.

Before implant insertion, the metacarpal is prepared for radial collateral ligament repair. Repair is mandatory to restore joint alignment and improve stability during pinch. Two 0.035-inch (0.89 mm) Kirschner wires are drilled through the dorsal radial metacarpal cortex at the distal end of the cut bone. A braided 3-0 permanent suture is passed through these holes and left untied (▶ Fig. 8.8). This suture is used later to reattach the radial collateral ligament to the metacarpal.

A temporary implant sizer is selected based on the largest broach size used. The sizer is oriented so that the cavity of the barrel faces volarly. The proximal stem is inserted first into the metacarpal, then the distal stem into the proximal phalanx. The stems should fit easily into the broached medullary canals and the implant should not compress or buckle during motion. If this occurs, the implant may be too large or the broached canal too short. More bone may need to be resected from the metacarpal. If the fit is adequate, the sizer is removed and the final implant is opened. After verifying the correct orientation, the implant is inserted in the same sequence using two clean, smooth forceps and a no-touch technique (▶ Fig. 8.9). Flexion and extension are tested intraoperatively.

The joint is held in extension while the soft tissues are repaired. The radial collateral ligament is imbricated using the suture previously placed through the metacarpal. When the radial collateral ligament is severely attenuated and repair is not possible, a distally based flap of the volar plate is elevated and anchored to the metacarpal. The joint capsule is repaired using a braided 3-0

8

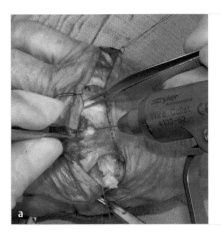
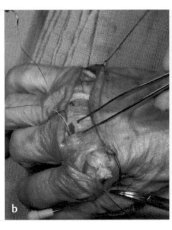

Fig. 8.8 (a, b) Preparations for repair of the radial collateral ligament. A permanent suture is placed through holes drilled in the dorsal radial metacarpal cortex.

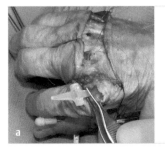
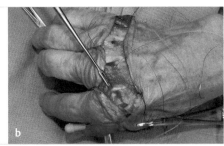

Fig. 8.9 (a, b) Insertion of the silicone metacarpophalangeal joint (MCPJ) implant.

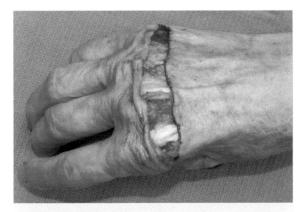

Fig. 8.10 Centralization of the extensor tendon and repair of the radial sagittal band.

permanent suture. Tight repair of the radial collateral ligament and joint capsule with the finger extended limits the flexion arc by 10 to 20 degrees but stabilizes the joint.

Lastly, the extensor tendon is centralized to prevent recurrence of ulnar drift. In longstanding deformity, the ulnar sagittal band becomes fibrotic and requires release. The radial aspect of the extensor hood is imbricated to the radial sagittal band (▶ Fig. 8.10). The MCPJ is passively flexed and extended to ensure the extensor tendon remains centralized through the arc of motion.

The skin is closed using 4–0 nylon sutures and the patient is splinted with the MCPJs extended.

8.3.7 Postoperative Care

Patients are seen in the office 2 weeks after surgery for suture removal. Dynamic, short-arm extension splinting with the wrist extended at 20 degrees and the MCPJs fully extended and radially deviated continues for 6 weeks. After 6 weeks, patients are allowed to increase activity (▶ Fig. 8.11).

8.3.8 Expected Outcomes

Silicone MCPJ arthroplasty is effective in correcting ulnar drift and improving hand appearance in rheumatoid patients.[7] Posttraumatic and osteoarthritis patients report good pain relief.[8] Patients can expect improved finger extension with a total arc of motion of 30 to 40 degrees.[9,10] Patients are typically satisfied despite minimal gains in grip and pinch strength.[11]

Long-term studies show a progressive increase in complications as the implant fatigues and cracks (characteristically at the stem-hinge junction).[1,12] The rate of implant fracture is approximately 10% at 7 years.[10] Fracture does not necessarily impair range of motion but is correlated with recurrent ulnar drift of the fingers, pain, and decreased patient satisfaction.[4]

8.4 PIP Joint Arthroplasty

Many of the principles in small joint silicone arthroplasty are similar for the MCP and PIP joints. Differences in

8

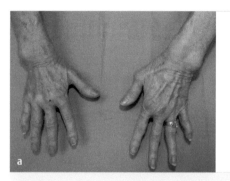
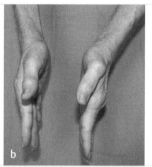
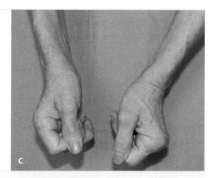

Fig. 8.11 (a–c) Three months after right second to fifthmetacarpophalangeal joint (MCPJ) silicone arthroplasty.

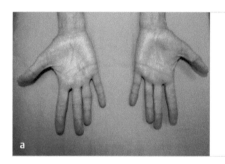
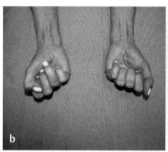

Fig. 8.12 (a, b) Preoperative evaluation of 56-year-old female patient with right ring finger proximal interphalangeal joint (PIPJ) osteoarthritis. Note reduced range of motion at PIPJ.

indications, technique, and outcome for PIPJ arthroplasty are described below.

8.4.1 Indications

Silicone PIPJ arthroplasty is considered in patients with severe pain, loss of motion, or deformity of the PIPJ who have failed nonoperative treatment. Inflammatory, degenerative, and posttraumatic arthritis can be effectively treated with silicone joint replacement.

8.4.2 Contraindications

Silicone PIPJ arthroplasty is contraindicated when infection, ligamentous instability, angular deformity of the bone, or significant periarticular bone loss is present. In active patients, arthrodesis is preferred for the index finger PIPJ due to lateral stress on the joint during key pinch. For low demand patients, PIPJ arthroplasty of the index finger may be considered.

8.4.3 Preoperative Evaluation

The fingers are inspected for collinearity and symmetry (▸ Fig. 8.12). Active and passive arcs of motion are evaluated and the PIPJ is stressed to assess for ligamentous stability. Implant stability is dependent upon the existing soft tissue envelope—an extremely unstable joint is better treated with a fusion.

Standard, three-view radiographs of the affected joint are obtained. Articular damage, loss of joint space, and joint incongruity are evaluated. Bone quality is assessed for its ability to accept and support an implant (▸ Fig. 8.13).

8.4.4 Surgical Anatomy

The PIPJ is a gliding hinge joint composed of the bicondylar head of the proximal phalanx and the concave base of the middle phalanx. The volar plate, collateral ligaments, and extensor mechanism stabilize the joint on all sides (▸ Fig. 8.14).

8.4.5 Approach

Dorsal, lateral, and volar approaches to the PIPJ are possible. The dorsal approach offers rapid, wide exposure to the joint but risks attenuating the central slip and often results in extensor lag. In the lateral approach, the collateral ligaments are divided to expose the joint; few articles describe this technique and the outcome is uncertain.[13,14,15] Recent studies[16,17,18,19] show favorable results with the volar approach—this is the authors' preferred technique. The neurovascular bundles, flexor tendons, and volar plate must be negotiated; however, the integrity of the extensor mechanism is maintained. Early postoperative motion is permitted, which reduces adhesions and joint contracture.

8.4.6 Authors' Preferred Technique

A Bruner incision is designed centered at the PIPJ (▸ Fig. 8.15). A flap of skin and subcutaneous tissue is

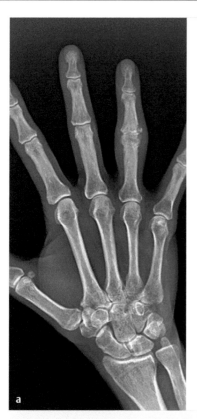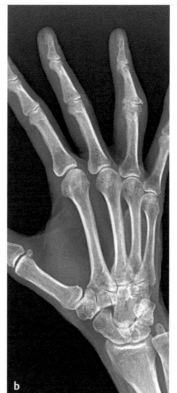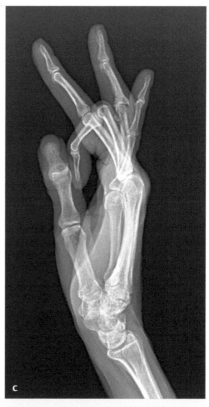

Fig. 8.13 (a–c) Standard three-view radiographs show degeneration of right ring finger proximal interphalangeal joint (PIPJ).

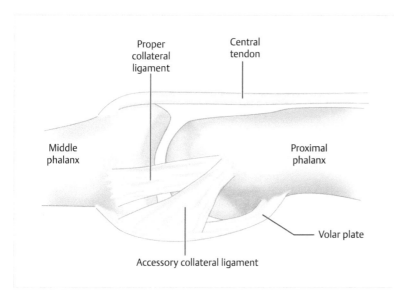

Fig. 8.14 Anatomy of the proximal interphalangeal joint. (Reproduced with permission from Saito T., Chung K. C., Haase S. C. Dynamic External Fixation of Fracture-Dislocation of Proximal Interphalangeal Joint (Suzuki Frame). In: Operative Techniques: Hand and Wrist Surgery. (Ed: Chung K. C.). Elsevier; 2018.)

elevated at the level of the flexor tendon sheath while protecting the neurovascular bundles. The A2, A3, and A4 pulleys are identified. A2 and A4 pulleys are preserved to prevent flexor tendon bowstringing. The A3 pulley is incised longitudinally along its lateral aspect, and the flexor tendons are retracted to expose the volar plate. The volar plate is incised proximally while the collateral

ligaments are maintained, if possible (▸ Fig. 8.16). A shotgun approach to the PIPJ is usually unnecessary for joint exposure.

A narrow sagittal saw is used to remove the articular surface of the proximal phalanx proximal to the flare of condyle. The cut must be perpendicular to the phalangeal shaft to prevent angulation of the joint once the implant

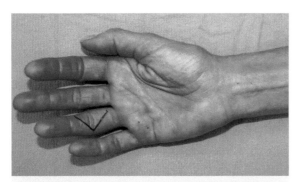

Fig. 8.15 Incision design for volar approach to the proximal interphalangeal joint (PIPJ).

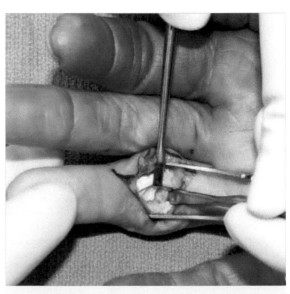

Fig. 8.16 Incise A3 pulley, retract flexor tendons, release volar plate from proximal phalanx to expose the proximal interphalangeal joint (PIPJ).

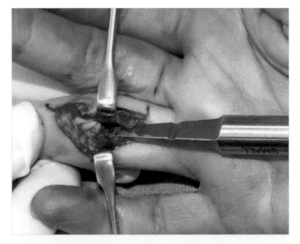

Fig. 8.17 Broaching the medullary cavity of middle phalanx.

is placed. A rongeur is used to remove any remaining osteophytes.

The broaching process is similar to that described above for MCPJ arthroplasty. The middle phalanx has a smaller medullary canal and is reamed first to determine the size of the implant. An awl is centered on the articular surface of the middle phalanx base. The smallest broach is inserted straight into the medullary canal to its full depth with the numbered side parallel to the dorsal cortex (▶ Fig. 8.17). Broaches are increased in size until the desired implant size is reached. Typical implant size is 00 for a small hand, 0 for an average hand, and 1 for a large hand.

The process is repeated for the proximal phalanx using the proximal awl and broaches—separate broaches for the proximal and distal joint surfaces match the stems of the implant. Broaches are sequentially inserted to their full depth until the implant size is reached.

A temporary implant sizer is selected. The sizer is oriented so that it hinges volarly. The distal stem is inserted first into the middle phalanx, then the proximal stem into the proximal phalanx. Fit is checked through the arc of motion and adjustments are made as needed. If the fit is adequate, the sizer is removed and the final implant is

inserted. Flexion and extension are tested with the final implant in place. Patients typically have an arc of motion from 0 to 90 degrees intraoperatively, although some of this is lost postoperatively because of scarring and procedure-related pain.

If the collateral ligaments were fully released to expose the joint, they are repaired with a 4–0 absorbable suture. The volar plate is repaired with a 4–0 absorbable suture. The flexor tendons are relocated centrally and the A3 pulley is repaired with a 4–0 absorbable suture. The skin is closed with 4–0 nylon sutures and the finger is placed in a dorsal blocking splint with the PIPJ in slight flexion (▶ Fig. 8.18).

8.4.7 Postoperative Care

The patient remains splinted for the first 2 to 3 days after surgery, then begins a supervised active motion protocol with a certified hand therapist (▶ Fig. 8.19). Sutures are removed at 2 weeks. After 6 weeks, patients are allowed to increase activity (▶ Fig. 8.20).

8.4.8 Expected Outcomes

Patients can expect about 60 degrees of motion, modestly increased grip and pinch strength, and excellent pain relief after silicone PIPJ arthroplasty using a volar approach. Long-term studies show a 6% revision rate at 41 months and an 11% risk of implant failure at 5 years.[20] Rheumatoid patients generally have poorer overall outcomes compared to patients with degenerative, posttraumatic, or idiopathic arthritis.[21] Women tend to have better results than men.[21]

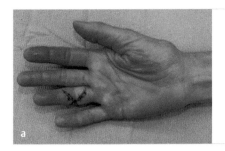
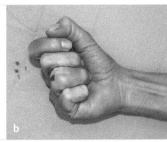

Fig. 8.18 (a, b) Intraoperative arc of motion 0 to 90 degrees at proximal interphalangeal joint (PIPJ).

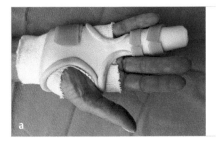
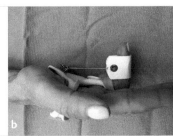

Fig. 8.19 (a, b) Postoperative splinting for ring finger proximal interphalangeal joint (PIPJ).

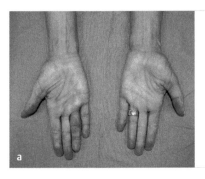
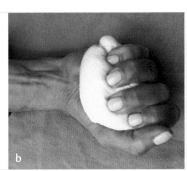

Fig. 8.20 (a, b) Nine weeks after right ring finger proximal interphalangeal joint (PIPJ) silicone arthroplasty.

8

References

[1] Swanson AB. Implant resection arthroplasty of the proximal inter-phalangeal joint. Orthop Clin North Am. 1973; 4(4):1007–1029

[2] Swanson AB. Silicone rubber implants for replacement of arthritis or destroyed joints in the hand. Surg Clin North Am. 1968; 48(5):1113–1127

[3] Swanson AB. Finger joint replacement by silicone rubber implants and the concept of implant fixation by encapsulation. Ann Rheum Dis. 1969; 28(5) Suppl:47–55

[4] Goldfarb CA, Stern PJ. Metacarpophalangeal joint arthroplasty in rheumatoid arthritis:a long-term assessment. J Bone Joint Surg Am. 2003; 85(10):1869–1878

[5] Rettig LA, Luca L, Murphy MS. Silicone implant arthroplasty in patients with idiopathic osteoarthritis of the metacarpophalangeal joint. J Hand Surg Am. 2005; 30(4):667–672

[6] Feldon P, Belsky MR. Degenerative diseases of the metacarpophalan-geal joints. Hand Clin. 1987; 3(3):429–447

[7] Chung KC, Kowalski CP, Myra Kim H, Kazmers IS. Patient outcomes following Swanson silastic metacarpophalangeal joint arthroplasty in the rheumatoid hand: a systematic overview. J Rheumatol. 2000; 27(6):1395–1402

[8] Goldfarb CA, Dovan TT. Rheumatoid arthritis: silicone metacarpopha-langeal joint arthroplasty indications, technique, and outcomes. Hand Clin. 2006; 22(2):177–182

[9] Elhassan B, McNeal D, Wynn S, Gonzalez M, Amirouch F. Experimen-tal investigation of finger dynamics before and after metacarpopha-langeal joint arthroplasty. J Hand Surg Am. 2006; 31(2):228–235

[10] Chung KC, Kotsis SV, Burns PB, et al. Seven-year outcomes of the sili-cone arthroplasty in Rheumatoid Arthritis Prospective Cohort Study. Arthritis Care Res (Hoboken). 2017; 69(7):973–981

[11] Waljee JF, Chung KC. Objective functional outcomes and patient satis-faction after silicone metacarpophalangeal arthroplasty for rheuma-toid arthritis. J Hand Surg Am. 2012; 37(1):47–54

[12] Boe C, Wagner E, Rizzo M. Long-term outcomes of silicone metacar-pophalangeal arthroplasty: a longitudinal analysis of 325 cases. J Hand Surg Eur Vol. 2018; 43(10):1076–1082

[13] Stahlenbrecher A, Hoch J. Proximal interphalangeal joint silicone arthroplasty: comparison of Swanson and NeuFlex implants using a new evaluation score. Handchir Mikrochir Plast Chir. 2009; 41(3):156–165

[14] Merle M, Villani F, Lallemand B, Vaienti L. Proximal interphalangeal joint arthroplasty with silicone implants (NeuFlex) by a lateral approach: a series of 51 cases. J Hand Surg Eur Vol. 2012; 37(1):50–55

[15] Hage JJ, Yoe EP, Zevering JP, de Groot PJ. Proximal interphalangeal joint silicone arthroplasty for posttraumatic arthritis. J Hand Surg Am. 1999; 24(1):73–77

[16] Proubasta IR, Lamas CG, Natera L, Millan A. Silicone proximal inter-phalangeal joint arthroplasty for primary osteoarthritis using a volar approach. J Hand Surg Am. 2014; 39(6):1075–1081

[17] Lautenbach M, Kim S, Berndsen M, Eisenschenk A. The palmar approach for PIP-arthroplasty according to Simmen: results after 8 years follow-up. J Orthop Sci. 2014; 19(5):722–728

[18] Lin HH, Wyrick JD, Stern PJ. Proximal interphalangeal joint silicone replacement arthroplasty: clinical results using an anterior approach. J Hand Surg Am. 1995; 20(1):123–132

[19] Bouacida S, Lazerges C, Coulet B, Chammas M. Proximal interphalangeal joint arthroplasty with Neuflex® implants: relevance of the volar approach and early rehabilitation. Chir Main. 2014; 33(5): 350–355

[20] Yamamoto M, Malay S, Fujihara Y, Zhong L, Chung KC. A systematic review of different implants and approaches for proximal interphalangeal joint arthroplasty. Plast Reconstr Surg. 2017; 139 (5):1139e–1151e

[21] Takigawa S, Meletiou S, Sauerbier M, Cooney WP. Long-term assessment of Swanson implant arthroplasty in the proximal interphalangeal joint of the hand. J Hand Surg Am. 2004; 29(5):785–795

8

9 Surface Gliding Implants for the Metacarpophalangeal Joints

Marco Rizzo

Abstract

Surface gliding implants for metacarpophalangeal joint arthritis serve as an alternative to their predecessor, silicone spacers. These metal-plastic and pyrocarbon implants are modular and therefore provide less inherent stability than the hinged silicone implants. However, they have material properties that are stronger and more durable than silastic joints. Patients with good bone quality and competent soft-tissue stabilizers of the MCP joint are the ideal candidates for these implants. Results with these implants have been favorable in the setting of non-inflammatory arthritis.

Keywords: surface replacement arthroplasty, pyrocarbon, metacarpophalangeal joint, osteoarthritis, inflammatory arthritis

9.1 Introduction

A healthy, pain-free, and functional metacarpophalangeal (MCP) joint is critical for good hand function. Arthritis of the MCP joint can lead to significant pain, disability, and deformity. The joint is commonly affected in inflammatory arthritis; it is also not uncommon for patients with posttraumatic and primary osteoarthritis to be affected. Conservative treatments include activity modification, splinting, topical, and oral anti-inflammatory medications and injections. Surgery is considered for continued pain, limited function, and deformity of the hand in patients who fail conservative measures.

While arthrodesis remains an option in the surgical treatment of MCP arthritis (and is an excellent option for thumb MCP arthritis), fusion is generally less well tolerated in the surgical management of MCP arthritis of the fingers. In addition to the loss of flexion and extension of the joint and the inability to abduct and adduct the digits can result in frustration with hand use, especially when more than one digit is fused.

Silicone MCP arthroplasty, introduced by Swanson in 1962, has remained the gold standard in surgical management of MCP arthritis, especially in patients with rheumatoid arthritis.[1] However, over the last two to three decades, the introduction of surface gliding implants has become an alternative to the traditional silicone implants. The primary choices in the United States include Pyrocarbon (Integra Life Sciences, Austin, TX) and the metal-plastic surface replacement arthroplasty (Stryker, New Jersey). These implants have favorable material properties compared to silicone. However, they are modular and nonconstrained and require more competent softtissues to help maintain joint stability.

The aim of this chapter is to review the indications, technique, and outcomes of surface gliding implants in the surgical management of MCP joint arthritis.

9.2 Characteristics of Surface Gliding Implants

9.2.1 Pyrocarbon

Pyrolytic carbon, or pyrocarbon, is a unique material. It has been utilized in replacement of heart valves for many years.[2] Its material properties are favorable in many ways. The elastic modulus is very similar to cortical bone. This allows the implant to favorably share the load with bone and minimize stress shielding. It is biologically inert and does not invite an immune-mediated reaction as seen with silicone and polyethylene. The wear characteristics of the articulation are also very favorable. Studies have demonstrated minimal particulate debris from repetitive cyclic loading. Unfortunately, the stems of these implants have no osseous ingrowth and depend primarily on appositional growth of the bone around the implant to help provide stability. Due to its favorable material properties, pyrocarbon has promise when utilized as a hemiarthroplasty. Canine studies have demonstrated that, when compared to cobalt chrome, pyrocarbon yielded no inflammatory response, and generated less surface cracks and promoted more fibrocartilage regeneration against its exposed articulation than cobalt chrome.[3]

Pyrocarbon was introduced as a small joint replacement in 1979.[4] The implant design has been modified from its original design, particularly the stems. The current design is a ball-and-socket joint that mimics the anatomy of natural MCP joints (▶ Fig. 9.1). Kinematically, the design is similar to that of the native MCP joint, maintaining the arc of curvature and center of rotation.

The surgical technique for insertion is similar to that of silicone implants. A dorsal or transverse incision can be utilized. In patients with inflammatory arthritis, I prefer to expose the joint radial to the extensor tendons through the radial sagittal band, which allows for plication and centralization of the extensor tendons at closure. The capsule is split longitudinally and allows for joint exposure. The MCP joint can then be flexed and the metacarpal head exposed. At the dorsal one-third point of the metacarpal head, a K-wire is inserted longitudinally down the canal of the metacarpal. It helps identify the start point for the alignment and cutting guide of the metacarpal. Fluoroscopy is used to confirm the appropriate insertion point for the guide. Following insertion of the guide, the cutting attachment is placed and the dorsal metacarpal cut is made. The guide is then removed and the rest of the cut is made freehand. The cut is designed to be oblique and protect the collateral ligaments. Resection of the metacarpal head allows visualization of the volar plate and softtissues and release can be performed

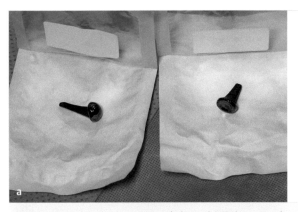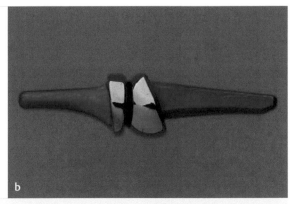

Fig. 9.1 The pyrocarbon metacarpophalangeal (MCP) joint implant. **(a)** The implants coming out of their packages. **(b)** Figure demonstrating how the implant articulates.

at this time, if indicated. Following the metacarpal preparation, the proximal phalanx cut can be performed. The alignment/cutting guide is inserted in the canal at the dorsal third junction. Again, a K-wire, followed by fluoroscopic evaluation, helps confirm the appropriate placement of the alignment guide. The cut at the proximal phalanx is perpendicular to the longitudinal axis. The cut is initiated with the guide in place and completed freehand after removal of the guide.

Broaching is performed up to the largest size that fits the canals. The use of a side-cutting burr can be helpful in preparing the canals to optimize fit. Following broaching, the implant is trialed. At this point, stability can be assessed in both coronal and sagittal planes. Adjustments to the softtissues, such as tightening of collateral ligaments and further volar release, if indicated, can then be performed and prepared for after insertion of the definitive implants. In addition, if the joint is not stable enough following trialing with the surface gliding trials, the system has silicone trials that match the bony cuts as a fallback option. Following placement of the final components, the motion and stability are reassessed. Softtissue balancing is then completed and the extensor tendon centralized.

In patients with osteoarthritis, it is uncommon to perform more than one or two implants in the same setting. Thus, a longitudinal incision is performed. A tendon-splitting approach can generally be utilized. The rest procedure are similar to the above technique, except that softtissue balancing is typically not as necessary.

9.2.2 Surface Replacement Arthroplasty (SRA) MCP joint

The SRA implant pre-dates the pyrocarbon joint. It was designed by Dr. Ronald Linscheid and has been used extensively. Like the pyrocarbon design, it is meant to be anatomic and duplicate the anatomy of the MCP joint. In addition, the bone preparation to fit the implant preserves the ligament and allows for repair/plication/release when indicated. It is a ball-and-socket design that mimics the native force transmission, and aims to maximize joint motion and tendon excursion. In addition, the metacarpal head design is such that it has an offset that helps provide stability with MCP flexion and laxity with extension. Finally, there are radial-ulnar flares that help provide coronal plane stability.

The SRA implant is a metal-polyethylene articulation (▶ Fig. 9.2). The metacarpal component is a cobalt chrome head with a titanium stem. The entire distal component is made of polyethylene. The metacarpal component can be cemented or uncemented; the distal component requires cementation.

The technique is similar to that of the pyrocarbon implants. A dorsal transverse (multiple digits) or longitudinal (single or two digits) incisions can be used. The collateral ligaments are preserved or reflected for later repair. If the collaterals are released for plication, then either the origin or K-wires holes in the dorsal distal metacarpal can be used to tighten the ligament following insertion of the final components. The metacarpal head is resected perpendicular to its axis in a similar manner as cuts would be for silicone systems. However, a second chamfer cut is made to remove the distal volar aspect of the metacarpal. The proximal phalanx cut is perpendicular to its long axis with care taken to protect the volar plate and insertions of the collateral ligaments. The canals are broached to the best fit. The implants are trialed and stability is assessed. The components can then be inserted. The distal component is cemented first and the proximal component is then placed. The ligaments are then advanced, the joint capsule reapproximated, and the tendon centralized.

Rehabilitation protocols vary based on the diagnosis. In patients with rheumatoid arthritis, in the first 3 to 4 weeks following surgery, the MCP joints are immobilized in extension, while allowing for PIP motion. Thereafter, a low profile static splint is made for the patient and an

9

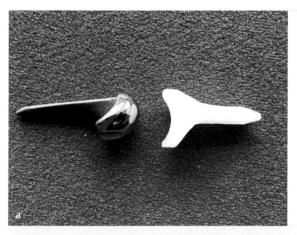
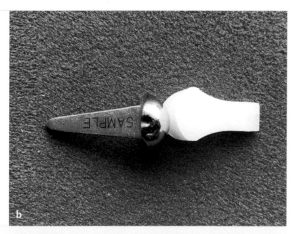

Fig. 9.2 The surface replacement arthroplasty. (a) An articulating view and (b) the view in the coronal plane.

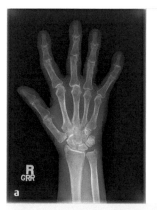
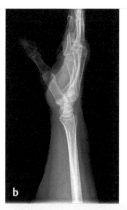
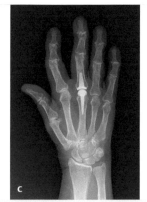
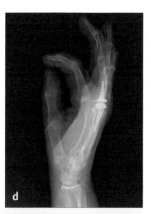

Fig. 9.3 A 69-year-old right-hand dominant female with severe metacarpophalangeal (MCP) osteoarthritis and pain of the right long finger. (a) Posteroanterior (PA) and (b) lateral radiographs demonstrate the arthritis. Postoperative (c) PA and (d) lateral X-rays at 6 months postoperative demonstrate a well seated and stable implant.

MCP motion protocol is initiated. At 8 to 12 weeks postsurgery, the patient may begin strengthening.

Patients with osteoarthritis tend to have more reliable softtissue stabilizers and therefore are able to progress with therapy sooner. Depending on joint stability and the status of the collateral ligaments, early motion can begin. If collateral ligament tightening is necessary, then a longer period of immobilization (closer to that of patients with inflammatory arthritis) should be utilized.

9.3 Indications/Contraindications

The surface gliding implants are an excellent option for the management of noninflammatory MCP joint arthritis. Given the modular nature of these designs, there is an inherent demand on the patient's native softtissue stabilizers to maintain a stable joint. Many patients with non-inflammatory arthrosis have the softtissues capable of successfully supporting their MCP arthroplasty. ▶ Fig. 9.3

and ▶ Fig. 9.4 illustrate two cases successfully treated with a pyrocarbon implant.

However, most patients who present with MCP arthritis have inflammatory arthritis. In this population, the role of unconstrained surface gliding MCP implants is less clear. Patients with well-controlled rheumatoid arthritis are likely to be better candidates.

Contraindications to surface gliding MCP arthroplasty include patients with poorly controlled inflammatory arthritis, those with significant deformities, a history of infection (relative), muscle incompetence, neurologic compromise, poor bone stock/quality, and incompetent softtissues.

Like all joints undergoing arthroplasty, preoperative radiographs are important in helping determine the feasibility of surface gliding implants. Subluxation and frank dislocation of the MCP joints, as seen in cases of severe inflammatory arthropathy, are usually not candidates for surface gliding MCP arthroplasty. In addition to frank instability, there is often significant bone loss along the

9

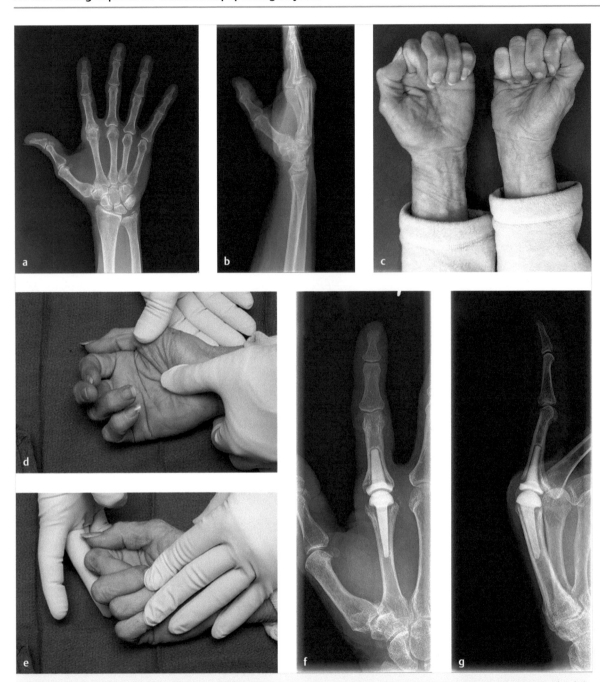

Fig. 9.4 A 65-year-old female with significant osteoarthritis of the index metacarpophalangeal (MCP) joint and malrotation and radial collateral insufficiency. Preoperative **(a)** PA and **(b)** lateral radiographs show advance arthritis and intraoperative **(c–e)** positional photos demonstrate the malrotation secondary to subluxation and radial collateral ligament insufficiency. These can be challenging to treat in both the primary and revision surgery setting. With a radial collateral ligament plication is often necessary and prolonged immobilization of 4 weeks of the MCP joint, a successful outcome can be achieved. **(f)** PA and **(g)** lateral radiographs at 2 years following surgery demonstrate stable implant. She also maintained excellent correction of her malrotation.

dorsal aspect of the base of the proximal phalanx. In addition, significant ulnar drift of the MCP joints is linked to radial collateral ligament and sagittal band insufficiency which compromise the success of gliding implants.

Because of its favorable biologic properties and wear characteristics, an additional indication for the use of pyrocarbon MCP arthroplasty in the setting of acute/subacute trauma. In these settings it can serve as both a total joint replacement as well as a hemiarthroplasty. In fact, even in the setting of arthrosis, pyrocarbon hemiarthroplasty has been shown to be an effective option at a variety of joints including wrist, shoulder, and thumb base as well as the finger.[5,6,7,8,9,10,11]

9.4 Results in the Literature

9.4.1 Pyrocarbon

Since the initial publication by Cook et al,[12] there have been numerous reviews of outcomes with pyrocarbon MCP arthroplasty.[13,14,15,16,17,18,19] Cook et al examined 71 MCP pyrocarbon arthroplasties in 26 patients at an average 12-year follow-up period.[12] Multiple degenerative etiologies were treated, but the most common was inflammatory arthritis. Kaplan–Meier analysis reviewed an 82% five-year and 81% 10-year survivorship, with a predicted 2% failure per year. Overall motion of the MCP joint was improved by an average of 13 degrees and extension (elevation) of the arc improved 16 degrees, providing the patients a more extended posture and improved hand function. Radiographic outcomes were available in 53 of 71 fingers. Ninety-four percent of the joints maintained their reduction. There was however a notable trend toward recurrent ulnar drift over time, but at the most recent follow-up, the drift was not worse than preoperative measurements. Pain relief overall was excellent. The authors concluded that pyrocarbon was biologically and biomechanically compatible and durable material for arthroplasty of the MCP joint.

Subsequent series have also reported encouraging outcomes, especially for patient with osteoarthritis. Parker et al examined a large series of 130 MCP primary pyrocarbon arthroplasties, of which 116 were available for radiographic analysis, with a mean follow-up of 17 months.[14] The rheumatoid arthritis group comprised 96 joints while the osteoarthritic patients included 20 joints. Clinical results were generally excellent, with 99% survivorship in this preliminary study. Pain relief was predictable. The ranges of motion and strength were also improved in both groups. Patient satisfaction was greater than 90% at a mean follow-up of 1 year. There were 6% minor and 9% major complications among the cohorts. A 10% major complication rate was seen in the rheumatoid arthritis patients. The main noteworthy complications were two MCP subluxations, two cases of hand dysfunction and drift requiring repeat softtissue balancing, one patient with a dislocation, and one case of stiffness that underwent manipulation under anesthesia. The osteoarthritis group had two "major" complications: one was an extensor tendon disruption; and another was for persistent pain that required explant of the prosthesis. The osteoarthritis group had generally stable overall radiographic appearances with none of the implants demonstrating evidence of loosening. However, the radiographic analysis for the rheumatoid/inflammatory arthritis patients was more worrisome, especially after 1 year. While most were not revised either because the patient was asymptomatic or preferred not to, the dislocation rate increased to 14%. In addition, on the radiographic analysis at over 1 year, nearly all (95%) had an increased radiolucent seam, 55% had axial subsidence, and 45% were noted to have periprosthetic erosions.

Kopylov et al also examined their results of 40 pyrocarbon MCP joint arthroplasties in 14 patients with rheumatoid arthritis.[13] At a minimum follow-up of 3 years, all patients had improved pain relief, clinical outcomes, and motion. Two joints in one patient were revised secondary to excessive loosening. However, the study lacked the longer-term radiographic analysis when compared to that of Parker et al.

As previously mentioned, encouraging results have been seen with the use of pyrocarbon MCP arthroplasty for osteoarthritis. Nunez and Citron published a short-term review on the use of pyrocarbon MCP joints in patients with osteoarthritis.[19] The authors treated seven patients with ten MCP joints with a mean follow-up of 2.2 (range 1–4) years. Pain scores improved significantly from 68 to 3%. In addition, there was no evidence of implant failure or loosening. Overall, there were excellent patient satisfaction scores. They concluded that pyrocarbon MCP arthroplasty is a promising solution for osteoarthritis.

Wall and Stern reviewed 11 cases with a minimum 2-year follow-up (mean 4 years).[18] Pain relief was excellent and the range of motion improved. However, grip strength did not. All patients were able to return to their prior employment and patient outcome measures were excellent. One finger had subluxation of the extensor tendon and another was revised to arthrodesis secondary to persistent unexplained pain. Radiographically, there was a mean subsidence of 3 mm, but no implant migration, fracture, or dislocation. The authors concluded that pyrolytic carbon MCP arthroplasty was a good surgical option for patients with osteoarthritis.

Simpson-White and Chojnowski also reviewed 18 fingers in ten patients who underwent pyrocarbon MCP arthroplasty for osteoarthritis.[17] The mean follow-up interval was nearly 5 years (58.6 months). Pain, arc of motion, and patient-related outcome (QuickDASH) measures were all improved. All but one patient was satisfied. One case required revision to silastic implant secondary to altered pinch of their index finger. Similar to Wall and Stern's report, the authors noted radiographic subsidence of the implants (in some components up to 5 mm), but no dislocations or overt loosening. They concluded that they would continue to use pyrocarbon implants in the management of osteoarthritis of the MCP joint.

Finally, Dickson et al reviewed their experience with 51 fingers in 36 patients who underwent pyrocarbon MCP arthroplasty for osteoarthritis.[16] The mean follow-up period was 103 months. Preoperatively, no consistent pain, motion, or functional scores were measured. However, similar to prior studies, the clinical outcomes were generally excellent. Postoperatively, the mean VAS (1–10) pain score was 0.9 (range 0–7). The MCP joint arc of motion was a mean of 54 degrees (range 20–80) and grip strength was a mean of 25 (range 11–45) kg. The QuickDASH and Patient Evaluation Measures (PEM) scores were a mean of 28.9 (range 0–56.8) and 26.5 (range 10–54), respectively. Overall implant survivorship was 88% at 10 years. The overall complication rate was 20%; four were defined as "early" and five as "late." Among the early complications, one patient developed complex regional pain syndrome and three had a dislocation. The early dislocations underwent further interventions: one was stable following closed reduction, second was revised to a silicone arthroplasty, and the third was "up-sized" to larger components. Among the late complications there were two cases of stiff MCP joints which underwent manipulation and percutaneous softtissue releases. There was one prosthetic stem fracture and another aseptic loosening occurred; both of these cases were revised to a silicone MCP arthroplasty. Finally, one case of subluxation of the MCP joint was corrected with up-sizing of the components. Interestingly, all implant revisions were performed within the first 18 months following surgery, suggesting of technical issues rather than inherent problems with the implants. The authors conclude that pyrocarbon MCP arthroplasty provides good pain relief, motion, and satisfaction for patients with noninflammatory arthritis.

As previously mentioned, the durability, material properties, and biomechanical characteristics of pyrocarbon lend itself to be used in younger patients and as a hemiarthroplasty. A novel indication for the use of pyrocarbon MCP arthroplasty is to address posttraumatic problems. Houdek et al reviewed the outcome of pyrocarbon MCP arthroplasty and hemiarthroplasty following injuries with non-reconstructable cartilage loss.[6] Ten fingers in seven patients were identified that underwent MCP arthroplasty within 24 hours of trauma leaving the joint cartilage either partially or completely damaged. The mechanism of injury in all cases was a saw. Six patients underwent hemiarthroplasty (four distal metacarpal and two proximal phalangeal replacements) and four total MCP joint replacements. The mean follow-up period was 4 years. Clinical outcomes demonstrated a mean arc of MCP motion of 56 degrees (range 30–70). Most patients had no or minimal pain. Since all cases had concomitant softtissue and tendon injuries that also required treatment, approximately half of the patients required a tenolysis 3 to 18 months following the index surgery. No cases of revision, loosening, infection, or dislocation occurred. This study demonstrates that pyrocarbon can be safely utilized to help reconstruct the MCP joints in select cases of trauma resulting in nonrepairable cartilage or joint injury.

9.4.2 Surface Replacement Arthroplasty (SRA)

While the metal-plastic SRA is a more established option for MCP reconstruction than pyrocarbon, there are no peer-reviewed published results available regarding experience with this implant.

The large experience at our institution has been with the use of SRA implants for treating patients with rheumatoid arthritis. We have reviewed 80 fingers in 27 patients with a mean follow-up of 9.5 years. Pain relief and arc of motion were significantly improved. Thirteen fingers (16%) underwent revision and 29 (36%) required reoperation. Kaplan–Meier analysis for 1-, 5-, 10-, and 20-year survival was 100%, 95%, 85%, and 69%, respectively. For reoperations, the analysis was worse, with 1-, 5-, 10-, and 20-year survival from overall reoperation rates were 89%, 80%, 65%, and 46%, respectively. Complications were common. Functional instability and/or subluxation occurred in 31% of digits. Less common complications included: delayed wound healing, tendon/ligament rupture, ligament laxity, heterotopic bone formation, and synovitis.

In noninflammatory arthritis, we reviewed 18 digits in 15 patients with SRA implants at a mean follow-up of 6.9 years. Pain and ranges of motion improved significantly. Three digits required revision surgery and five required reoperation. The most common indication for reoperation was stiffness. Kaplan–Meier analyses for 2-, 5-, 10-, and 15-year survivorship was 89%, 89%, 76%, and 76%, respectively. The analyses for reoperations at 2, 5, 10, and 15years was 72%, 72%, 62%, and 62%, respectively. Overall, patient satisfaction was 72%.

9.5 Personal Experience (Pearls/Pitfalls)

Most of my experience relates to pyrocarbon implants. My preference is to avoid cementing in finger arthroplasty, and the SRA implant requires cement for at least the distal component.

Patient selection is critical in the use of these implants. I have seen numerous difficulties and failures when used in patients with inflammatory arthritis. The lack of competent softtissue stabilizers in this population invites recurrent instability, subluxation, and deformity. However, in patients with noninflammatory arthritis, I find this implant to be very reliable. My experience mimics that of the literature.

Technically, I like to remove the minimum amount of bone. It helps protect the collateral ligaments and preserves bone stock. I try and identify the bone–cartilage interface along the dorsal distal metacarpal and use that as a starting point for the bone cuts. Care needs to be taken to remove the osteophytes prior to making this assessment as it may result in excessive bone resection. When making the metacarpal cut, care needs to be taken to protect the collateral ligaments. Following removal of the metacarpal head, releasing the volar plate (if it is tight) will help facilitate stability, especially in patients with volar subluxation of the MCP joint. I try to remove only 2 to 3 mm of bone off the proximal phalanx. Recognizing the collaterals attach more volar at the proximal phalanx base will help protect them. I broach to the largest size that fits the canals. When inserting the trials, if the best fit is between sizes, I prefer to err on the side of the smaller implant as overstuffing the joint can cause limited extension/motion and occasionally pain. Assessing stability following insertion of the trials is essential. The surgeon needs to be sure there is good gliding of the joint without impingement, especially into flexion, as occasionally volar osteophytes will limit flexion or deviate the finger as it flexes. I prefer to be able to hyperextend the MCP joint at least 5 degrees with passive extension, as this reassures me that the implant is not overstuffed. If the fit is poor, either more bone resection or placement of larger implants may be needed. A side cutting burr can be used to enlarge the medullary canals to allow for placement of larger components. Impaction bone grafting into the canals, using bone from the resected metacarpal head, can help improve fit and alignment of the components. When necessary, the collateral ligaments can be reinforced/tightened through K-wire holes in the dorsal metacarpal or through the footprint of the origin of the collateral ligament. The sutures for plication of the ligament, of which I prefer to use, include a 3–0 mersilene, 2–0 ticron, or 3–0 vicryl (depending on the tissue quality and degree of laxity). These should be set in place prior to placement of the final components for tightening after placement.

The index finger can pose challenges as the loads across that joint due to lateral pinch may invite instability. Care should be taken at the preoperative assessment of these digits and intraoperative stability following implant placement. Radial collateral ligament reinforcement is often valuable in my experience, and my threshold for immobilizing the MCP joint for longer is low. ▶ Fig. 9.4 illustrates a patient who had index finger radial collateral laxity and malrotation. She was successfully treated with surface replacement arthroplasty, radial collateral ligament reinforcement, and prolonged (4 weeks) MCP joint immobilization.

Through the guidance of our occupational and hand therapy team, rehabilitation has been simplified over the years. Depending on the stability of the joint intraoperatively, I typically immobilize the MCP in extension, allowing for PIP motion for 1 to 2 weeks following surgery. The patient can then graduate to a removable splint that also holds the MCP joint in extension and can initiate a short arc type of protocol, progressively increasing active

motion 10 to 15 degrees weekly until 75 to 80 degrees. Strengthening can start at 3 months postoperatively.

9.6 Conclusion

Surface gliding implants in the treatment of MCP joint arthritis have become a viable alternative to silicone, especially in patients with noninflammatory arthritis. With designs that mimic the native joint and stronger and more favorable material properties, they have the potential to become the preferred option. In my practice it has already become the case for patients with osteoarthritis. Longer-term follow-up studies will further define their role.

References

[1] Swanson AB. Flexible implant resection arthroplasty. Hand. 1972; 4(2): 119–134

[2] Haubold AD. On the durability of pyrolytic carbon in vivo. Med Prog Technol. 1994; 20(3–4):201–208

[3] Kawalec JS, Hetherington VJ, Melillo TC, Corbin N. Evaluation of fibrocartilage regeneration and bone response at full-thickness cartilage defects in articulation with pyrolytic carbon or cobalt-chromium alloy hemiarthroplasties. J Biomed Mater Res. 1998; 41(4):534–540

[4] BeckenbaughRD. Pyrolytic carbon implants.In: Simmen, ed. Hand Arthroplasties.London: Martin Dunitz;2000:323–327

[5] Garret J, Harly E, Le Huec JC, Brunner U, Rotini R, Godenèche A. Pyrolytic carbon humeral head in hemi-shoulder arthroplasty: preliminary results at 2-year follow-up. JSES Open Access. 2018; 3(1):37–42

[6] Houdek MT, Wagner ER, Rizzo M, Moran SL. Metacarpophalangeal joint arthroplasty in the setting of trauma. J Hand Surg Am. 2015; 40(12):2416–2420

[7] Kim K, Gong HS, Baek GH. Pyrolytic carbon hemiarthroplasty for avascular necrosis of the metacarpal head: a case report. J Hand Surg Asian Pac Vol. 2018; 23(1):140–143

[8] Pettersson K, Amilon A, Rizzo M. Pyrolytic carbon hemiarthroplasty in the management of proximal interphalangeal joint arthritis. J Hand Surg Am. 2015; 40(3):462–468

[9] Santos FL, Ferreira A, Grazina R, Sá D, Canela P, Lemos R. APSI scaphoid hemiarthroplasty: long-term results. Rev Bras Ortop. 2018; 53(5): 582–588

[10] Vitale MA, Hsu CC, Rizzo M, Moran SL. Pyrolytic carbon arthroplasty versus suspensionplasty for trapezial-metacarpal arthritis. J Wrist Surg. 2017; 6(2):134–143

[11] Bigorre N, Saint Cast Y, Cesari B, Rabarin F, Raimbeau G. Intermediate term evaluation of the Eclypse distal radio-ulnar prosthesis for rheumatoid arthritis. A report of five cases. Orthop Traumatol Surg Res. 2016; 102(3):345–349

[12] Cook SD, Beckenbaugh RD, Redondo J, Popich LS, Klawitter JJ, Linscheid RL. Long-term follow-up of pyrolytic carbon metacarpophalangeal implants. J Bone Joint Surg Am. 1999; 81(5):635–648

[13] Kopylov P, Tagil M. Ascension MCP metacarpophalangeal nonconstrained pyrolytic carbon prosthesis in rheumatoid arthritis. J Hand Surg [Br]. 2005; 30B:61

[14] Parker WL, Rizzo M, Moran SL, Hormel KB, Beckenbaugh RD. Preliminary results of nonconstrained pyrolytic carbon arthroplasty for metacarpophalangeal joint arthritis. J Hand Surg Am. 2007; 32(10): 1496–1505

[15] Syed MA, Smith A, Benjamin-Laing H. Pyrocarbon implant fracture after metacarpophalangeal joint arthroplasty: an unusual cause for early revision. J Hand Surg Eur Vol. 2010; 35(6):505–506

9

[16] Dickson DR, Badge R, Nuttall D, et al. Pyrocarbon metacarpophalangeal joint arthroplasty in noninflammatory arthritis: minimum 5-year follow-up. J Hand Surg Am. 2015; 40(10):1956–1962

[17] Simpson-White RW, Chojnowski AJ. Pyrocarbon metacarpophalangeal joint replacement in primary osteoarthritis. J Hand Surg Eur Vol. 2014; 39(6):575–581

[18] Wall LB, Stern PJ. Clinical and radiographic outcomes of metacarpophalangeal joint pyrolytic carbon arthroplasty for osteoarthritis. J Hand Surg Am. 2013; 38(3):537–543

[19] Nuñez VA, Citron ND. Short-term results of the ascension pyrolytic carbon metacarpophalangeal joint replacement arthroplasty for osteoarthritis. Chir Main. 2005; 24(3–4):161–164

9

10 Vascularized Toe Joint Transfers for Proximal Interphalangeal and Metacarpophalangeal Joint Reconstruction

Gilles Dautel

Abstract

In children or young adults, vascularized toe joint transfers are an alternative option to prosthetic implants, for proximal interphalangeal (PIP) or metacarpophalangeal (MCP) joint reconstruction. In children, reconstruction aims to restore both range of motion (ROM) and growth potential. The PIP joint of the second toe is the preferred donor site for PIP reconstruction and can also be used for MCP reconstruction when preservation of the donor toe is mandatory. These transfers are performed with a short vascular pedicle in order to reduce the dissection time and diminish the donor site morbidity. While these reconstructions provide a long-lasting result, the ROM achieved is always less than in a normal finger joint and slightly less than in artificial PIP joint replacement.

Keywords: toe transfers, toe joint transfers, microsurgery, proximal interphalangeal joint, metacarpophalangeal joint, vascularized joint transfers

10.1 Introduction

The indications for vascularized toe joint transplantation are the destruction of a functionally important joint in the fingers, such as the proximal interphalangeal (PIP) joint or metacarpophalangeal (MCP) joint of the fingers, either in a growing child or a young adult. Destruction of the distal interphalangeal (DIP) joint of the fingers or MCP joint of the thumb can be treated successfully by joint fusion. In children, joint reconstruction with a toe joint transfer aims to restore both the range of motion (ROM) of the affected joint and its ability to grow. In a young adult, the goal is to provide a longer-lasting reconstruction than typically provided by an implant arthroplasty.

10.2 Anatomical Bases for Joint Transfer to the Hand

10.2.1 Arterial Network

The arterial supply of the second toe and its joints is provided by branches of the dorsalis pedis artery, which is an extension of the anterior tibial artery. At the proximal end of the first intermetacarpal space, this artery gives off the first dorsal metatarsal artery (DMA1) and the first plantar metatarsal artery (PMA1). The DMA1 runs in the first intermetatarsal space at a variable depth. Several authors have described its anatomical variations. Gilbert[1] proposed a classification system based on its depth in the first space:

- Type 1 (66 % of cases): the artery runs superficially in the first space, either above the first dorsal interosseous muscle (type 1a) or in the body of this muscle (type 1b);
- Type 2 (22 % of cases): the artery runs under the first dorsal interosseous muscle deeply in the first space, then becomes superficial in the distal portion of the space by passing above the deep transverse intermetatarsal ligament;
- Type 3 (12 % of cases): the artery runs in a deep plantar location over its entire course; this plantar form is the most challenging to work with. When it is encountered, and a long pedicle is required, we typically resort to a bypass to obtain a useful pedicle length instead of performing a tedious and risky dissection through a dorsal approach.

When a second toe joint transfer is performed, it is vascularized by the medial (tibial) proper plantar digital artery of the second toe, which feeds a periarticular anastomotic circle at the level of the PIP joint.

While performed less often, transfer of the second metatarsophalangeal (MTP) joint is performed occasionally. The arterial supply is from the dorsal and plantar network of the metatarsal arteries of the first and second intermetatarsal spaces. These two networks supply an anastomotic circle at the level of the second metatarsal neck. During dissection, it is essential to preserve the continuity of the dorsal and plantar networks to preserve as many branches to the joint as possible. In particular, the second plantar metatarsal artery (PMA2) always contributes to MTP vascularization. Thus, the transfer will involve harvesting both the PMA2 and DMA1.

10.2.2 Venous Drainage of Toe Joint Transfers

The dorsal and plantar veins of the toe anastomose in the web space and drain into superficial and deep venous networks. The superficial network, derived from the middle of the venous arch, drains into the greater saphenous vein. The deep network consists of veins associated with the proper plantar digital arteries.

In clinical practice, the superficial venous network is used for the tissue transfer anastamoses. One or two veins are dissected, up to where they emerge from the skin paddle. Throughout the dissection, it is essential to preserve the existing connections between the skin paddle and the underlying joint, as they support the articular venous return. When dissecting the donor site, the surgeon must also keep in mind the very superficial, practically subdermal, location of the return veins, in the vicinity of the web space and beyond, especially during the skin incision and when the flaps are first developed for exposure. If the dissection is too deep, there is a risk of irreparable damage to this venous return network.

10.3 Indications for Toe Joint Transfers

Major destruction of a dominant joint (MCP or PIP) of a finger in a skeletally immature child is the most common indication for toe joint transfers. Thumb IP or MCP joint injuries in children are mostly treated by joint fusion.

In adults, the reconstruction of a finger joint by joint transfer is only indicated when fusion and arthroplasty are contraindicated. In this case also, it is almost only considered for dominant joints (PIP or MCP of the fingers) in young adults with high functional demands. In our practice, the mean age at the time of the transfer was 18.1 years highlighting the age limits we apply.

Some local conditions are also required in order to be allowed to achieve a good result after toe joint transfer. The flexor tendons should glide freely and the recipient finger should have good or normal sensory capacity.

Finally this very demanding surgery should only be performed in highly motivated patients, ready to go through a complex surgical protocol and a very prolonged and time consuming rehabilitation.

10.4 Surgical Technique for PIP Transfer from the Second Toe

10.4.1 Preparation of the Recipient Site

A dorsal approach is used from the base of the proximal phalanx (P1) to the distal third of the middle phalanx (P2). We prefer a straight-line incision over the involved joint. The extensor mechanism is exposed and can be released (tenolysis) where there are existing adhesions. Exposure of the palmar recipient artery is possible through this dorsal approach by reflecting the lateral slip of the extensor tendon. The PIP joint should be excised using two parallel osteotomies, performed with an oscillating saw with continuous saline irrigation to minimize thermal damage. The joint is resected en bloc, including the remnants of the volar plate. In order to reduce the length of the bone graft that will be required to fuse the donor PIP joint, we usually try to harvest the smallest possible transfer. However, in our experience it is not safe to harvest a transfer smaller than 15 mm. Measurements are taken of the ideal transplant length, i. e., the length of

the bones and joint, along with the appropriate lengths of blood vessels. It is never appropriate to plan to lengthen the recipient finger during joint reconstruction. After local instillation of lidocaine 1 % (to prevent arterial spasm), the site is covered with a moist bandage and the tourniquet released.

10.4.2 Dissection of Transplant (Donor Site)

Via a dorsal approach, a rectangular skin flap is outlined over the PIP joint of the second toe. This flap will be used postoperatively to monitor the transfer and will provide extra skin to facilitate closure of the recipient site. The flap incision is extended proximally via a zigzag incision. Exsanguination prior to tourniquet inflation should be partial, in order to make dissection of the vessels easier. During the dissection we recommend first finding the draining vein in the subdermal layer which is crucial to preserve the venous return of the transfer. The incision is extended distally on the lateral side of the skin paddle. The lateral proper plantar digital pedicle of the toe is located and carefully preserved as it will be the sole nutrient artery for the second toe. Then the medial proper plantar pedicle is located, and the artery meticulously separated from the nerve; the artery and its articular branches will remain in contact with the joint. The lateral plantar digital artery (the one on the peroneal side of the toe) is the only remaining nutrient vessel *for the second toe*, whereas the medial plantar artery (the one on the tibial side of the toe) is the nutrient vessel *for the harvested joint*. The extensor mechanism is divided beyond the insertion of the central slip, level with the osteotomy site, and the lateral plantar artery is cut between two clips at the same level. The plantar arcades are located and cut. The distal osteotomy is performed with an oscillating saw and continuous saline irrigation. The bone is lifted up, exposing the flexor tendon sheath, which is incised longitudinally, leaving its deep face next to the transplant and the plantar plate. The extensor tendon is incised at the level of P1 and lifted to expose the second osteotomy site, parallel to the first, isolating a transplant of the desired length. The flexor digitorum brevis tendon is cut while the flexor digitorum longus tendon is left intact. The transplant is thus isolated as an island on its medial arterial pedicle. Dissection of the nutrient artery is continued in a retrograde manner, if possible until the emergence of the proper lateral plantar digital artery of the hallux, which is left intact. At this point, the tourniquet is released to check the bleeding of the distal osteotomy cut and the skin paddle. The flap is finally divided by cutting the veins and arteries after double ligation. A 1.0-mm axial K-wire is inserted across the middle and proximal phalanges of the toe guided by an image intensifier to provide temporary stabilization of the toe.

10.4.3 In Situ Arrangement of Transplant

The tourniquet in the recipient limb is reinflated. The transplant is positioned, and the axial K-wire advanced with a drill until it crosses the DIP joint and is left outside the tip of the finger. At this point, the rotation alignment of the transplant is set. However, this is difficult because the PIP joint is held extended. The proximal end of the transplant is then reduced onto the proximal donor site bone, and the axial K-wire is driven into the base of the proximal phalanx, leaving the MCP free. Two antirotation K-wires are inserted at each osteotomy site. They can be positioned by hand and applied using a back-and-forth motion. The extensor tendons of the recipient finger and the transferred toe are trimmed as needed. An overlapping tendon suture is performed with maximal tension to account for the likely development of a PIP flexion deformity. If the native central slip is long enough it is linked to the transfer with a Pulvertaft weave aiming for maximal extension. The straight arthrodesis and tendon suturing in full extension both contribute to optimizing the final extension of the PIP joint. At this point, the transplant's feeder artery is slid into its tunnel under the lateral slip of the extensor tendon and anastomosed to a digital artery using a microscope. The first step is end-to-end anastomosis of the artery to the recipient proper palmar digital artery after adventitial stripping, mechanical dilation, heparinization, and recutting as needed. This is performed using interrupted 10–0 nylon sutures. Next, the veins are sutured end-to-end in the same way linking the donor veins to superficial digital or commissural veins. The tourniquet can be released at this point. Refilling of the skin paddle and blood flow in the return vein are evidence of good vascularization of the transplant. The skin is closed using interrupted 5–0 absorbable sutures. There, skin paddle needs to be sutured in loosely to avoid restricting the return flow in the vein. In doubt, a partial thickness skin graft is harvested from the hypothenar eminence harvested and sutured in place. Supportive dressings are applied in an intrinsic positive position including a volar plaster slab and carefully leaving a window over the skin paddle.

10.4.4 Reconstruction of Donor Site

It requires special attention, even if it is performed at the end of the procedure. It is essential to perform a bone graft, even when the piece of resected bone is as small as possible (about 15 mm long in adults). Shortening of the donor site would simplify this step, avoiding bone grafting and a skin flap; however, the resulting toe will be short, ugly, and uncomfortable when wearing shoes. Various sites can be used to harvest the bone graft. One option is to use the bone block removed from the recipient finger—a new harvest site would not be needed. This technique is particularly useful in situations where the transfer occurs in the context of a reversal of PIP fusion. When this is not possible, we prefer using a bicortical bone graft from the iliac crest. Another option is to harvest the graft from the tibial malleolus. The graft is shaped very carefully. In the ideal case, PIP fusion will be done in slight flexion instead of complete extension, in order to optimize function and appearance. The length is chosen to reproduce the initial length of the donor toe, although 1 mm of shortening is acceptable (depending on the initial length of the second toe).

Fixation at the recipient site consists of a combination of an axial K-wire and oblique antirotation K-wires.

Covering this bone graft with a skin flap is essential. It is important not to resort to local skin reconstruction to avoid a cross-toe flap. Given the harvesting of the skin paddle, and the preservation of the toe's length, this option is never sufficient and risks compromising both the skin's healing and the survival and incorporation of the underlying bone graft. For many years, we have used a reversed, de-epithelialized cross-toe flap. We now prefer using a cross-toe flag flap harvested from the third toe and tunneled under the web space skin between the second and third toes. This avoids the need to detach the flap on the 15th day. This flap is supplied by the dorsal arterial network and has always been reliable in our practice, even if capillary refill is slow when the tourniquet is released.

10.5 Surgical Technique for MTP Transfer from the Second Toe

Joint transfer for MCP reconstruction is much rarer. MTP movements mainly occur in hyperextension (dorsal flexion). To restore the flexion range of an MCP joint, the transplant must be reversed 180 degrees. After harvesting of the toe MTP joint, there are two reconstruction options. We prefer proximal amputation of the second ray; other surgeons prefer MTP fusion with an iliac crest bone graft. While PIP fusion at the second toe is typically well tolerated, MTP fusion is much less well tolerated in our experience. This need to amputate the proximal part of the donor toe is one of the reasons we have shied away from MTP joint transfer. MCP reconstruction can also be performed with a PIP transfer from the second toe. However, the limited ROM of the transferred PIP joint makes it more difficult to achieve a satisfactory clinical outcome.

10.6 Outcomes of Vascularized Toe Joint Transfers

Currently, our case series consists of 56 vascularized toe joint transfers, 13 for MCP joint reconstruction, and 43 for PIP joint reconstruction.[2,3,4,5]

10

10.6.1 PIP Joint Reconstruction (▶ Fig. 10.1a-l)

The mean age of this subgroup was 18.1 (range 5–40) years; 23 patients were less than 17 years of age at the time of the procedure. Two-thirds of patients were male. The PIP joint destruction was due to trauma in 80% of cases and due to an infection in 15%. The 5% were due to congenital anomalies or tumors. The donor site was the PIP joint of the second toe in all cases. More than half of these transfers were performed using the short pedicle technique, allowing a connection at the finger level. In three cases, the digital connection required rerouting to a healthy artery from an adjacent finger. Four patients required early revision for arterial ischemia; the reoperation resulted in full transplant survival. More than half of our patients required one or more secondary surgical procedures (tenolysis of extensor mechanism, arthrolysis of reconstructed PIP joint, defatting, correction of malunion).

There were five cases of functional failure: complete ankylosis of the transplant in two cases and septic complications in three cases leading to fusion or surgical amputation of the finger. In the latter three cases, the joint transfer was performed due to septic arthritis or an open intra-articular fracture. The active ROM of the remaining transfers was measured with a goniometer after a mean follow-up of 60 months. The mean range of motion was 45 degrees with an active flexion of 79 degrees (range 40–90 degrees) and an average extensor lag of 34 degrees (20–55 degrees).[2,3,4,5,6,]

10.6.2 MCP Reconstruction (▶ Fig. 10.2a-e)

The mean age of this subgroup was 21.3 years[2]; there were ten men and three women. The MCP joints destruction was posttraumatic in 11 cases and infective in 2. The donor site was always from the second toe: the PIP joint in 2 cases and MTP joint in 11 cases. The active ROM was a mean of 60 degrees (range 35–80 degrees) at a mean follow-up of 50 months.[4,5]

Excluding the cases of postoperative ankylosis, there were no cases of secondary deterioration on radiographs

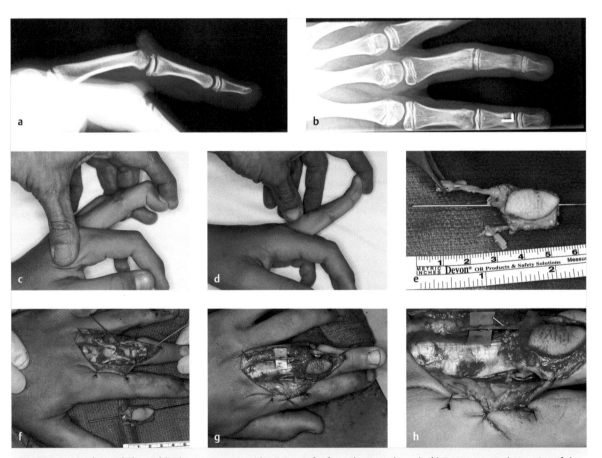

Fig. 10.1 Proximal interphalangeal (PIP) reconstruction with a PIP transfer from the second toe. **(a, b)** Posttraumatic destruction of the PIP joint of the middle finger in a teenager due to a roll over car accident. **(c, d)** Spontaneous fusion of the transferred PIP joint. **(e)** PIP compound transfer from the second toe, 15 mm long. **(f, g)** In situ insetting of the toe joint. **(h–k)** Clinical result.

(Continued)

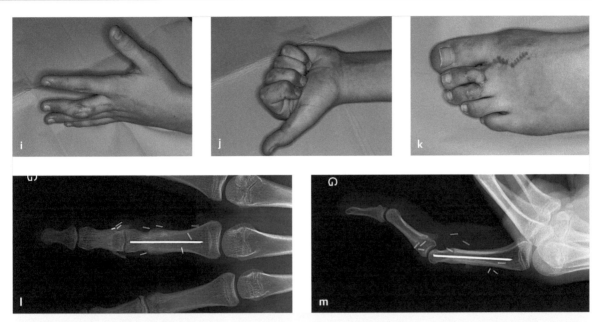

Fig. 10.1 (*Continued*) **(l, m)** Radiological result.

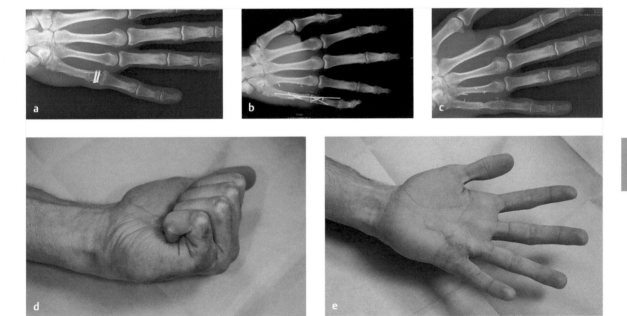

Fig. 10.2 Metacarpophalangeal (MCP) reconstruction with a proximal interphalangeal (PIP) transfer from the second toe. **(a)** Posttraumatic destruction of the MCP joint space in a young rock climber. The involved joint was very stiff and painful. **(b)** Bony fixation: The reconstructed joint was held in full extension for 6 weeks. **(c)** Result after removal of the K-wires. **(d, e)** Final range of motion.

after a mean follow-up of 50 months (range 3–126), indicating the long-term survival of the joint cartilage. In children operated upon before skeletal maturity, axial growth of the involved phalanx was confirmed radiologically indicating that the growth plate was intact. Early growth arrest was observed in two cases; but the cause was unclear.

10.7 Discussion

Over the years, we have not been able to improve the ROM following joint transfers. At the same time, the diversity of available arthroplasty implants has increased, as has their performance. Consequently—and now no more than before—the superiority of joint transfers cannot be based on the final ROM, which is not better than achieved with joint implants. The indications for joint transfer surgery continue to be limited to contraindications to arthroplasty. Instances of joint destruction in children or young adults continue to be appropriate indications in our opinion. Surgically, the latest technical advances that have advanced our practice include the use of short pedicle transfers and the reconstruction methods for the donor site.

The choice of a short pedicle, proposed by Yoshimura,[7] has many advantages. The dissection is simpler, faster, as extension into the dorsum of the foot is unnecessary, which means that variations in the arrangement of the proximal vascular network are no longer an issue, and just as reliable. The harvesting preserves the vascularization of the hallux and avoids an ugly scar on the dorsum of the foot.

In our early cases, we amputated the donor toe, as described in Foucher's benchmark paper.[8] This is no longer justifiable, since using toe joint transfer to reconstruct a finger is no longer accepted by patients or their family unless the donor site sequelae are minimized. Now, the donor toe is always preserved, with the primary procedure being PIP fusion, restoring the length of the donor ray. More recent use of a heterodigital dorsal island flap, harvested from the dorsal side of the third toe, provides an elegant single-stage procedure with limited consequences for the third toe.

There is widespread agreement that an extensor lag will occur. Various authors have reported extensor lags around 40 degrees: 39 degrees by Foucher[9]; 35 degrees by Chen[10]; and 41 degrees by Tsubokawa.[11] None of the technical tricks that we have used have prevented this.

In our case series, only one patient did not have an extensor lag; this case was very unusual because the dorsal side of the recipient finger was intact, and the damage was mainly on the volar side. This allowed us to preserve the physiological attachment of the central slip of the extensor mechanisms and to slide the transplant under this intact tendon. It is very rare to be able to perform PIP joint transfer when the central slip at the recipient site is completely intact. In a cadaver study, a Chinese team intentionally made the transplant shorter to reduce the extent of the extensor lag.[12] Mohan et al proposed shifting the reconstruction proximally by placing the reconstruction joint line more proximal than its anatomical location, believing that this will make finger curling and fingertip-to-palm contact easier to achieve.[13] Loh et al advocated customized reconstruction of the central slip of the extensor mechanism of the recipient finger,[14] while Lin et al suggest reinforcing the bone attachment of the central slip.[15] We believe the extensor lag is a direct consequence of the flexion–extension ROM of the donor joint, which is rarely the same as that of a finger PIP joint. There is currently no established way to get around this anatomical limitation.

Since a denervated joint could theoretically be the site of degenerative events that alter the joint space, authors such as Foucher[16] and Kuo[17] have proposed reinnervating the transplant by suturing one or more nerves; the benefits have not been proven. We have more than 25 years' follow-up of several of our patients. We have never observed any degenerative events that could be attributed to joint denervation.

The literature describing the outcomes of MCP joint reconstructions is sparser than for PIP joint reconstructions. The authors are divided on use of the toe PIP or MTP joints. The preoccupation with reducing morbidity now favors using the toe PIP joint; however in growing children, the need to take two active growth plates with the transplant (metatarsal neck and P1 base) forces us to transfer the MTP joint.

10.8 Conclusion

Vascularized toe joint transfers must remain in our armamentarium, providing rewarding and long-standing results in children or young highly motivated patients.

References

[1] Gilbert A. Vascular anatomy of the first web space of the foot. In: Landi A, ed. Reconstruction of the Thumb. 1st ed. London: Chapman and Hall Medical; 1989:199–204
[2] Pozzetto M, Dautel G. The vascularized articular transfers from the foot. Chir Main. 2010; 29 Suppl 1:S156–S171
[3] Dautel G, Merle M. Results of vascularized toe joints transfers. J Hand Surg. 1997; 22B: 492–498
[4] Dautel G, Gouzou S, Vialaneix J, Faivre S. PIP reconstruction with vascularized PIP joint from the second toe: minimizing the morbidity with the "dorsal approach and short-pedicle technique". Tech Hand Up Extrem Surg. 2004; 8(3):173–180
[5] Dautel G, Merle M, Prévot J. Toe transfers in traumatic mutilations of the hand in children. Solutions, techniques and results. Chirurgie. 1993–1994; 119(8):419–424
[6] Dautel G. Reconstruction articulaire par transferts vascularisés. In: Merle M, Dautel G, eds. La main traumatique, tome 2, chirurgie secondaire. 1st ed. Paris: Masson; 1995:29–45
[7] Yoshimura M. Toe-to-hand transfer. Plast Reconstr Surg. 1984; 73(5): 851–852
[8] Foucher G. Vascularized joint transfers. In: Green DP, ed. Operative Hand Surgery. New York: Churchill Livingstone; 1988:1271–1293
[9] Foucher G, Lenoble E, Smith D. Free and island vascularized joint transfer for proximal interphalangeal reconstruction: a series of 27 cases. J Hand Surg Am. 1994; 19(1):8–16
[10] Chen SH, Wei FC, Chen HC, Hentz VR, Chuang DC, Yeh MC. Vascularized toe joint transfer to the hand. Plast Reconstr Surg. 1996; 98 (7):1275–1284
[11] Tsubokawa N, Yoshizu T, Maki Y. Long-term results of free vascularized second toe joint transfers to finger proximal interphalangeal joints. J Hand Surg Am. 2003; 28(3):443–447
[12] Hsu CC, Loh CYY, Kao D, Moran SL, Lin YT. The impact of transferred vascularized toe joint length on motion arc of reconstructed finger proximal interphalangeal joints: a cadaveric study. J Hand Surg Eur Vol. 2017; 42(8):789–793
[13] Mohan R, Wong VW, Higgins JP, Katz RD. Proximalization of the vascularized toe joint in finger proximal interphalangeal joint reconstruction: a technique to derive optimal flexion from a joint with expected limited motion. J Hand Surg Am. 2017; 42(2):e125–e132

10

[14] Loh CY, Hsu CC, Lin CH, et al. Customizing extensor reconstruction in vascularized toe joint transfers to finger proximal interphalangeal joints: a strategic approach for correcting extensor lag. Plast Reconstr Surg. 2017; 139(4):915–922

[15] Lin YT, Loh CY. A novel technique for correcting extensor lag in vascularized toe PIP joint transfers. Tech Hand Up Extrem Surg. 2016; 20 (3):104–107

[16] Foucher G, Sammut D, Citron N. Free vascularized toe-joint transfer in hand reconstruction: a series of 25 patients. J Reconstr Microsurg. 1990; 6(3):201–207

[17] Kuo ET, Ji ZL, Zhao YC, Zhang ML. Reconstruction of metacarpophalangeal joint by free vascularized autogenous metatarsophalangeal joint transplant. J Reconstr Microsurg. 1984; 1(1):65–74

10

Section 2B

PIP and DIP Arthroplasty

11 The Treatment Strategy in PIP Arthroplasty

Daniel B. Herren

Abstract

Proximal interphalangeal joint (PIP) arthroplasty is gaining increasing popularity. Besides the optimization of the surgical technique and the rehabilitation, new implants have been developed in order to improve the treatment results. Thus, the options in the treatment modalities have become more differentiated and should be tailored to the individual situation.

This chapter will discuss the anatomical features of the PIP joint related to implant arthroplasty, touch on the conservative treatment of PIP joints affections, and focus mainly on prosthetic joint replacement. Based on a case discussion, a flow chart for the different surgical treatment possibilities is presented. It should act as a possible guideline for the indications and choice of PIP arthroplasty.

Keywords: proximal interphalangeal joint, surgical treatment, implant arthroplasty, indication, silicone implants, surface replacement

11.1 Introduction

11.1.1 Anatomical Considerations for PIP Arthroplasty

Anatomically, the distal (DIP) and the proximal interphalangeal (PIP) joints are very similar; the main difference is the dimension and the reduce mobility at the DIP joint level.

In contrast to the metacarpophalangeal (MCP) joint, the osseous shape of the PIP and DIP plays an important role in joint stability.[1] The head of the phalanx has a trapezoidal shape with an intercondylar groove which increases from dorsal to volar. There are no significant differences between the ulnar and the radial condyles. The counterpart to the head of the proximal phalanx is the base of the middle and the distal phalanges. The joint is not a perfect hinge allowing some degree of freedom for abduction and adduction as well as for joint rotation. There is, therefore, no constant center of rotation but rather an instantaneous rotational axis.[2]

There are slightly different radii of curvature between the radial PIP joints and the ulnar joints. The radial joints need greater lateral stability and the ulnar joints more mobility in order to function correctly. These anatomical features are only partially mimicked by the different types of implant arthroplasty available.

11.1.2 Evaluation of PIP Joint Problems

Destruction of a PIP joint is either a result of an inflammatory/degenerative process or is posttraumatic. It is a clinical diagnosis and is confirmed with conventional radiographic examination. Patients classically present with swollen, tender PIP joints, with a diffuse, swollen appearance and a fusiform joint contour. Joint stiffness is almost always present and often correlates with the degree of swelling. In posttraumatic PIP joint arthritis, a CT scan may be useful to determine whether a joint preserving procedure is warranted, such as an intra-articular osteotomy or joint reconstruction.

Most authors, especially in the rheumatology and arthritis literature, use a modification of the Kellgren and Lawrence scale,[3] initially described for patellofemoral arthritis, for radiographic classification:

- Grade 1: doubtful narrowing of joint space and possible osteophytic lipping.
- Grade 2: definite osteophytes, definite narrowing of joint space.
- Grade 3: moderate multiple osteophytes, definite narrowing of joint space, some sclerosis, and possible deformation of bone contour.
- Grade 4: large osteophytes, marked narrowing of joint space, severe sclerosis, and definite deformation of bone contour

As always in the evaluation of a joint destruction, the grade of radiographic destruction does not predict the symptoms of an individual joint.

11.1.3 Nonoperative Treatment of PIP Destruction

Nonoperative treatment for advanced destruction of finger joints should be the first line of treatment both for inflammatory disease or osteoarthritis (OA). Treating affected joints with OA does not, to date, alter the appearance of OA in unaffected joints, or delay the progression of OA elsewhere. In the pathophysiology of the disease, catabolic cytokines and anabolic growth factors play key roles in the destruction of the cartilage.

Conventional treatment includes analgesics and nonsteroidal anti-inflammatory drugs. Intra-articular visco-supplementation with hyaluronic acid has been shown to be effective in terms of pain relief and improved disability. In comparison with intra-articular corticosteroids, it seems to have a longer benefit,[4] especially in the knee joint. However, this has not been reproduced in the hand literature and is not supported with personal experience.

Glucosamine and chondroitin are important components of the normal cartilage. Like visco-supplementation, the efficiency of glucosamine and chondroitin in the treatment of OA has been documented best in the knee joint.[5] They seem to reduce the need for anti-

11

inflammatory drugs and improve functionality.[6] Few side effects have been reported. Most authors recommend a combination of the two, at a dosage of 1500 mg glucosamine and 1200 mg chondroitin daily. Since the onset of the effects is slow and takes at least 4 weeks, most authors recommend either 3 months' therapy twice a year or continuous treatment.[6] There is no literature supporting its efficacy in the hand. Disease modifying drugs, used mainly in patients suffering from rheumatoid arthritis, are good candidates for suppressing the destructive inflammatory process in OA as well. Besides the classic systemic application of this drug, an intra-articular treatment with injection showed a possible disease modifying action of intra-articular Infliximab in erosive OA of the hands in a pilot study.[7]

The PIP joint reacts well to intra-articular corticosteroid injections. The most common side effect is atrophy of the skin and subcutaneous tissue, which is more of an aesthetic than a functional problem. No known correlation exists between the radiographic appearance of the joint and the effectiveness of intra-articular steroid administration, and is typically self-limiting. There are different techniques for PIP infiltration: the author finds injecting into the dorsal recess of the joint, similar to a knee joint, is the easiest to perform.

Splints for painful inflamed joints might be effective, but their regular use limits hand function and lowers patient satisfaction.[8] Modification of activity may be beneficial in limiting articular inflammation. Joint protection devices may relieve the joints and help to prevent further irritation of the affected joints.

The effects of ultrasound, laser, and electrotherapy in the treatment of OA in the fingers are not well documented. Experience has shown limited effects, typically only short term, with an often inappropriate cost–efficiency ratio.

11.2 PIP Joint Replacement

11.2.1 General Remarks

PIP joint arthroplasty is a widely accepted procedure in joints with either OA or in posttraumatic arthritis. In inflammatory conditions like rheumatoid arthritis, the indication depends on the disease activity and on the pattern of bone and joint destruction. Prerequisites are intact tendons and at least some residual joint stability. Although no exact degree of instability can be defined, lateral deviation beyond 30 degrees are difficult to treat successfully; they are likely to fail.

PIP arthroplasty has a shorter history than MCP joint replacement. For decades, joint arthrodesis was the standard procedure for painful PIP joint destruction, and the functional results of this procedure were generally reported to be good.[9] Pellegrini and Burton[10] reviewed a number of patients who had undergone different procedures for PIP joint destruction. They observed that arthrodesis in the radial digits brought an improvement in the lateral pinch, while arthroplasty in the ulnar digits gave reasonable functional mobility with good pain relief. Based on this analysis, the authors were not able to make a definitive recommendation on the optimal procedure for destroyed PIP joints. Since that publication, however, several authors have advocated the concept of reserving PIP arthroplasty for ulnar digits and treating the index finger, which is the main partner for pinching with the thumb, with PIP joint fusion.

Contraindications to PIP joint replacement include the classic criteria of insufficient bone stock, missing or dysfunctional tendons, and severe tendon imbalance, especially contracted boutonnière and swan-neck deformities. In severely contracted joints with a long-standing history of immobility, PIP joint fusion in a functional position may be a better choice than implant arthroplasty. Severe joint instability and deformity of more than 30 degrees is extremely difficult to correct with an implant and is a relative contraindication to arthroplasty.

11.2.2 Choice of Implants

The choice of implant and the surgical approach used are the two most frequently discussed issues in PIP arthroplasty. A variety of implants is available, but only a few series with adequate long-term follow-up have been published. Silicone implants (▶ Fig. 11.1), introduced by Swanson in the early 1960s, are still the gold standard for newer generations of implants with respect to functional performance, revision rate, and long-term outcomes. Silicone joint spacers carry a risk of implant breakage and, much less commonly, silicone synovitis. Overall, the silicone spacer produces fairly consistent results with good pain relief and reasonable function, with an arc of motion of 40 to 60 degrees. Silicone synovitis is not a hallmark of PIP joint arthroplasty as it has been historically with wrist implants. Only a few cases of silicone synovitis have been reported and, although implant failure is seen, it does not necessarily lead to revision.[11,12,13,14] No randomized controlled trials with series of different silicone implants in the PIP joint are available, and analysis of the

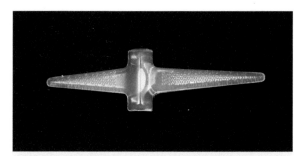

Fig. 11.1 Classical proximal interphalangeal (PIP) silicone implant in the original Swanson design.

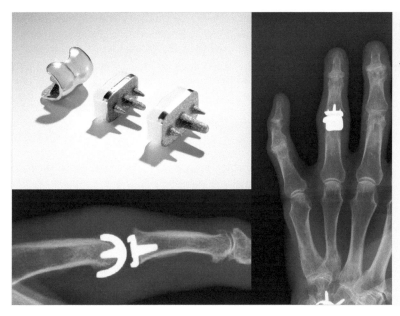

Fig. 11.2 Resurfacing implant (CapFlex, KLS Martin Group, Tuttlingen, Germany), with modular components. The fixation is provided with a cement-free very short stems.

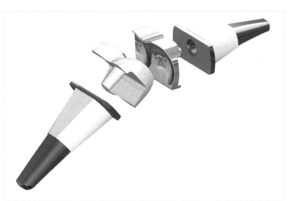

Fig. 11.3 Tactys proximal interphalangeal (PIP) prosthesis (Stryker USA). The four different components can be modularly mixed.

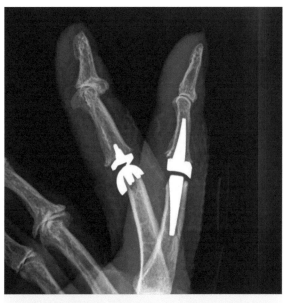

Fig. 11.4 Two different types of two-component implants: the CapFlex and the Tactys prosthesis.

different case series suggests similar results for most of the Silicone implant designs.

The newer generations of PIP joint implants follow the principles of surface replacement with a two-component concept.[15,16,17] The proximal component replaces the bicondylar head of the proximal phalanx and the distal component has a convex surface, which articulates with the head. Most of these implants do not represent a real resurfacing concept, since a significant amount of bone must be resected and long stems for both components are needed to provide adequate bone fixation. However, the newest generation of implants provides a real surface replacement with a very short-stem subchondral bone fixation (CapFlex, KLS Martin Group, Tuttlingen, Germany) (▶ Fig. 11.2 and ▶ Fig. 11.4).

Several material combinations are available, from the classic chrome cobalt/polyethylene to ceramic/ceramic and pyrocarbon/pyrocarbon. Although pyrocarbon has excellent biocompatibility and gliding characteristics, problems have been reported, with difficulty achieving osseous stability and reports of joint squeaking.[18,19,20,21,22] Similar problems have been observed with ceramics on ceramics. The most frequently used combination is still metal on polyethylene. According to the often-cited recommendation that the polyethylene should be on the concave side, most implants follow that principle. However there are implants on the market which have reversed this principle. The Tactys (Stryker USA) (▶ Fig. 11.3 and ▶ Fig. 11.4) implant has the implant head

11

made out of polyethylene and shows no adverse effects in the midterm results.[16,23]

Most of these implants can be used without cement, although some of them require cementing for primary fixation in the bone. The majority of surgeons prefer non-cemented implants, since revision is easier, and removal of the implant causes less damage and bone loss. Overall, the newer generation of PIP implants based on the resurfacing concept seems a logical development in PIP arthroplasty, but most of them have not yet stood the test of time and long-term studies are still lacking for most implant designs.

The concept of resection–interposition arthroplasty, with a volar plate for example, similar to what has been described by Tupper for the MCP joint, is reported only for traumatic or posttraumatic conditions.[24,25] Depending on the existing condition and the soft tissue configuration, this technique has an inherent danger of producing an unstable PIP joint, especially in the radial digits.

The choice of implant depends on several factors, including the surgeon's experience, the local anatomical situation, especially the bone stock, and the surgical approach. Silicone devices, which act as joint spacers, are by far the most forgiving implants. They provide reproducible results even in cases with difficult bone stock and with limited surgical experience. They can be implanted easily using different surgical approaches. More complex, two-component joints need adequate bone stock; no large cystic defects can be allowed to exist with implants, as they must be inserted without cementing. Correct placement, with the goal of restoring the biomechanical center of rotation, needs some experience. Some of these implants are supplied with resection guides, which can be used only with a dorsal approach. In addition, some prostheses need more space for implantation, which also means that a dorsal or lateral approach is required.

11.2.3 Combination of Different Interventions

Since osteoarthritis affects different joints, it is necessary to think about different combined interventions at the same time, according to the patient's symptoms.

If cases of several painful PIP joints it may be appropriate to operate on multiple joints at a single operation. During rehabilitation the fingers are typically mobilized together, so it is helpful to have neighbor fingers, which tolerate buddy splinting. Every different combination is possible as long as the rehabilitation program is not compromised as this can cause marked adverse outcomes.

The combination of DIP surgery, most often joint fusion, and PIP arthroplasty at the same finger or in the same hand is appropriate. Although the finger will have more postoperative swelling, the immobilization of the DIP and the movement of the PIP joint are complimentary.

Combining thumb base surgery and PIP joint arthroplasty is not so reliable. They are often better treated separately. Typically, the most symptomatic joint needs then to be addressed first.

11.3 Strategies and Indications in the Treatment of PIP Joint Destruction

In this chapter, our current philosophy, based on published literature, own research data and experience, will be discussed. It does not imply that these are the only options but they should highlight possible strategies and practical approaches to PIP joint arthroplasty.

11.3.1 Case Example (▶ Fig. 11.5)

Extensive destruction of the small finger joints in the index of the right dominant hand in a 65-year-old male. There is progressive disease involving multiple fingers. He had three intra-articular steroid injections over the previous 2 years. Each brought significant pain relief for several months, but the last injection only helped for under 6 weeks. The DIP joint is significantly deformed but no longer painful and barely mobile. There are no significant comorbidities.

The radiographs show a significant bone defect of the base of the middle phalanx. There is a severe inflammatory reaction in the joint, which has already reached the medullary canal mainly of the middle phalanx. The DIP joint is also destroyed with multiple osteophytes.

Clinically, the PIP joint is inflamed, swollen, and painful. There is a residual flexion/extension arc of movement of 60/20/0 degree. The DIP joint is deformed and very stiff but painless.

What are the options?

The schematic flow chart in ▶ Fig. 11.6 summarizes the different treatment options for surgical PIP treatment under different joint conditions.

PIP Destruction with Intact Tendons, Good Bone Stock, and Stable Joint Condition

▶ Fig. 11.7 shows the different techniques available to address PIP joint destruction if the bone condition is still good and the architecture of the joint largely preserved.

The index and the middle fingers are subject to marked shearing forces while pinching with the thumb. Silicone arthroplasty have shown to have their limits in resisting these forces, leading to instability and probable long-term implant failure.

For this reason, we recommend a two-component implant for index or middle finger PIP joint arthroplasty. With their more anatomical joint shape, they offer better

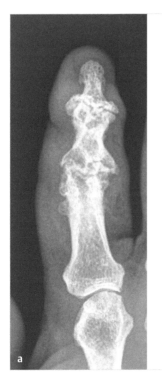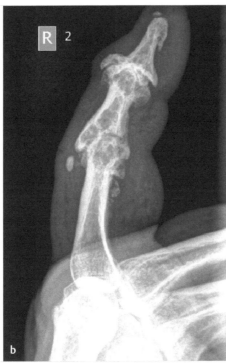

Fig. 11.5 (a, b) X-rays of the dominant index proximal interphalangeal (PIP) joint in a 65-year-old patient suffering from osteoarthritis.

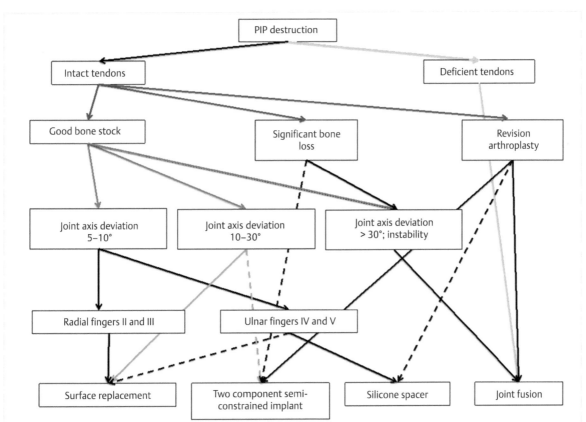

Fig. 11.6 Summary of the different indications and treatment options in proximal interphalangeal (PIP) joint destruction.

11

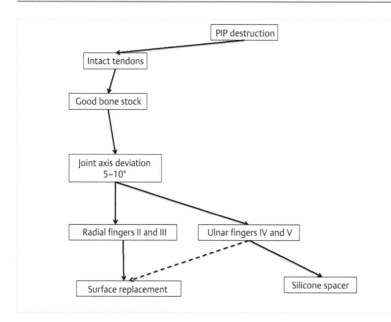

Fig. 11.7 Proximal interphalangeal (PIP) joints with good bone stock and minimal deformation.

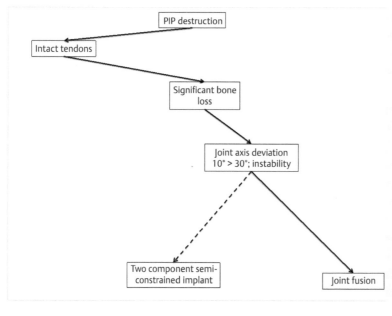

Fig. 11.8 Proximal interphalangeal (PIP) joints with significant bone defect and instability.

stability and even the possibility of restoring joint alignment (CapFlex Publication). So in this case (see also ▶ Fig. 11.7) we would recommend a surface replacement arthroplasty.

PIP Destruction with Intact Tendons, Significant Bone Stock Deficiency, and Joint Instability

In cases of significant bone loss (▶ Fig. 11.8), a surface replacement might be difficult to fix to the bone. In such cases medullary bone fixation, with or without cement is likely to be preferable.

Implants like the Tactys or the SR PIP (both from Stryker) offer this fixation mode. However, despite the modular character of these implants, there are limits of overcoming significant bone defects; careful preoperative planning is needed.

If the bone defect is too extensive, a joint fusion, with or without bone graft, is often the better choice. The fusion angle needs to be chosen according to the needs. Suitable fusion positions are usually 15 to 20 degrees of flexion angle in the radial digits and 25 to 40 degrees in the ulnar joints. Intraoperative trial positioning is performed with a temporary K-wire in order to optimize the surgical outcome.

11.3.2 Revision of Failed PIP Arthroplasty

Revision of a failed PIP arthroplasty remains a challenge. Bone defects, scarring, poor soft tissues, stiffness, or instability are common. In cases of tendon deficiency and multiple surgical interventions, a PIP joint fusion is almost always the best solution. Since implant removal leaves a significant bone defect, a bone graft is always needed in order to avoid excessive finger shortening. A combination of medullary cancellous bone impaction with a block of cortical bone to bridge the defect is recommended. Autografts, allografts, or a combination can be used. Smaller defects can be filled with bone from the distal radius, preferably from volar side since there is more bone stability. Bigger defects might require harvesting from the iliac crest.

Little information about revision PIP arthroplasty is available. In two series from the Mayo Clinic,[26,27] revision arthroplasty was associated with a 70% 5-year survival but with a high incidence of complications. Instability was associated with worse outcomes. In this series, silicone and metal-polyethylene implants had lower rates of implant failure and postoperative complications than pyrocarbon implants. In the series of Herren et al[28] revision surgery after failed silicone PIP joint arthroplasty was most successful in patients with severe postoperative stiffness. Patients with a restricted range of motion as the indication for revision had a considerably increased flexion of 71 degrees following revision, compared with 33 degrees before revision surgery. Pain was relieved to a level of 1.6 on a visual analog scale (VAS) after revision surgery. Ulnar deviation could not be corrected completely and showed a high recurrence. Overall, patients were fairly satisfied with the results of the revision when pain or restricted motion were the prime indications.

In most cases it is possible to convert a two-component PIP arthroplasty into a silicone implant, especially if the components are not cemented. The conversion of a failed silicone in a two-component arthroplasty is very difficult, since the bone loss is often significant. In selected cases it might be possible especially if there is no significant synovial reaction around the joint or bone canals (▶ Fig. 11.9a, b; ▶ Fig. 11.10).

11.3.3 Discussion of the Case Example

A man is suffering from severe pain in a badly damaged index finger PIP joint of his dominant hand. Since there is still a functional range of motion, we would like to retain some motion.

A silicone implant can almost always be inserted. But in the index finger there is a high likelihood of long-term instability. One compromise would be to splint the joint for longer postoperatively for example after 4 weeks. The aim would be to achieve more soft tissue stability in order to protect the implant.

Alternatively, a two-component implant like the Tactys might be recommended. Due to the high modularity of the implant, the bone defect can be more easily addressed. Intramedullary fixation should be achievable possibly supplemented with impaction bone grafting.

PIP joint fusion is always an option but the decision has to be made before the bone cuts are performed and even more bone is missing. In this particular case, we recommended a Tactys prosthesis, but reserving the option of recommending a fusion once the joint is exposed perioperatively.

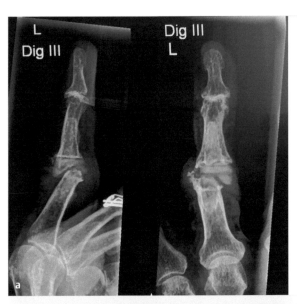
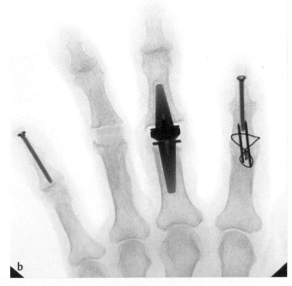

Fig. 11.9 **(a)** Failed silicone arthroplasty with broken implant and significant joint instability. **(b)** Same finger after revision with a Tactys implant. Due to the high modularity, the missing bone could be compensated with the implant components.

11

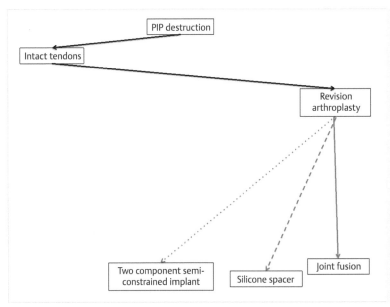

Fig. 11.10 Possibilities for revision proximal interphalangeal (PIP) arthroplasty.

References

[1] Pang EQ, Yao J. Anatomy and biomechanics of the finger proximal interphalangeal joint. Hand Clin. 2018; 34(2):121–126

[2] Dumont C, Albus G, Kubein-Meesenburg D, Fanghänel J, Stürmer KM, Nägerl H. Morphology of the interphalangeal joint surface and its functional relevance. J Hand Surg Am. 2008; 33(1):9–18

[3] Kellgren JH, Lawrence JS. Radiological assessment of osteo-arthrosis. Ann Rheum Dis. 1957; 16(4):494–502

[4] Strauss EJ, Hart JA, Miller MD, Altman RD, Rosen JE. Hyaluronic acid viscosupplementation and osteoarthritis: current uses and future directions. Am J Sports Med. 2009; 37(8):1636–1644

[5] Huskisson EC. Glucosamine and chondroitin for osteoarthritis. J Int Med Res. 2008; 36(6):1161–1179

[6] Uebelhart D. Clinical review of chondroitin sulfate in osteoarthritis. Osteoarthritis Cartilage. 2008; 16 Suppl 3:S19–S21

[7] Fioravanti A, Fabbroni M, Cerase A, Galeazzi M. Treatment of erosive osteoarthritis of the hands by intra-articular infliximab injections: a pilot study. Rheumatol Int. 2009; 29(8):961–965

[8] Ikeda M, Ishii T, Kobayashi Y, Mochida J, Saito I, Oka Y. Custom-made splint treatment for osteoarthritis of the distal interphalangeal joints. J Hand Surg Am. 2010; 35(4):589–593

[9] Uhl RL. Proximal interphalangeal joint arthrodesis using the tension band technique. J Hand Surg Am. 2007; 32(6):914–917

[10] Pellegrini VD, Jr, Burton RI. Osteoarthritis of the proximal interphalangeal joint of the hand: arthroplasty or fusion? J Hand Surg Am. 1990; 15(2):194–209

[11] Herren DB, Simmen BR. Palmar approach in flexible implant arthroplasty of the proximal interphalangeal joint. Clin Orthop Relat Res. 2000(371):131–135

[12] Takigawa S, Meletiou S, Sauerbier M, Cooney WP. Long-term assessment of Swanson implant arthroplasty in the proximal interphalangeal joint of the hand. J Hand Surg Am. 2004; 29(5):785–795

[13] Iselin F, Conti E. Long-term results of proximal interphalangeal joint resection arthroplasties with a silicone implant. J Hand Surg Am. 1995; 20(3 Pt 2):S95–S97

[14] Swanson AB, de Groot Swanson G. Flexible implant resection arthroplasty of the proximal interphalangeal joint. Hand Clin. 1994; 10 (2):261–266

[15] Schindele SF, Hensler S, Audigé L, Marks M, Herren DB. A modular surface gliding implant (CapFlex-PIP) for proximal interphalangeal joint osteoarthritis: a prospective case series. J Hand Surg Am. 2015; 40(2):334–340

[16] Athlani L, Gaisne E, Bellemère P. Arthroplasty of the proximal interphalangeal joint with the TACTYS® prosthesis: Preliminary results after a minimum follow-up of 2 years. Hand Surg Rehab. 2016; 35 (3):168–178

[17] Jennings CD, Livingstone DP. Surface replacement arthroplasty of the proximal interphalangeal joint using the SR PIP implant: long-term results. J Hand Surg Am. 2015; 40(3):469–473.e6

[18] Herren DB, Schindele S, Goldhahn J, Simmen BR. Problematic bone fixation with pyrocarbon implants in proximal interphalangeal joint replacement: short-term results. J Hand Surg [Br]. 2006; 31(6):643–651

[19] Wagner ER, Weston JT, Houdek MT, Luo TD, Moran SL, Rizzo M. Medium-term outcomes with pyrocarbon proximal interphalangeal arthroplasty: A study of 170 consecutive arthroplasties. J Hand Surg Am. 2018; 43(9):797–805

[20] Ceruso M, Pfanner S, Carulli C. Proximal interphalangeal (PIP) joint replacements with pyrolytic carbon implants in the hand. EFORT Open Rev. 2017; 2(1):21–27

[21] Tägil M, Geijer M, Abramo A, Kopylov P. Ten years' experience with a pyrocarbon prosthesis replacing the proximal interphalangeal joint. A prospective clinical and radiographic follow-up. J Hand Surg Eur Vol. 2014; 39(6):587–595

[22] Watts AC, Hearnden AJ, Trail IA, Hayton MJ, Nuttall D, Stanley JK. Pyrocarbon proximal interphalangeal joint arthroplasty: minimum two-year follow-up. J Hand Surg Am. 2012; 37(5):882–888

[23] Griffart A, Agneray H, Loubersac T, Gaisne E, Bellemère P. Arthroplasty of the proximal interphalangeal joint with the Tactys® modular prosthesis: results in case of index finger and clinodactyly. Hand Surg Rehab. 2019; 38(3):179–185 [published online ahead of print March 19, 2019]

[24] Gong HS, Chung MS, Oh JH, Lee YH, Lee YK, Baek GH. Ligament reconstruction and tendon interposition for advanced posttraumatic arthritis of the proximal interphalangeal joint: 3 case reports. J Hand Surg Am. 2008; 33(9):1573–1578

[25] Ostgaard SE, Weilby A. Resection arthroplasty of the proximal interphalangeal joint. J Hand Surg [Br]. 1993; 18(5):613–615

[26] Wagner ER, Luo TD, Houdek MT, Kor DJ, Moran SL, Rizzo M. Revision proximal interphalangeal arthroplasty: an outcome analysis of 75 consecutive cases. J Hand Surg Am. 2015; 40(10):1949–1955.e1

[27] Pritsch T, Rizzo M. Reoperations following proximal interphalangeal joint nonconstrained arthroplasties. J Hand Surg Am. 2011; 36 (9):1460–1466

[28] Herren DB, Keuchel T, Marks M, Schindele S. Revision arthroplasty for failed silicone proximal interphalangeal joint arthroplasty: indications and 8-year results. J Hand Surg Am. 2014; 39(3):462–466

12 Second-Generation Surface Gliding Proximal Interphalangeal Joint Implants (Metal, Pyrocarbon, and Ceramic)

Athanasios Terzis, Florian Neubrech, Lukas Pindur, Nikolai Kuz, and Michael Sauerbier

Abstract

Arthroplasty of the proximal interphalangeal (PIP) joint of the finger remains an established surgical treatment option for the arthritic and painful PIP joint. Various materials and surgical approaches have been used. The first generation arthroplasty consisted of silicone spacers. Outcomes of this type of PIP joint arthroplasty generally showed very good pain relief. Several complications were reported though, including implant fracture or loosening. This led to the concept of resurface replacement arthroplasty (second generation), which aims to relieve pain, restore range of motion and maintain stability of the PIP joint. Understanding of current biomaterials and the complex PIP joint anatomy and biomechanics resulted in introducing new implants, which could achieve very good pain relief and good range of motion of the PIP joint, compared to arthrodesis. In this chapter these second generation implants are introduced.

Keywords: arthroplasty, resurfacing, proximal interphalangeal joint, pyrocarbon, titanium, ceramic

12.1 Introduction

Osteoarthritis of the proximal interphalangeal (PIP) joint is a frequent cause of pain and loss of function of the hand. Pain relief and preservation of a satisfactory range of motion (ROM) are the goals of arthroplasty of the PIP joint as an alternative to arthrodesis. Over the past four decades silicone implant arthroplasty has become a standard procedure in the surgical treatment of PIP joint osteoarthritis.[1,2,3] The main complications of silicone implants, such as poor long-term ROM and implant fractures (▶ Fig. 12.1a, b), can, in theory, be avoided using new resurfacing implants.[5,16,19]

12.2 Characteristic of Implant or Technique

High rates of loosening, implant breakage, and restricted ROM with silicone and semiconstrained implants have led to new treatment strategies.[8] The development of the new PIP joint implant by Avanta (San Diego, USA) with its first clinical application at the Mayo Clinic (Rochester, USA) in the early 1980s signaled the birth of second-generation surface gliding PIP joint implants.[18]

12.2.1 SR-PIP Prosthesis

The surface replacement PIP (SR-PIP) joint arthroplasty implant consists of a distal titanium shaft with biconcave joint surface made of ultrahigh-molecular-weight polyethylene (UHMWPE) and a matching proximal component consisting of a titanium shaft and core, as well as a joint surface made of a cobalt chrome alloy (▶ Fig. 12.2). The matched opposing joint surfaces help create lateral stability and congruity. The shape of the shaft is similar to the shape of the medullary cavity and has a slight dorsal convexity. The implant can be cemented (polymethylmethacrylate; PMMA) or inserted using a press-fit technique. The implant system is available in five different sizes.

12.2.2 Pyrocarbon Prosthesis

This implant (Ascension, Plainsboro/New Jersey, USA) is made of pyrocarbon, a wear-resistant graphite alloy created from hydrolysis of hydrocarbon gas (▶ Fig. 12.3). It has a similar bicondylar design as the SR-PIP implant. The key advantages of pyrocarbon implant include its biocompatibility, due to its inert properties, and the material's high level of resistance and high load-bearing capacity. The implant consists of separate proximal and distal components, which are available in five different sizes. It is implanted exclusively using a press-fit technique.

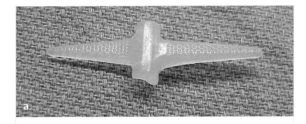

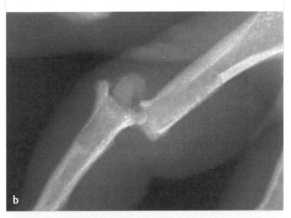

Fig. 12.1 (a) Silicone implant for the proximal interphalangeal (PIP) joint. (b) Complication after silicone arthroplasty of the PIP joint with implant fracture.

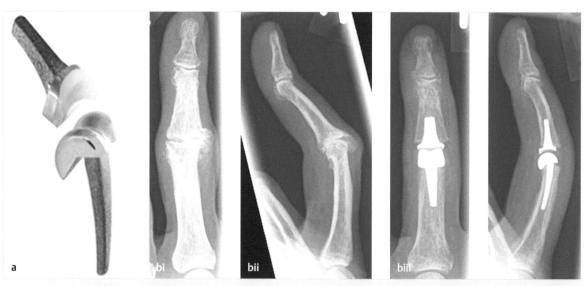

Fig. 12.2 (a) SR-PIP implant, **(b)** posttraumatic osteoarthritis of the PIP joint and postoperative result after PIP joint arthroplasty with the SR-PIP implant.

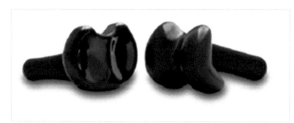

Fig. 12.3 Pyrocarbon implant.

12.2.3 Ceramic Prosthesis

An unconstrained, ceramic prosthesis (▶ Fig. 12.4) PIP arthroplasty has been manufactured by the MOJE company (Petersberg/Germany); it is now being offered in its third generation. It has a similar bicondylar design. It has a volar tilt of 8 degree of the proximal and distal components, longer conical stems as well as a slope of 2 degree in the proximal and 6 degree in the distal component. The purpose of this new prosthesis was to more closely imitate the normal anatomy and physiology of the PIP joint as it preserves the collateral ligaments. The components are made of zirconium oxide ceramic with an additional bioceramic hydroxyapatite coating. The conical implant shafts have grooves to increase surface area for an optimal osseous integration. It is implanted using a press-fit technique.

12.3 Indication and Contraindication

The indication for PIP joint arthroplasty is joint destruction as a result of osteoarthritis, posttraumatic arthritis, or rheumatoid arthritis.[6] If pain persists after appropriate

conservative management or if joint instability leads to functional impairment, operative treatment is indicated. The main treatment options are arthrodesis, arthroplasty, or vascularized joint transfer.[4] While both arthrodesis and arthroplasty typically give good pain relief and improvement in stability, the benefits of an arthrodesis are achieved at the cost of lost motion. This is a significant drawback especially for active patients. In contrast, the arthroplasty aims to maintain or improve the range of PIP joint motion while reducing pain, thus improving the hand function. In the published literature, the total ROM in the PIP joint after successful arthroplasty is expected to be around 50 to 60 degrees.[8,9] The ROM is dependent in part on the preoperative ROM; the greater the ROM preoperatively, the greater it will be postoperatively. The choice of the surgical treatment will also depend upon which finger is affected. PIP arthroplasty is mainly performed in the middle, ring, and small finger in order to improve grip function. In the index finger, lateral stability of the PIP joint is essential for the key pinch strength. In cases of severe deformity and instability, some hand surgeons may prefer joint fusion for the index finger, as the capacity to correct these through arthroplasty is limited.

The contraindications to arthroplasty are severe chronic boutonniere or swan-neck deformities, insufficient bone stock for example after infection, insufficiency of the collateral ligaments, or long-lasting advanced joint contracture. However, there is a clear trend in favor of arthroplasty in recent years as even limited mobility of the PIP joint may improve overall hand function. Generally, the second-generation implants show promising results in short-term follow-up data. The definitive role of each individual implant, however, is yet to be established.

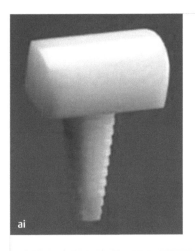
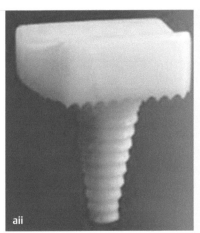

Fig. 12.4 (a, b) Ceramic implant.

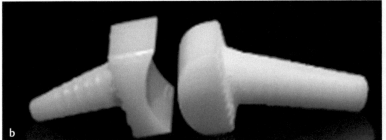

12.4 Results in the Literature

12.4.1 Results for SR-PIP

One of the first studies to investigate long-term outcomes after arthroplasty with the SR-PIP implant was by Sauerbier et al.[2,18] They reported on 82 implants in 60 patients with a mean follow-up of 64 months. The PIP joint ROM increased from 31 to 47 degrees postoperatively; over 70% of patients were pain-free. Similar results were reported by Vogt et al. They reviewed 66 implants in 53 patients. Surgery could improve ROM at approximately 20 degrees and led to a substantial reduction in pain.[7] Murray et al reported similar results in 67 implants in 47 patients at a mean follow-up at 8.8 (range 0.1–31.8) years. They reported significant improvement in ROM and pain. Their mean ROM increased to a mean of 40 degrees (range 0–160) and the mean VAS (visual analog scale) pain score was 3 out of a maximum of 100.[8] Of note, they reported that the rate of complications was significantly higher for the volar as opposed to the dorsal approach. The reported revision rate for SR-PIP implants due to loosening, dysfunction of the extension apparatus, or insufficiency of collateral ligaments was around 26% at a mean of 9.3 years in a study of 39 implants in 21 patients (▶ Fig. 12.5).[9]

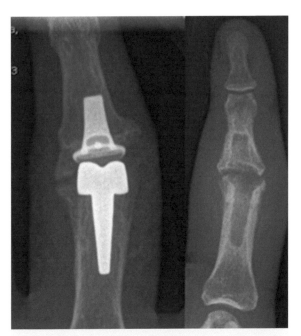

Fig. 12.5 Complication after SR-PIP arthroplasty with implant loosening which eventually led to explantation.

12

A successful SR-PIP implant gives good pain relief and ROM but with a high failure rate.

12.4.2 Results for Pyrocarbon PIP Arthroplasties

Several studies on the results of arthroplasty using the pyrocarbon implant have been published since its introduction in 2001 (▶ Fig. 12.6).[10,11,12,13,14,17] Most authors presented the outcomes in short- or medium-term follow-up studies. The vast majority of the studies have shown good pain relief and maintained or slightly improved ROM. However, reduced ROM compared to preoperatively was demonstrated over a longer follow-up of 10 years.[10] The rates of complications and revision surgery are very variable in the literature with some studies suggesting relatively low complications, satisfactory implant survival rates, and overall good patient satisfaction while others demonstrated unfavorable results.[12,13,17] The most frequently encountered problem was migration of the implant due to instability at the bone–implant interface as the implant stem does not osseointegrate; at best, the bone will grow up to the stem achieving a stable interface. The high rate of implant loosening and malalignment led some hand surgeons to abandon the use of pyrocarbon PIP arthroplasties. In a large study, Wagner et al analyzed the outcome of 170 PIP arthroplasties with a mean follow-up of 6 (range 2–14) years.[14] The study confirmed the previous series that in cases not requiring revision surgery, pain relief was good and ROM satisfactory.

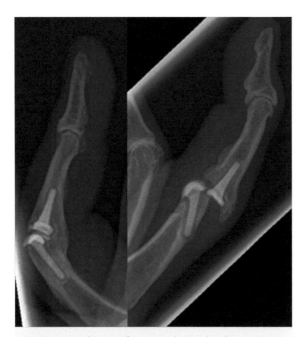

Fig. 12.6 Complication after pyrocarbon arthroplasty with dislocation and heterotopic ossification.

Overall when successful the pyrocarbon PIP arthroplasties give good outcomes but the concerns over failure of stability of the stems and secondary problems has led to hand surgeons moving away from their use.

12.4.3 Results for the Ceramic PIP Arthroplasty

Only few studies investigated the mid- and long-term outcomes of ceramic PIP arthroplasties.[20,21,22] Pettersson et al reported a prospective study of 20 prostheses in 13 patients at a follow-up of 12 months. They reported an improvement of mean ROM from 43 to 60 degrees and grip strength from 46 to 60 N as well as significant pain relief from 7.2 to 3 on the VAS 0–10.[20] In 2008 a retrospective study of 20 ceramic prostheses in 12 patients[21] reported high revision rates and poor functional outcomes, which led to the lead author no longer using these implants. In another retrospective study Wesemann et al reported on 21 ceramic prostheses in 15 patients at a mean follow-up of 12.9 months.[22] The noted moderate functional outcomes and patient satisfaction, but high complication (loosening of the proximal component, subluxation, and fracture) and revision rates.

Overall, it appears that these implants are not reliable enough to be recommended for most surgeons.

12.5 Authors' Own Experience and Preferred Technique: Tips and Tricks

The implantation can be performed via a dorsal, palmar, or lateral approach. We prefer the Chamay approach via a curved dorsal skin incision raising a distally based triangle of extensor tendon over the PIP joint (▶ Fig. 12.7).[15] The collateral ligaments are preserved if possible; if resection of the accessory collateral ligament is necessary, this must be reinserted at the end of the procedure. Next, the PIP joint is opened. After determining the limits of bone resection, the joint surfaces are removed using an oscillating saw, carefully protecting the collateral ligaments, palmar plate, and extensor tendon center slip when resecting the base of the middle phalanx. The medullary cavities of the proximal and middle phalanges are broached to receive the implants. After inserting the trial implants, the passive mobility and stability of the finger are assessed clinically and radiologically, and when satisfactory the final implants are inserted in press-fit technique. Radiographs are performed again to confirm correct implant positioning. Then the extensor tendon is reconstructed with braided nonabsorbable suture and the skin closed.

Postoperatively, a forearm-finger plaster cast is applied in the intrinsic-plus position. This is worn for a few days to help reduce postoperative swelling and pain. Thereafter, active and passive mobilizations start without load

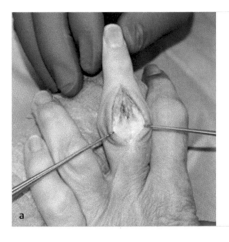

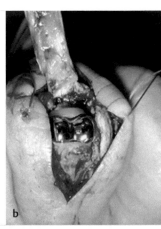

Fig. 12.7 (a, b) Dorsal approach to the proximal interphalangeal (PIP) joint with release of the tractus intermedius according to Chamay.

bearing under the guidance of hand-and-occupational therapy. A protective forearm thermoplastic splint is used at night. Sometimes in order to improve ROM a splint to the adjacent finger can be worn. After 6 weeks, bone–implant stability is assessed radiologically and free mobilization may begin.

References

[1] Deb R, Sauerbier M, Rauschmann MA. History of arthroplasty for finger joints. Orthopade. 2003; 32(9):770–778

[2] Sauerbier M, Cooney WP, Berger RA, Linscheid RL. Complete superficial replacement of the middle finger joint: long-term outcome and surgical technique. Handchir Mikrochir Plast Chir. 2000; 32(6):411–418

[3] Bales JG, Wall LB, Stern PJ. Long-term results of Swanson silicone arthroplasty for proximal interphalangeal joint osteoarthritis. J Hand Surg Am. 2014; 39(3):455–461

[4] Dautel G. Vascularized toe joint transfers to the hand for PIP or MCP reconstruction. Hand Surg Rehab. 2018; 37(6):329–336

[5] Schindele S. Arthroplasty at the proximal interphalengeal joint. Orthopade. 2019; 48(5):378–385

[6] Herren DB. Current European practice in the treatment of proximal interphalangeal joint arthritis. Hand Clin. 2017; 33(3):489–500

[7] Vogt R, Aerni M, Ampofo C, Schmelzer-Schmied N. Proximal interphalangeal (PIP) finger prosthesis: what have we learnt? Experiences over 10 years. Handchir Mikrochir Plast Chir. 2012; 44(5):293–299

[8] Murray PM, Linscheid RL, Cooney WP, III, Baker V, Heckman MG. Long-term outcomes of proximal interphalangeal joint surface replacement arthroplasty. J Bone Joint Surg Am. 2012; 94(12):1120–1128

[9] Jennings CD, Livingstone DP. Surface replacement arthroplasty of the proximal interphalangeal joint using the SR PIP implant: long-term results. J Hand Surg Am. 2015; 40(3):469–473.e6

[10] Reissner L, Schindele S, Hensler S, Marks M, Herren DB. Ten year follow-up of pyrocarbon implants for proximal interphalangeal joint replacement. J Hand Surg Eur Vol. 2014; 39(6):582–586

[11] Bravo CJ, Rizzo M, Hormel KB, Beckenbaugh RD. Pyrolytic carbon proximal interphalangeal joint arthroplasty: results with minimum two-year follow-up evaluation. J Hand Surg Am. 2007; 32(1):1–11

[12] Herren DB, Schindele S, Goldhahn J, Simmen BR. Problematic bone fixation with pyrocarbon implants in proximal interphalangeal joint replacement: short-term results. J Hand Surg [Br]. 2006; 31(6):643–651

[13] Chung KC, Ram AN, Shauver MJ. Outcomes of pyrolytic carbon arthroplasty for the proximal interphalangeal joint. Plast Reconstr Surg. 2009; 123(5):1521–1532

[14] Wagner ER, Weston JT, Houdek MT, Luo TD, Moran SL, Rizzo M. Medium-term outcomes with pyrocarbon proximal interphalangeal arthroplasty: a study of 170 consecutive arthroplasties. J Hand Surg Am. 2018; 43(9):797–805

[15] Chamay A. A distally based dorsal and triangular tendinous flap for direct access to the proximal interphalangeal joint. Ann Chir Main. 1988; 7(2):179–183

[16] Takigawa S, Meletiou S, Sauerbier M, Cooney WP. Long-term assessment of Swanson implant arthroplasty in the proximal interphalangeal joint of the hand. J Hand Surg Am. 2004; 29(5):785–795

[17] Daecke W, Kaszap B, Martini AK, Hagena FW, Rieck B, Jung M. A prospective, randomized comparison of 3 types of proximal interphalangeal joint arthroplasty. J Hand Surg Am. 2012; 37(9):1770–9.e1, 3

[18] Luther C, Germann G, Sauerbier M. Proximal interphalangeal joint replacement with surface replacement arthroplasty (SR-PIP): functional results and complications. Hand (N Y). 2010; 5(3):233–240

[19] Linscheid RL, Murray PM, Vidal MA, Beckenbaugh RD. Development of a surface replacement arthroplasty for proximal interphalangeal joints. J Hand Surg Am. 1997; 22(2):286–298

[20] Pettersson K, Wagnsjö P, Hulin E. Replacement of proximal interphalangeal joints with new ceramic arthroplasty: a prospective series of 20 proximal interphalangeal joint replacements. Scand J Plast Reconstr Surg Hand Surg. 2006; 40(5):291–296

[21] Field J. Two to five year follow-up of the LPM ceramic coated proximal interphalangeal joint arthroplasty. J Hand Surg Eur Vol. 2008; 33(1):38–44

[22] Wesemann A, Flügel M, Mamarvar M. Moje prosthesis for the proximal interphalangeal joint. Handchir Mikrochir Plast Chir. 2008; 40(3):189–196

12

13 Third-Generation PIP Joint Arthroplasty: Tactys

Michaël Y. Papaloïzos

Abstract

This chapter describes the development of the anatomically designed, unconstrained Tactys total joint proximal interphalangeal (PIP) replacement, as well as its particularities and clinical results, both in the literature and in the experience of the author and the developers. The operative procedure is described in detail, together with caveats and surgical tips and tricks.

Keywords: PIP joint, surface arthroplasty, proximal interphalangeal joint, prosthesis, implant

13.1 Introduction

There are three main types of surgery for functionally disabling degenerative arthritis of the proximal interphalangeal (PIP) joint: denervation, arthrodesis, and arthroplasty. Whatever the choice, they all aim to alleviate pain while preserving a useful level of function, not only for the finger itself, but for the hand as a whole. The final decision is based upon the general needs of the patient, any specific requirements, and the state of all the fingers both symptomatic and asymptomatic. Bone stock and quality in the symptomatic finger may be further considerations.

Among the implant arthroplasties, silicone spacers have long been the only solution and are still in use and often considered the gold standard.[1] In addition to their simplicity and ease of implantation, they give relatively consistent results, but their usage is most commonly recommended for low-demand patients. Meanwhile, implants made of various more rigid materials have been developed in order to improve the outcomes.[2] Anatomically designed metallic, ceramic, or pyrocarbon implants

have been developed to improve ranges of motion, stability, and longevity.[3,4,5] However, due to the delicate balance of forces, PIP prosthetic replacement is fraught with complications.[6,7] The Tactys implant was designed to address these issues.

13.2 Development

The Tactys modular prosthesis (Stryker–Memometal, Bruz, France) is a total gliding, unconstrained, modular surface replacement prosthesis with an anatomic design. Started in 2008 by a group of hand surgeons from Belgium, France, and Switzerland together with engineers of the Memometal company, it was set out to imitate the condylar surfaces of the proximal phalanx and the concavities at the base of the middle phalanx, as well as the subtle incongruency and tribological peculiarities as found in nature (▶ Fig. 13.1). The development focused on anatomical premises and studies regarding the size of the phalanges, the form of the condyles,[8] the natural surface incongruency between them and the base of the middle phalanx, as well as the tribology and lubrication.

Our fundamental hypothesis was that a prosthesis anatomically and physiologically as close as possible to the natural model would achieve the best results. Special attention was paid to the morphology and dimensions of the joint surfaces.[9,10]

The second major concern is fixation of the implant to bone to achieve early implant stability and long-term fixation including in cases of deficient bone stock. Press-fit fixation was chosen.

Some modularity was considered essential to be able to treat different fingers in different sized hands in men and women.

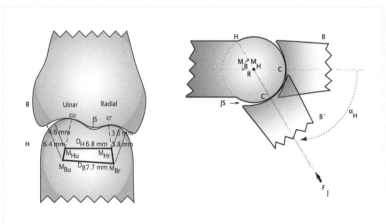

Fig. 13.1 Natural surface incongruency of the proximal interphalangeal joint in the frontal and sagittal plane. (Reproduced with permission from Dumont et al[8].)

13

13.3 Characteristics of the Implant

The Tactys prosthesis is made of four components (▶ Fig. 13.2). The proximal and distal medullary components are made of titanium partially coated with hydroxyapatite in the metaphyseal region in order to ensure secondary bony fixation without making subsequent revision too difficult if required. The stems are designed to be relatively short, especially the distal stem, in order to allow

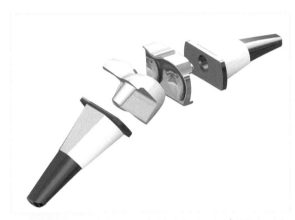

Fig. 13.2 The four components of the Tactys implant (from left to right: proximal medullary component, high-density polyethylene proximal joint surface, distal chrome-cobalt distal joint surface, and a distal medullary component).

for distal interphalangeal (DIP) joint arthrodesis. The proximal convex joint surface is made of ultrahigh-density polyethylene while the distal concave surface is made of chrome-cobalt alloy. The four components (two stems and two articulations) are available in four different sizes for considerable surgical flexibility (▶ Fig. 13.3).

13.3.1 Surgical Technique

The surgery is performed under axillary block with a tourniquet. Via a dorsal curvilinear incision over the PIP joint, the joint is accessed through a longitudinal transtendinous approach with the central slip detached from the base of the middle phalanx. A synovectomy is performed and peripheral osteophytes removed. While preserving the collateral ligaments, the condyles are removed from the head of the proximal phalanx with a thin oscillating saw resecting perpendicular to the long axis of the proximal phalanx. The cartilage remnants and the underlying sclerotic bone at the base of the middle phalanx are removed sparingly either with a saw or a drill aiming to create a flat surface strictly perpendicular to the long axis of the middle phalanx (▶ Fig. 13.4). The gap approximator (▶ Fig. 13.5) is inserted between the two phalanges to estimate the gap width, thus defining the size and the thickness of the distal surface component. Resection can be adjusted if necessary. Proximal and middle phalanges are then reamed to the appropriate stem

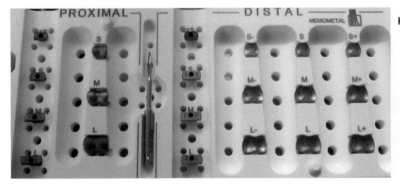

Fig. 13.3 The set with the modular trials.

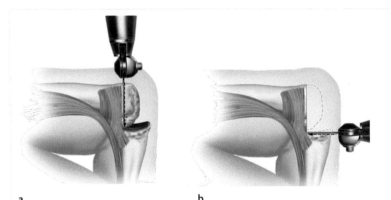

Fig. 13.4 Removing the condyles from the proximal phalanx (**a**) and the base of the middle phalanx (**b**).

a b

13

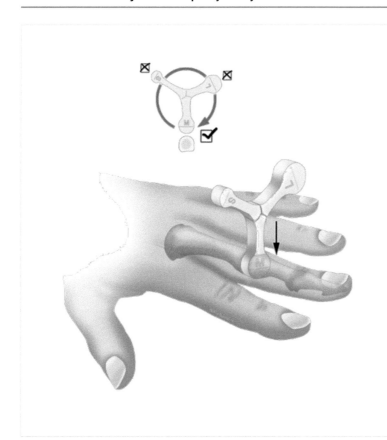

Fig. 13.5 Measuring the gap between the phalanges with the gap approximator.

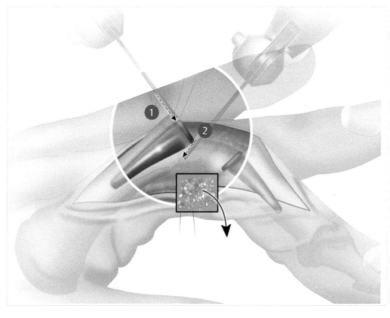

Fig. 13.6 Resecting the volar aspect and dorsal ridge of the proximal condyles in order to fit the bone by the proximal resurfacing component.

13

size as measured with the stem gauge. Proximally the entry point is placed slightly dorsally, whereas it is strictly central in the middle phalanx. For the less experienced surgeon, preinserted pins and fluoroscopic control are mandatory to achieve the correct alignment. Both stems should be inserted so that their articular ends lie flush with the bone surfaces. Using the dedicated palmar cutting guide, the volar edge of the condyles is removed with a saw, taking care to protect the volar plate. Two millimeters of the dorsal cortical ridge over the stem must be removed for the polyethylene component to fit well against the end of the proximal phalanx (▶ Fig. 13.6).

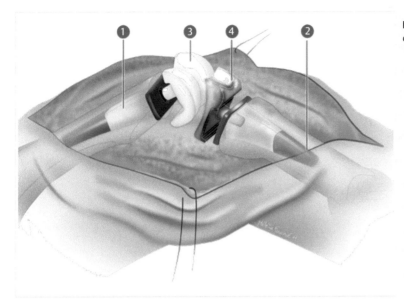

Fig. 13.7 The placement order of the definitive components.

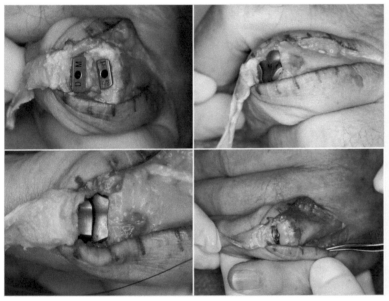

Fig. 13.8 Intraoperative views. Medullary trials in place. Condylar (right) and base of the middle phalanx trials in place (lateral and from above views). Definitive implants in place.

The proximal and distal resurfacing components can then be selected to fit the size of the bone surfaces aiming to be slightly smaller/larger than the bone ends. The thickness of the implants is adjusted so that the joint is stable laterally without excessive tension axially. The tenodesis effect should ideally be restored (passive PIP extension in full wrist flexion and PIP flexion in full wrist extension). When the four trials are in place the finger is assessed fluoroscopically. The trials are removed and replaced by the final implants in the following order: proximal stem, distal stem, proximal polyethylene surface, distal chrome-cobalt surface (▶ Fig. 13.7). The joint is carefully washed out and all bone debris removed. The central slip is sutured with interrupted slow-absorbable stitches (4–0 suture) with or without bone reattachment at the base of the middle phalanx. A clinical case (middle finger) is shown intraoperatively (▶ Fig. 13.8) and the postoperative 1-year course is shown in ▶ Fig. 13.9.

A palmar plaster slab is applied holding the metacarpophalangeal (MCP) joint in flexion and the PIP joint in extension for 2 to 3 days. Self-mobilization is started after the first dressing is changed. The finger is protected by a removable thermoformed splint for 3 to 4 weeks postoperatively.

13.3.2 Indications/Contraindications

The main indication is primary or secondary degenerative osteoarthritis with functional impairment or a painful PIP joint and inflammatory arthritis (although that is much

13

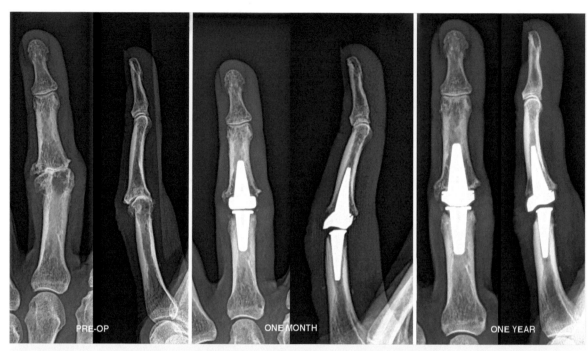

Fig. 13.9 A clinical case: preoperative, 1 month, and 1 year postoperative radiographs of the middle finger. Ulnar deviation is corrected and maintained. Note the ossification on the side of the implant. Active range of motion at 1 year 85–0-0 degree.

less commonly treated because of the disease-modifying drugs) not resolved adequately by conservative treatments. The index finger and frontal deviation up to 15 degrees are not definitive contraindications, provided the collateral ligaments are intact. Caution is mandatory in case of marked ligamentous laxity and in the presence of large subchondral cysts, which might require an additional bone graft.

13.4 Results in the Literature

▶ Table 13.1 shows the number of implanted Tactys prostheses in European countries from 2014 to 2018. Over 2000 were implanted in 2017 with a slight decrease in 2018. The differences between the countries are striking: an overwhelming number were implanted in France. The numbers implanted in Germany, the United Kingdom, Denmark, Spain, and Belgium are only two-thirds of the numbers in France.

Only three scientific papers have been published on the Tactys prosthesis from 2016 to 2019; two of them from the same group including the senior author involved in the development of the implant.[11,12,13] The three papers report on a total of 90 implants in 81 patients (with some of them possibly counted twice, as they are from the same group during a similar period). The follow-up periods were means of 34, 21, and 30 months, respectively.

The two first papers report similar results with significant reductions in pain measured on the visual analog

Table 13.1 Number of Tactys prostheses implanted in European countries during the last 5 years

	2014	2015	2016	2017	2018
Austria	12	–	–	–	–
Belgium	98	115	100	101	108
Denmark	33	112	105	141	116
Finland	8	56	71	90	31
France	590	750	940	1111	1110
Germany	171	241	156	164	164
Norway		4	33	40	39
Portugal	16	8	4	4	4
Spain	16	94	136	116	123
Sweden	13	22	23	28	4
Switzerland	60	34	30	19	51
United Kingdom	129	158	103	143	76
Total	**1150**	**1594**	**1641**	**1957**	**1826**

Source: Data from Stryker Europe Ltd.

scale (VAS), improved ranges of motion of 35 and 45% increase from the preoperative measurements, and improved functional scores. In the first paper, 4 of 22 cases (22 patients) had secondary procedures in the first series (22 cases), but no implants were revised.[11] In the second paper, 4 (of 33) implants (27 patients) were also reoperated for similar reasons: stiffness, a swan-neck deformity, and periarticular ossifications (seen in 13 cases).[12] No loosening or implant migration was reported. The third publication focused on the index finger in cases with ulnar deviation as this is usually considered as a contraindication for PIP prostheses. The PIP range of motion was improved by a mean of 5 degrees (range 57–62 degrees). The ulnar deviation improved from a mean of 7 degrees (range 5–30 degrees) preoperatively to a mean of 1.4 degree (range 0–20 degrees) at a mean follow-up of 2.6 years (range 1–6.3 months). Otherwise, patient satisfaction, overall results, and complications were similar to the previous two publications. The authors concluded that ulnar deviation of the index finger PIP joint of more than 5 degrees is no longer an absolute contraindication to an arthroplasty when using the Tactys.

13.5 Author's Own Experience

In my experience the Tactys is a very useful and flexible implant because of its modularity. That does not mean it is the only implant I use; there is still a role for silastic implants. Particular problems are postoperative swan-neck deformities and reducing ranges of motion with time.

13.6 Tips and Tricks

This is *not* an easy procedure. There is no place for improvisation and no way to make it twice—these are tiny and sometimes fragile bones. Careful preparation following every step of the technique is essential to ensure a good outcome.

Protecting the collateral ligaments can be difficult. In doubt, the radial collateral ligament is the more important ligament to preserve. The Tactys provides some intrinsic stability. If both collateral ligaments cannot be maintained for any reason, it is important to ensure that the volar plate is functioning and it is necessary to splint the joint laterally, resisting ulnar deviation for 4 to 6 weeks postoperatively between rehabilitation sessions.

Tensioning the joint is paramount, particularly avoiding "overstuffing" the joint and making it too tight. As a consequence, special attention should be paid first to the bone resection and second to the thickness of the distal surface replacement (see ▶ Fig. 13.3, ▶ Fig. 13.4, and ▶ Fig. 13.5), in order to achieve smooth-and-full motion with all implant spacers in place.

It is important to ensure correct implant alignment along the long axis of the finger by careful bone preparation and use of perioperative radiographs.

I recommend careful washout of the joint to reduce the risk of postoperative ossification around the joint.

Although reattachment of the central slip is not considered necessary, it might contribute to the swan-neck deformity, so if easily doable I recommend reattachment of the central slip to the base of the middle phalanx with a slow resorbable suture.

Acknowledgments

Thanks to Ph. Bellemère, X. Martinache, and P. Siret for sharing their experience.

References

[1] Branam BR, Tuttle HG, Stern PJ, Levin L. Resurfacing arthroplasty versus silicone arthroplasty for proximal interphalangeal joint osteoarthritis. J Hand Surg Am. 2007; 32(6):775–788

[2] Moutet F, Guinard D, Gerard P, De Soras X, Ranc R, Moreau C. A new titanium-carbon finger joint implant: apropos of 15 initial cases. Ann Chir Main Memb Super. 1994; 13(5):345–353

[3] Nunley RM, Boyer MI, Goldfarb CA. Pyrolytic carbon arthroplasty for posttraumatic arthritis of the proximal interphalangeal joint. J Hand Surg Am. 2006; 31(9):1468–1474

[4] Jennings CD, Livingstone DP. Surface replacement arthroplasty of the proximal interphalangeal joint using the PIP–SRA implant: results, complications, and revisions. J Hand Surg. 2008; 33A:1565e1–1565e11

[5] Schindele SF, Hensler S, Audigé L, Marks M, Herren DB. A modular surface gliding implant (CapFlex-PIP) for proximal interphalangeal joint osteoarthritis: a prospective case series. J Hand Surg Am. 2015; 40(2):334–340

[6] Herren DB, Schindele S, Goldhahn J, Simmen BR. Problematic bone fixation with pyrocarbon implants in proximal interphalangeal joint replacement: short-term results. J Hand Surg [Br]. 2006; 31(6):643–651

[7] Luther C, Germann G, Sauerbier M. Proximal interphalangeal joint replacement with surface replacement arthroplasty (SR-PIP): functional results and complications. Hand (N Y). 2010; 5(3):233–240

[8] Dumont C, Albus G, Kubein-Meesenburg D, Fanghänel J, Stürmer KM, Nägerl H. Morphology of the interphalangeal joint surface and its functional relevance. J Hand Surg Am. 2008; 33(1):9–18

[9] Ash HE, Unsworth A. Proximal interphalangeal joint dimensions for the design of a surface replacement prosthesis. Proc Inst Mech Eng H. 1996; 210(2):95–108

[10] Lawrence T, Trail IA, Noble J. Morphological measurements of the proximal interphalangeal joint. J Hand Surg [Br]. 2004; 29(3):244–249

[11] Athlani L, Gaisne E, Bellemère P. Arthroplasty of the proximal interphalangeal joint with the TACTYS® prosthesis: preliminary results after a minimum follow-up of 2 years. Hand Surg Rehabil. 2016; 35 (3):168–178

[12] Degeorge B, Athlani L, Dap F, Dautel G. Proximal interphalangeal joint arthroplasty with Tactys®: clinical and radiographic results with a minimum follow-up of 12 months. Hand Surg Rehabil. 2018; 37 (4):218–224

[13] Griffart A, Agneray H, Loubersac T, Gaisne E, Bellemère P. Arthroplasty of the proximal interphalangeal joint with the Tactys® modular prosthesis: results in case of index finger and clinodactyly. Hand Surg Rehabil. 2019; 38(3):179–185

13

14 Third-Generation PIP Arthroplasty: CapFlex-PIP

Martin Richter

Abstract

The CapFlex-PIP surface replacement is an unconstrained modular system with different sizes made of cobalt-chrome coated with titanium and one polyethylene gliding surface. Advantages of this new implant are minimal primary bone resection and high lateral stability of the prosthesis. The preferred implantation technique is from dorsal. The technique and aftercare are explained in detail. The results are promising. In the author's own series (n = 23), there was a mean ROM of 71 degrees for the PIP joint after 1 year and no signs of loosening.

Keywords: proximal interphalangeal joint, replacement, arthroplasty, cementless, surface gliding implant, prosthesis, CapFlex implant

14.1 Introduction

The surgical treatment of symptomatic proximal interphalangeal (PIP) osteoarthritis has been a challenge for hand surgeons for many years. The history of total joint replacement of the PIP joint began in 1966 with the introduction of the silicone spacer. Prosthetic fractures, collateral ligament instability, and silicone synovitis have caused recurring problems with these prostheses. The next generation of prostheses was introduced by Linscheid and Dobyns in 1979.[1] The unconstrained anatomically shaped PIP prosthesis with stems for the medullary cavity was first made of cobalt-chromium type, next titanium, and finally pyrocarbon. The shape remains largely unchanged. Loosening, migration, and dislocation were the main complications.

As part of the third generation, the CapFlex-PIP prosthesis (KLS Martin Group, Tuttlingen, Germany) is also a surface prosthesis; however, the stems reaching into the shaft are minimal and bone resection is less.

14.2 Characteristic of Implant

The CapFlex prosthesis consists of two unconstrained components shaped to match the ends of the contiguous proximal and middle phalanges (▶ Fig. 14.1). The proximal component is made of a cobalt-chromium alloy with polished distal articular surface replicating "normal" condylar anatomy. The proximal part of the component head is roughened and coated with titanium to encourage osteointegration.[2] Schindele et al confirmed osteointegration in a CapFlex prosthesis removed in 2016 due to soft tissue complications.[3] For stabilization prior to osteointegration, the proximal component has two small ministems that secure the metal cap on the head of the proximal phalanx.

The distal component is made of three different materials: the proximal gliding surface is made of ultra-high-molecular-weight polyethylene (UHMWPE) sitting on a cobalt-chrome body coated distally with roughened titanium.

The CapFlex prosthesis is a modular system with three different sizes for each component: small, medium, and large. They can be linked in seven different combinations: each size with its equivalent, e. g., small with small of one size different, i. e., small with medium or medium with small or large. The commonest combination is a medium (M) proximal component and a medium (M) or large (L) distal (middle phalanx) component. The distal components are available in three different thicknesses: 2.1 mm, 3.0 mm, and 4.4 mm. The different thicknesses help balance the joint soft tissues at the end of the procedure.

Due to the limited bone resection, the collateral ligaments can "always" be preserved, which helps maintain joint stability.

The prosthesis can be inserted via a dorsal or a volar approach. The instruments are designed for both approaches.

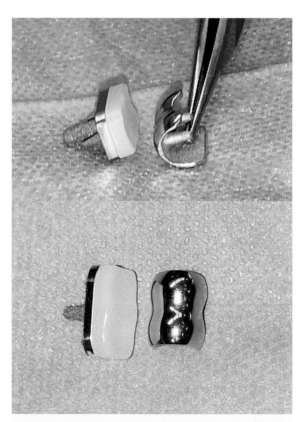

Fig. 14.1 The CapFlex prosthesis consists of two anatomically shaped unconstrained components.

14.3 Indication and Contraindication

The main indication for the CapFlex prosthesis is degenerative osteoarthritis.[3] Good bone quality is a prerequisite for the use of the prosthesis, as the small components need bony support. The modern antirheumatic medication, which often leads to osteoarthritis-like progressions in rheumatoid arthritis (RA) patients, may increase the indications in patients with RA. I have treated a patient with RA with a CapFlex prosthesis in their index finger PIP joint which already had a Swanson MCP joint arthroplasty.

There is likely to be role in treating posttraumatic arthritis but it is less common and the results are likely to be worse.

Intact functioning collateral ligaments are essential as the implants have only limited joint stability on their own. If there is some instability, then one or both collateral ligaments can be shortened or re-sited. This is often necessary in cases with primary deviations of the joint. In the group of our patients the results regarding the straight finger axis were encouraging, since due to the good bone support there is probably little tension on the shortened collateral ligaments.

As with PIP prostheses in general, it should be noted that the actual indication is the relevant pain, as a normal range of motion is not to be expected. Whether an expected improvement of 10 to 40 degrees for the patient justifies the operation should be examined in each individual case. I used a CapFlex prosthesis with a musician who had an almost stiff, nonpainful PIP joint of the index finger due to degenerative osteoarthritis. After surgery the patient was able to play again her clarinet due to the improvement of motion, so that she was satisfied with the treatment. However, these are individual decisions!

14.4 Results in the Literature

Since the CapFlex prosthesis is still quite new on the market and no aggressive but cautious introduction was made, only a few studies and results are available. The greatest experience for the CapFlex prosthesis is certainly in the Schulthess Klinik in Zurich (Switzerland), where the prosthesis was codeveloped. A publication from 2017 refers to 50 cases with a follow-up of 1 year. The motion of the PIP joint improved during this period from 43.4 to 55.9 degrees on average. The pain measured with the VAS (0–10) decreased from 6.5 to 2.2 points. There was one revision surgery due to radial collateral ligament instability and four secondary tenolyses.[4]

In 100 patients with 104 fingers, 1 year after surgery they found decreasing pain at rest from 4.3 to 1.3 on the VAS and during activities from 6.5 before to 2.3 points on the VAS after surgery. A minimal important change (MIC) of 1.2 for pain at rest and 2.8 for pain during activities was estimated for patients being satisfied with the procedure.[5] The brief MHQ increases after 1 year from 45 to 71 points.[5]

Comparing the approach using the CapFlex prosthesis 2 years after surgery in 100 patients, they found the best results for the dorsal tendon split approach with increase of active PIP-ROM from 40 to 61 degrees which corresponds to an improvement of 21 degrees compared with the preoperative value.[6]

14.5 Author's Own Experience and Preferred Technique

In our department, the CapFlex prosthesis has been implanted since the end of the year 2015. By July 2019, we had implanted 43 prostheses in 38 patients.

14.5.1 Author's Preferred Technique

All our patients were operated from a dorsal approach. In my opinion, this gives the best view and allows for accurate implant alignment which is very important to optimize function and avoid instability such as a swan-neck deformity. I use a dorsal, slightly curved off, longitudinal incision centered over the PIP joint. The joint is opened via a longitudinal tendon-splitting incision raising the central slip tendon off the base of the middle phalanx in two halves (▶ Fig. 14.2). The incision begins distally in the tendon-free triangle beyond the central slip insertion and runs proximally to the middle of the proximal phalanx. After exposing the joint by reflecting the divided halves of the tendon laterally I remove osteophytes to better define the joint margin which needs to be exposed fully especially volarly. Around 3 to 4 mm of the head of the proximal phalanx must be resected so the distal part of the origin of the collateral ligaments must be released carefully with a scalpel. A small elevator is now used to create a blunt canal volar to the proximal phalanx, effectively deep to the volar plate, to insert the saw gauge for head resection. The extent of bony resection can be set in mm, typically 3 to 4 mm. The saw cut should be performed perpendicular to the long axis of the proximal phalanx (▶ Fig. 14.3) if anything aiming slightly volar to help optimize PIP joint flexion; a dorsally angulated cut may increase the risk of a swan-neck deformity.

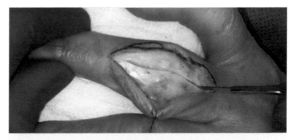

Fig. 14.2 Dorsal approach with central split of the extensor tendon.

14

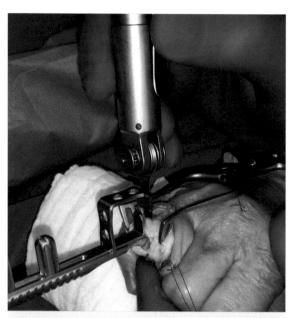

Fig. 14.3 Resection of 3 to 4 mm of the head of the proximal phalanx using the adjustable saw guide.

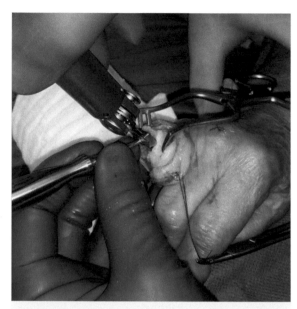

Fig. 14.4 Saw guide for the 45-degree saw cuts of the head of the prominal phalanx.

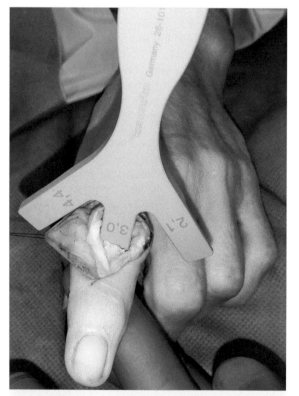

Fig. 14.5 Measuring the height of the distal component.

The size of the proximal component is then determined. In order not to irritate the collateral ligaments, a "as small as possible" component is preferred. An appropriate instrument allows for sizing and creation of small

holes for the implant ministems. After that a 45-degree volar and dorsal angulated saw cut are made with the help of another saw guide to accommodate the shape of the proximal implant (▶ Fig. 14.4). Because there is limited bone these cuts need to be performed with great care, not least to avoid introducing a rotational deformity. The corresponding trial prosthesis can then be inserted. Like the subsequent prosthesis, it is hammered in place and confirmed with perioperative radiographs. If the first is not optimal, it should be corrected. In my experience, a well-aligned proximal implant is extremely important for the later result.

The preparation for the insertion of the distal component begins with the planar resection of the joint surface of the base of the middle phalanx. I typically use a ronguer for this step. Next I measure the depth of the distal component (▶ Fig. 14.5). The depth should not be too great leading to tightness, as this increases the risk of swan-neck deformity although it is tempting to put in a thick implant to maximize the stability. The instrument used to determine the height should be placed in the resection space without much tension. Now the size of the distal implant is determined, usually one size larger than the proximal implant. The instrument to measure the size of the implant aids preparation of the three holes for the ministems of the distal component. The appropriate trial component is now hammered into the base of the middle phalanx (▶ Fig. 14.6) and is checked radiologically. Once satisfied, the definitive prostheses are hammered into place for a press-fit (▶ Fig. 14.7).

If the collateral ligament is loose on one side, as is typical if there is preoperative coronal deviation of the PIP joint, the lax collateral ligament is tightened with a

14

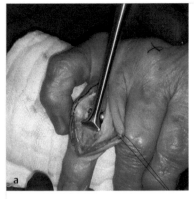

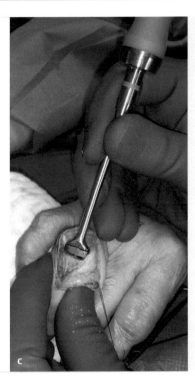

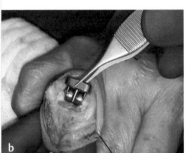

Fig. 14.6 (a–c) Inserting the distal trial component.

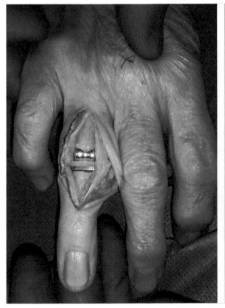

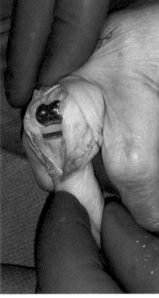

Fig. 14.7 After replacement with the original prosthesis components.

suture. I insert an "X"-shaped 4×0 PDS suture centered on the PIP joint line (▶ Fig. 14.8). This technique allows the ligament to be tensioned without restricting the range of motion. I use a continuous 4×0 PDS crisscross suture to appose the two halves of the extensor mechanism. I usually release the tourniquet and wait for some minutes until most of the bleeding stops, helped by electrocautery aiming to minimize the postoperative swelling. The operated finger is immobilized with a neighboring finger on an "intrinsic plus splint."

14.5.2 After-Care

During the postoperative dressing changes, the patient may already perform careful limited movements. If the soft tissue situation permits, the Intrinsic plus splint is replaced between 7 and 14 days after surgery with a thermoplastic splint that immobilizes only the affected finger in a straight position. In the second postoperative week, the patient may then remove the finger from the splint during the day for exercises. After 2 weeks, the

14

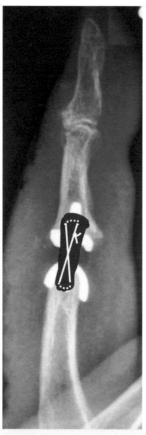

Fig. 14.8 Suture technique for shortening/tensioning the collateral ligament (in purple).

finger splint may be removed during the day and a compression tube bandage is applied during the day to stabilize the finger and to have an antiedematous effect. At night, the thermoplastic finger splint is worn as a positioning splint. After 4 weeks, provided the radiographs are satisfactory, the patient is allowed to mobilize freely but without loading and without splintage. Full use is permitted after 3 months, provided radiographs are satisfactory.

14.5.3 Author's Own Results

Regarding our patients treated with this technique, we excluded from the follow-up two patients with posttraumatic cases. In July 2019, we were able to review 25 patients treated for primary degenerative osteoarthritis with a minimum follow-up of at least 1 year. We excluded two patients: one after failed treatment of a fracture of the base of the middle phalanx; and one with a failed resection arthroplasty who did not want to get an arthrodesis.

The ranges of motion improved from a mean of 52 degrees (0–14–66 degree) to a mean of 71 degrees (0–1–72 degree). Pain at rest measured on a VAS (0–10) improved from a mean of 1 and under load a mean of 3. Radiographs after a year showed no signs of loosening or malalignment (▶ Fig. 14.9, ▶ Fig. 14.10, ▶ Fig. 14.11).

The results are comparable to the reports of Herren and Schindele,[4,5,6] who achieved a smaller range of motion but their patients also had less good preoperative motion.

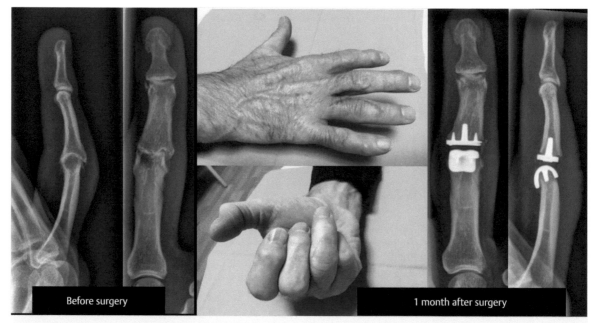

Fig. 14.9 Result, ring finger 1 month after surgery.

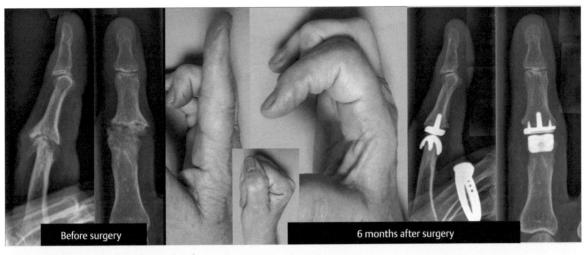

Fig. 14.10 Result, index finger 6 months after surgery.

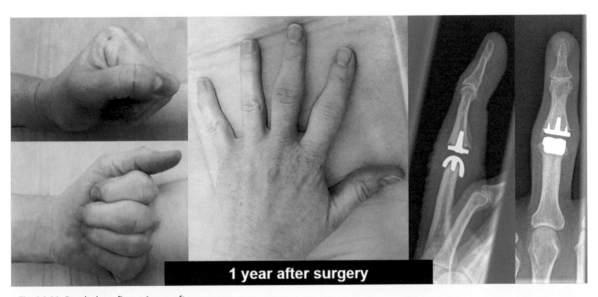

Fig. 14.11 Result, long finger 1 year after surgery.

References

[1] Linscheid RL, Dobyns JH. Total joint arthroplasty: the hand. Mayo Clin Proc. 1979; 54(8):516–526

[2] Daecke W, Veyel K, Wieloch P, Jung M, Lorenz H, Martini AK. Osseointegration and mechanical stability of pyrocarbon and titanium hand implants in a load-bearing in vivo model for small joint arthroplasty. J Hand Surg Am. 2006; 31(1):90–97

[3] Schindele SF, Sprecher CM, Milz S, Hensler S. Osteointegration of a modular metal-polyethylene surface gliding finger implant: a case report. Arch Orthop Trauma Surg. 2016; 136(9):1331–1335

[4] Schindele SF, Altwegg A, Hensler S. Surface replacement of proximal interphalangeal joints using CapFlex-PIP. Oper Orthop Traumatol. 2017; 29(1):86–96

[5] Marks M, Hensler S, Wehrli M, Schindele S, Herren DB. Minimal important change and patient acceptable symptom state for patients after proximal interphalangeal joint arthroplasty. J Hand Surg Eur Vol. 2019; 44(2):175–180

[6] Bodmer E, Marks M, Hensler S, Schindele S, Herren DB. Comparison of outcomes of three surgical approaches for proximal interphalangeal joint arthroplasty using a surface-replacing implant. J Hand Surg Eur Vol. 2019:1753193419891382

14

15 Third-Generation PIP Arthroplasty: The PIP-R

Chris Williams and Timothy Hardwick

Abstract

This chapter describes the unique features of the Mat-Ortho PIP-R implant designed for replacing an arthritic proximal interphalangeal (PIP) joint of a finger. The design and background to it will be described along with the indications for the use of the device. The published results will be presented from both the principal designer's unit along with our own results and complications. Tips and tricks for the use of this implant will also be discussed based on the authors' experience along with a suggested rehabilitation protocol.

Keywords: Arthroplasty, finger joint, proximal interphalangeal, PIP-R

15.1 Design Rationale

The PIP-R (MatOrtho, Leatherhead, United Kingdom) is a two-part cobalt-chromium and polyethylene joint replacement for the proximal interphalangeal (PIP) joints of the fingers. It came about as a result of a photographic study of the morphology of cadaveric PIP joints which had been finely sectioned in two planes. This suggested that the effect of the radial or ulna tilt of the condyles coupled with a different radius of curvature in each digit leads to a degree of axial rotation of the middle phalanx relative to the proximal phalanx as the digit flexed.[1] Other designs of PIP replacement at the time did not allow for this, leading the authors to suggest that this might be the reason for the variability in outcomes following replacement surgery. As a result, the senior author of the paper was involved in the design of the PIP-R.

15.2 Design Features

The implant initially came as three parts: a proximal stem, a distal stem, and the polyethylene insert, which had to be assembled onto the middle phalanx component at the time of insertion. This changed to a preassembled middle phalanx component soon after due to difficulties in carrying out this maneuver in the operating theater under sterile conditions. The implant comes in a box containing both components packed separately. There are five sizes, from a size 7 component on both sides to a size 11 on both sides based on the radio-ulna width of the articular surface. There are "intermediate" combinations allowing for differing sizes on both sides of the joint, with the larger part proximally (7/8, 8/9, 9/10, and 10/11) giving nine possible combinations.

The proximal component has a bicondylar bearing surface with a greater degree of surface anteriorly copying the natural joint to potentially allow over 90 degrees of flexion. It is also flared anteriorly as is the native proximal phalangeal head. The stem is anatomically shaped to fit the medullary canal of the proximal phalanx based on the data from the aforementioned study. The stem is coated in calcium hydroxyapatite to allow for bone ongrowth for long-term stability, and early stability is provided by the press fit into the prepared medullary canal and the cut end of the proximal phalanx (▶ Fig. 15.1).

The distal component has a smaller thinner stem than the other contemporary implants, again based on the morphological study. It is also coated in hydroxyapatite. This component is designed to sit on the subchondral cancellous bone within the cortical rim of the middle

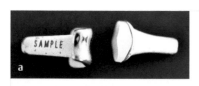
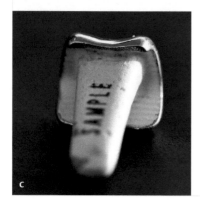
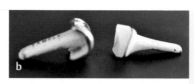
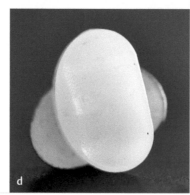

Fig. 15.1 Views of the PIP-R. The proximal component is on the left. **(a)** The dorsal view with the bicondylar articular surface visible. **(b)** The lateral view with the shape of the stems shown. **(c)** Proximal view of the proximal component with the anterior flare of the articular surface evident. **(d)** Proximal view of the distal component with the rotating polyethylene part turned approximately 75 degrees anticlockwise.

15

phalanx in order to avoid impinging on the collateral ligaments which can be better preserved during surgery. An added benefit of this is that any defect in the middle phalangeal base can be bone grafted, if contained by the cortical margin (▶ Fig. 15.1).

The polyethylene articular surface is contoured to the proximal component providing a large contact area to reduce the contact loads. It also rotates on the middle phalangeal component allowing for the rotation that is seen to occur in the PIP joint during flexion of the digit. It can rotate through 360 degrees but this is not of clinical relevance. This rotation also compensates for any unintentional malrotation of either component at the time of implantation, which may be caused by a previous fracture, etc. (▶ Fig. 15.1).

The implant entered clinical use in 2006, with the first joints being implanted at Wrightington Hospital, United Kingdom by the principal designer. The PIP-R can be inserted by a dorsal, lateral, or volar approach, with the instrumentation working well to prepare the bones via all three approaches. The only exception is that the device used to check the flexion and extension gaps which has a handle dorsally gets in the way of the extensor tendon falling into place in the lateral approach and cannot be used with the volar approach at all.

15.3 Indications

The implant is designed for the replacement of the PIP joint of the fingers in cases of osteoarthritis. It can also be used for posttraumatic arthritis where the alignment is maintained. The soft tissue envelope (collateral ligaments, central slip, and volar plate) need to be in good condition. Preoperative radial or ulna deviation deformities can be accommodated if the bone loss is not too great. If any defect is contained in the base of the middle

phalanx, bone grafting can be carried out but not on the proximal phalangeal side as the cutting of the phalangeal head removes the cortical shell. This is not usually a problem because although initially the implant has bone under the articular surface a degree of stress shielding occurs (▶ Fig. 15.2). For cases of inflammatory arthritis, the same limitations apply.

15.4 Contraindications

The implant is unlinked so will sublux or dislocate if the soft tissues are not competent. If the radial collateral ligament is ruptured or attenuated we would not carry out the procedure. Ulna deviation is not necessarily a contraindication if it is due to bone loss but if the deformity is severe the radial collateral ligament is often attenuated and may rupture following surgery (▶ Fig. 15.3). If the tendons are nonfunctional then the implant should not be used. Preoperative stiffness can limit the postoperative recovery but not in all cases.

15.5 Published Results

In 2015 a paper was published looking at the wear characteristics of this implant. They found that there was minimal wear of the articulating surfaces between the proximal component and the polyethylene component and between this and the metal part of the distal component (backside wear).[2]

The only published clinical results of this implant in the English literature are from the principal designer's institution in 2015 describing 100 joints in 50 patients followed up for 2 to 6.5 years. Implant survival was 85% from 4 years onwards. There were 13 revisions in the first year for stiffness, instability, and component disassembly. A further seven cases had to have removal of bone

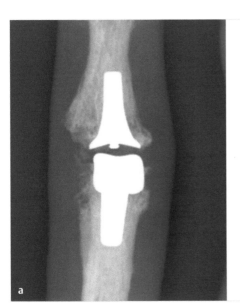
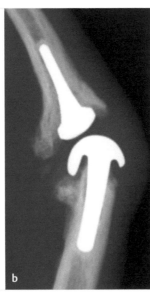

Fig. 15.2 Radiographs of an implant **(a)** soon after the procedure and **(b)** showing stress shielding at 6 months. There is resorption of bone from under the articular surface of both implants with trabecular growth of bone onto the stems. (The stud holding the polyethylene component on is seen in **[a]**).

15

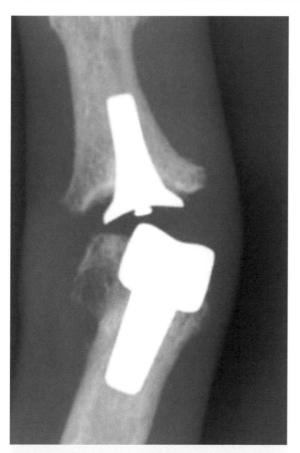

Fig. 15.3 Radiograph with subluxation of the implant due to rupture of the radial collateral ligament.

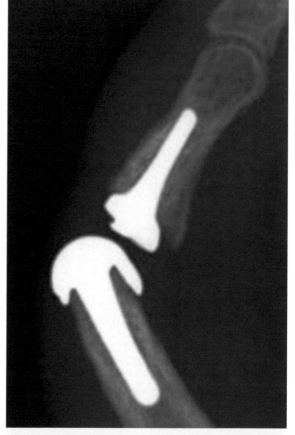

Fig. 15.4 Radiograph of a patient with a rupture of the central slip.

overgrowth or a manipulation carried out. They describe good or excellent results in two-thirds of the patients, noting that stiff or deformed joints did not do as well.[3]

A second paper, in preparation from the same unit, reports the outcomes at a minimum of 2 years for prostheses implanted via the lateral approach describing 33 implants in 19 patients. They reported six revisions to other implants or to fusion and one tenolysis. The results suggested a better arc of motion via the lateral approach when compared to the previous study.[4]

15.6 Author's Results

We reported our early results from 2009 to 2011 at the British Society for Surgery of the Hand meeting in November 2011. This included 9 patients with 11 joints with a mean range of motion of 10 to 50 degrees operated upon through a dorsal approach. Two patients achieved an arc of motion of full extension to 80 degrees of flexion. One patient required arthrolysis for persistent stiffness and another required surgery for a central slip detachment (▶ Fig. 15.4).

Our recent review (in preparation) of 65 joints in 50 patients, with follow-up between 1.5 and 10 years, has a mean arc of motion of 54 degrees (range 10–90 degrees) with ten patients achieving a full range of movement. We have had to carry out 15 secondary soft tissue procedures: seven for central slip failure and dislocation and eight soft tissue releases for persistent stiffness/deformity. A further six patients have been revised to fusions for stiffness or loosening and collapse (▶ Fig. 15.5). Overall 40 of the arthroplasties performed (62%) have required no further treatment.

15.7 How We Do the Procedure and Tips

We usually use an ulna-sided approach for all digits preserving the radial collateral ligament but have used the dorsal approach previously. Once the joint is dislocated and the osteophytes removed, we tend to prepare the middle phalanx first. This is because the medullary canal is often smaller than that in the proximal phalanx and if the disparity is large then there may be a two-size mismatch between the implants required which will not be tolerated. When reaming the middle phalanx with the starter awl, it is very important to take great care to

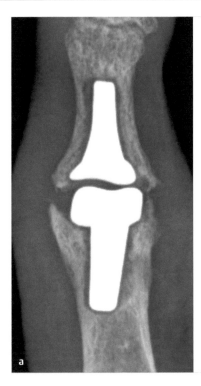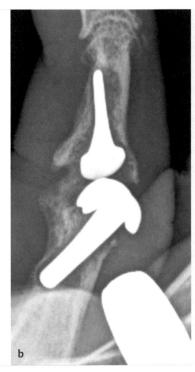

Fig. 15.5 Radiographs of a loose implant. **(a)** PA view with lucent lines around the components and subsidence. **(b)** Lateral view.

ensure that as the subchondral bone is breached the reamer does not sink into the softer cancellous bone. We tend to leave the ossified central slip insertion alone. The bone on the head of the proximal phalanx is often quite hard so a small bone rongeur is used to excise the intercondylar area for ease of access and to allow correct alignment within the medullary canal to be achieved. This also prevents an intercondylar split occurring when the reamers are inserted. We prefer the joint tension to be slightly loose after the implants are inserted.

15.8 Rehabilitation

Postoperatively the patient is left in a splint in extension from theater and sees the therapist within 2 to 3 days when gentle active and passive arc of motion exercises start from full extension up to 30 degrees of flexion. If the central slip attachment remains in a good condition this is progressed at 10 days up to 45 degrees and further

as comfort allows at 3 weeks. This is slowed if the central slip is in poor condition. A resting day-and-night splint is provided to reduce the risk of a flexion contracture developing and this is left off during the day from 6 weeks but continued at night for 3 to 6 months.

References

[1] Lawrence T, Trail IA, Noble J. Morphological measurements of the proximal interphalangeal joint. J Hand Surg [Br]. 2004; 29(3):244–249

[2] Naylor A, Talwalker SC, Trail IA, Joyce TJ. In vivo wear testing of a CoCR-UHMWPE finger prosthesis with Hydroxyapatite coated CoCr stems. Lubricants.. 2015; 3(2):244–255

[3] Flannery O, Harley O, Badge R, Birch A, Nuttall D, Trail IA. MatOrtho proximal interphalangeal joint arthroplasty: minimum 2-year follow-up. J Hand Surg Eur Vol. 2016; 41(9):910–916

[4] Trail IA. MatOrtho proximal interphalangeal joint arthroplasty via lateral approach: minimum 2 year follow up. Personal communication. 2019

16 Surgical Approaches for PIP Joint Arthroplasty

Massimo Ceruso, Sandra Pfanner, and Giovanni Munz

Abstract

There are three possibilities to approach the proximal interphalangeal joint when planning a PIP arthroplasty: dorsal, volar, and lateral. The chosen incision must respect the complex anatomy of tendons, ligaments, nerves, and vessels surrounding the joint and preserve skin flaps vascularity; it must also allow an early mobilization of the operated joint without the wound itself coming into tension in the postoperative rehabilitation. Whatever access the surgeon prefers, it is advisable to be familiar with the different options available in order to better address specific PIP joint deformities and the possible coexisting problems caused by periarticular soft tissue damage.

Keywords: PIP arthroplasty, PIP surgical approach, PIP joint lesion, finger joint reconstruction, finger joint implants

16.1 Introduction

The surgical approach to the proximal interphalangeal (PIP) joint matters. The key issue is the complex anatomy of the soft tissues surrounding the joint: the extensor and flexor tendons which are closely related to the articular heads and the ligamentous structures stabilizing the PIP joint. In particular, the extensor apparatus is most critical; it is fragile and very liable to adhesions. The chosen incision must respect the vascularization of the skin flaps; it must also allow an early mobilization of the operated joint without the wound itself coming into tension in the postoperative rehabilitation. There are three possibilities: dorsal, volar (palmar), and lateral.

16.2 Dorsal Approach

This is the most used approach to the PIP joint. It provides safe access and wide exposure to the joint which makes

planning easier for the bone cut at implant arthroplasty. Moreover, the alignment and cutting guides for most prostheses are designed for use through a dorsal exposure.[1]

16.2.1 Dorsal Skin Incision

The skin incision is most commonly performed following a curved line that does not centrally cross the dorsal aspect of the PIP joint (▶ Fig. 16.1a). This incision is preferred to a central longitudinal rectilinear one in order to reduce the traction on the surgical wound at an early postoperative mobilization. Avoiding skin sutures directly over the extensor apparatus could prevent adhesions with the tendon on the dorsal median line. The skin flap should be sharply elevated, keeping intact the connection between the cutaneous and the subcutaneous fat layer in order to preserve the vascularity of the latter.

16.2.2 Dorsal Tenotomy to the PIP Joint

Once the flap is raised, there are different ways of handling the extensor apparatus. The key question is whether to respect, or not, the insertion of the central band.[2] It may be preserved carrying out an incision either between the transverse retinacular ligament and the volar margin of one of the lateral bands or, alternatively, the incision can be made on the midline, splitting the lateral bands up to the central band.[2] A third option is the Chamay tenotomy; it is carried out by raising a distally based triangular flap extending into the proximal extensor tendon with its apex at the level of the proximal third of the proximal phalanx (▶ Fig. 16.1b).[3] This approach gives a good exposure of the articular surfaces by rotating the tendon flap distally and dislocating the lateral bands volarly when flexing the joint (▶ Fig. 16.1c). The major drawback comes from the intratendinous suture that is needed to relocate the flap; this can be fragile in the early mobilization, with elongation of the tendon scar reducing the function of

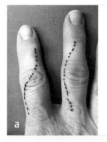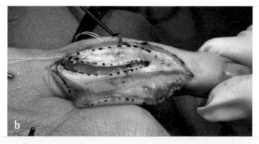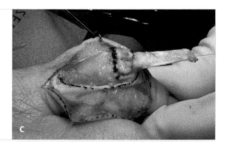

Fig. 16.1 **(a)** Curvilinear incisions for dorsally based approaches. **(b)** Dorsal approach: Chamay tenotomy. **(c)** Dorsal approach: Distal rotation of the Chamay flap and dislocation of the proximal interphalangeal (PIP) joint.

the extensor mechanism. Yet if immobilized for long it can lead to major adhesions and stiffness.

Other authors prefer to detach the central band from its insertion on the base of middle phalanx obtaining a wide mobilization of the tendon; the tendon can be then fixed back to the base of middle phalanx using transosseous sutures or left unattached where it seems to function well.[2,4]

16.3 Lateral Approach

The skin incision is performed on the lateral side of the distal half of the proximal phalanx and is then curved dorsally over the middle phalanx (▶ Fig. 16.2a). The skin flap is elevated in order to achieve an adequate exposure of the radial and ulnar aspects of the PIP joint as well as of the extensor apparatus and the flexor sheath (▶ Fig. 16.2b). The neurovascular bundle is protected by the Cleland's ligament.[2] The retinacular ligament is incised and the lateral band of the extensor tendon is mobilized, while the insertion of the central band is preserved (▶ Fig. 16.2c). The collateral ligament is then elevated as a proximally based triangular flap (▶ Fig. 16.2d, e). This is performed through a V-shaped incision whose longitudinal branch corresponds to the dorsal margin of the collateral ligament, while the anterior-oblique incision separates the collateral and accessory collateral ligaments from the phalangoglenoidal ligament fibers that run obliquely from the base of the middle phalanx (P2) to the lateral margin of the volar plate and the corresponding annular pulley (▶ Fig. 16.2f).[5] The dorsal capsule and the

homolateral proximal insertion of the volar plate are then released in order to laterally dislocate the joint with the opposite collateral ligament complex as a pivot point (▶ Fig. 16.2g, h). An ulnar lateral approach is generally preferred, particularly for the index and middle fingers, in order to keep the radial collateral ligament intact so as to maintain stability in pinch with the thumb.[6]

As the arthroplasty is completed, the joint is reduced and the collateral ligament complex is sutured back to the phalangoglenoidal fibers (▶ Fig. 16.2i). The extensor apparatus is repaired suturing the retinacular ligament to the lateral band (▶ Fig. 16.2j). Joint stability and passive ranges of motion (ROM) are tested.

The PIP joint is splinted in slight flexion and immediate gentle active joint mobility is allowed. On the third postoperative day a dorsal custom-made static splint is applied, which limits PIP extension to 5 degrees and prevents lateral deviation away from the side of the surgical approach. Four weeks postoperatively, activities of daily living (ADL) are permitted with buddy-taping to the adjacent finger on the side of the approach.[5]

16.4 Volar Approach

Schneider[7] described a volar approach in which the pulley system and the volar plate were opened separately. In addition, the main collateral ligament origin had to be released completely. To provide immediate functional rehabilitation with the best possible initial stability, Simmen and Herren[8,9,10] described a volar approach that leaves the main collateral ligaments intact, and also

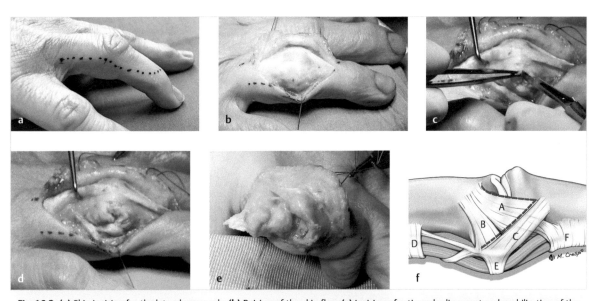

Fig. 16.2 (a) Skin incision for the lateral approach. (b) Raising of the skin flap. (c) Incision of retinacular ligament and mobilization of the lateral band. (d,e) Elevation of the collateral ligament with a proximally based triangular flap. (f) The collateral ligament complex consists of three parts: the collateral ligament (A), the accessory collateral ligament (B), and the phalangoglenoidal ligament (C), which is connected to the annular pulley system (D: A2 pulley; E: A3 pulley; F: A4 pulley).

(Continued)

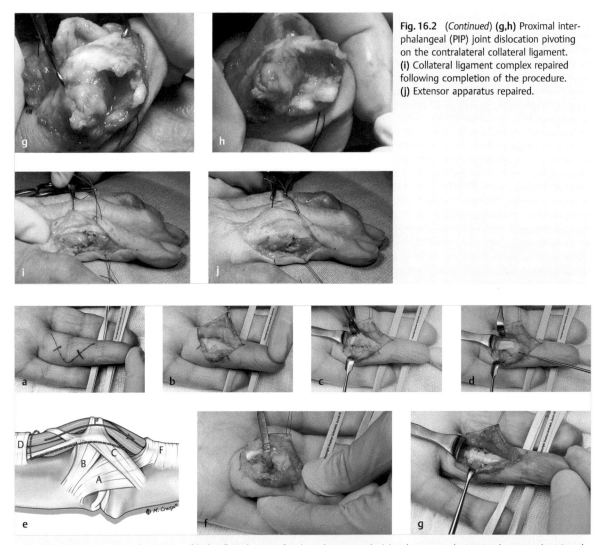

Fig. 16.2 (*Continued*) (**g,h**) Proximal interphalangeal (PIP) joint dislocation pivoting on the contralateral collateral ligament. (**i**) Collateral ligament complex repaired following completion of the procedure. (**j**) Extensor apparatus repaired.

Fig. 16.3 (**a**) Bruner-type volar incision. (**b**) Skin flap elevation for the volar approach. (**c**) Volar approach: Incision between the A2 and C 1 pulleys and the accessory collateral ligament. (**d**) Volar approach: The flexor apparatus and the volar plate are mobilized as a tubular sleeve. (**e**) Volar approach: The volar plate mobilized as a tubular sleeve (A: collateral ligament; B: accessory collateral ligament; C: phalangoglenoidal ligament; D: A2 pulley; E: A3 pulley; F: A4 pulley.). (**f**) Dislocation of the proximal interphalangeal (PIP) joint via a volar approach. (**g**) Volar approach: Repair of pulley system and volar plate. ([**a–d,f,g**] Courtesy Stephan Schindele, Zurich, Switzerland.)

developed a modified approach to the flexor pulley system and the volar plate.

After a Bruner-type volar incision forming a radially based triangular flap, the two neurovascular bundles are identified and protected (▸ Fig. 16.3a, b). The flexor tendon sheath is opened in the interval between the A2 and the C 1 pulleys with incision of the accessory collateral ligaments on either side (▸ Fig. 16.3c). The main collateral ligaments are left intact. The flexor pulley system and the volar plate are then mobilized as a tubular sleeve and retracted to the radial side (▸ Fig. 16.3d, e). The head of the proximal phalanx can be resected, leaving the origins of the main collateral ligaments intact. If necessary, osteophytes at the base of the middle phalanx are also resected.[9] After complete dislocation of the joint, the bone edges can be either remodeled or resected in order to ream the medullary canals and to insert the implant components (▸ Fig. 16.3f). The pulley system with the volar plate is then reattached with a few stitches of resorbable suture material 4-0 or 5-0 (▸ Fig. 16.3g). Functional rehabilitation is started on the first day after the operation, with active flexion and extension exercises three to four times per day. When needed, dynamic splinting is added after 3 to 4 weeks.[9]

16.5 Literature Review and Authors' Preferred Technique

The most popular approach for PIP arthroplasty is dorsal; it is technically the least demanding, except for the preservation of the extensor central slip, as previously described. It is generally preferred as the joint is exposed very clearly, with the least risk for the neurovascular bundles. Moreover, resection guides are commonly designed for this approach.[1,10]

The rationale behind the volar PIP approach is preservation of the main collateral ligaments and the central slip of the extensor tendon, allowing early active and passive mobilization and favoring a complete restoration of extension.[9] The venous drainage is spared theoretically leading to less swelling.[10,11] This approach may also be taken into consideration for rheumatic mild swan neck deformity, when repositioning and strengthening of the volar plate are indicated.[1,6,10,12] However, the volar approach is technically more demanding, it creates some risk to the digital neurovascular bundles and gives less good access for implantation of a prosthesis.[1] Major dorsal osteophytes may be difficult to resect and extensor tendon imbalance cannot be corrected.

The main advantage of the lateral approach is the preservation of both the extensor and flexor apparatuses. It is also not commonly performed by hand surgeons. Adopting this approach, Pritsch and Rizzo reported the lowest reoperation rate for implant arthroplasty,[13] Segalman reported no instability or second surgery with silastic spacers.[14] The interest in the lateral approach is growing. Flannery et al changed from the dorsal to the lateral approach in order to improve postoperative PIP joint ROM.[15] Furthermore, a lateral approach can be taken into consideration to remove osteophytes in a second surgery after volar approach.[16]

The surgical approach is also influenced by the choice of implants, with a clear distinction between silicone spacers and hard-bearing implant arthroplasties. Via a volar approach, silastic implants have been reported to achieve the best ROM, and least extension lag, while for hard-bearing implants the opposite occurs with worse ROM and greater extensor lag.[12] Furthermore the risk of failure of hard-bearing implant arthroplasties is reported to be higher rate using a volar rather than a dorsal approach, while silastic spacers had the lowest failure rate following surgery via a volar approach.[10,12] Another unsolved complication of the volar approach is the post-operative flexion contracture in implants reported by Shirakawa et al,[13,16,17] with development of osteophytes probably caused by intraoperative fracture or fragility of the central slip insertion.[16]

Currently the authors use the lateral approach as their first choice for implant arthroplasty, given the balance it offers between complexity, immediate postoperative stability, and tendon integrity.

Whatever access the surgeon prefers when planning an arthroplasty, it is advisable to be familiar with the different options available in order to better address specific PIP joint deformities and the possible coexisting problems caused by periarticular soft tissue damage.

References

[1] DeDeugd CM, Rizzo M. Surgical exposure of the proximal interphalangeal joint. Hand Clin. 2018; 34(2):127–138

[2] Cheah AE, Yao J. Surgical approaches to the proximal interphalangeal joint. J Hand Surg Am. 2016; 41(2):294–305

[3] Chamay A. A distally based dorsal and triangular tendinous flap for direct access to the proximal interphalangeal joint. Ann Chir Main. 1988; 7(2):179–183

[4] Linscheid RL, Murray PM, Vidal MA, Beckenbaugh RD. Development of a surface replacement arthroplasty for proximal interphalangeal joints. J Hand Surg Am. 1997; 22(2):286–298

[5] Ceruso M, Pfanner S, Carulli C. Proximal interphalangeal (PIP) joint replacements with pyrolytic carbon implants in the hand. EFORT Open Rev. 2017; 2(1):21–27

[6] Merle M, Villani F, Lallemand B, Vaienti L. Proximal interphalangeal joint arthroplasty with silicone implants (NeuFlex) by a lateral approach: a series of 51 cases. J Hand Surg Eur Vol. 2012; 37(1):50–55

[7] Schneider LH. Proximal interphalangeal joint arthroplasty: the volar approach. Semin Arthroplasty. 1991; 2(2):139–147

[8] Simmen BR. Der palmare Zugang zur Arthroplastik des proximalen Interphalangeal-Finger-Gelenkes. Oper Orthop Traumatol. 1993; 5:112–123

[9] Herren DB, Simmen BR. Palmar approach in flexible implant arthroplasty of the proximal interphalangeal joint. Clin Orthop Relat Res. 2000(371):131–135

[10] Herren DB. Current European practice in the treatment of proximal interphalangeal joint arthritis. Hand Clin. 2017; 33(3):489–500

[11] Yamamoto M, Malay S, Fujihara Y, Zhong L, Chung KC. A systematic review of different implants and approaches for proximal interphalangeal joint arthroplasty. Plast Reconstr Surg. 2017; 139(5):1139e–1151e

[12] Murray PM, Linscheid RL, Cooney WP, III, Baker V, Heckman MG. Long-term outcomes of proximal interphalangeal joint surface replacement arthroplasty. J Bone Joint Surg Am. 2012; 94(12):1120–1128

[13] Pritsch T, Rizzo M. Reoperations following proximal interphalangeal joint nonconstrained arthroplasties. J Hand Surg Am. 2011; 36(9):1460–1466

[14] Segalman KA. Lateral approach to proximal interphalangeal joint implant arthroplasty. J Hand Surg Am. 2007; 32(6):905–908

[15] Flannery O, Harley O, Badge R, Birch A, Nuttall D, Trail IA. MatOrtho proximal interphalangeal joint arthroplasty: minimum 2-year follow-up. J Hand Surg Eur Vol. 2016; 41(9):910–916

[16] Shirakawa K, Shirota M. Post-operative contracture of the proximal interphalangeal joint after surface replacement arthroplasty using a volar approach. J Hand Surg Asian Pac Vol. 2016; 21(3):345–351

[17] Wagner ER, Luo TD, Houdek MT, Kor DJ, Moran SL, Rizzo M. Revision proximal interphalangeal arthroplasty: an outcome analysis of 75 consecutive cases. J Hand Surg Am. 2015; 40(10):1949–1955.e1

17 Joint Replacement of Osteoarthritic and Posttraumatic Distal Interphalangeal Joints

David Elliot, Maria Sirotakova, Adam Sierakowski, and Claire Jane Zweifel

17

Abstract

This paper reviews the management of painful degeneration of the distal interphalangeal (DIP) joint by Swanson prosthetic replacement in a single unit between 2004 and 2019. The earlier experience of 129 DIP joint replacements for painful osteoarthritis and two for ongoing pain after injury during the period from 2004 to 2009 was reported in a peer-reviewed publication in 2012. In the initial study, 37 arthroplasties (28 patients) were carried out with extensor tendon division and repair, and postoperative immobilization for 8 weeks. Ninety-four (60 patients) were then carried out without tendon division, allowing immediate mobilization. At assessment after a mean period of 57 months, the mean postoperative range of movement was 39°, and the mean extensor lag was 11°, with significant improvement of both in both operative groups. The severity of pain improved significantly following surgery. All but one patient were satisfied with the cosmetic result of replacement. The overall complication rate was 7/131 (5%). Three joints developed cellulitis and one developed osteomyelitis, requiring subsequent fusion. Two joints had subsequent fusions because of persistent lateral instability and marked ulnar deviation and one had a persistent mallet-type deformity, corrected by tendon shortening. This review describes minor modifications of the original technique to reduce infection and increase stability of the reconstructed joints and extension of the technique to replacement of the IP joint of the thumb over the subsequent 17 years.

Keywords: joint replacement, distal interphalangeal joint, Swanson prosthesis, osteoarthritis

17.1 Introduction

Degenerative changes of the distal interphalangeal (DIP) joints can be painful, disabling, and disfiguring. If nonoperative treatment fails to relieve the pain, arthrodesis is still considered by most surgeons to be the gold standard of operative treatment. Frequently ignored is the failure of fusion of this joint by conventional means, with reported rates of delayed union and nonunion from 0 to 20%,[1,2] and the need for the expensive extreme of compression screws to avoid this problem.[3,4] Patients are often unenthusiastic about losing movement of the DIP joints, particularly in the index and middle fingers, realizing that many finer functions of the hand rely on the rapid movement of these joints through a small range of motion. Therefore, they may perceive joint fusion as exchange of one disability for another.

17.2 Characteristic of Silicone Implants for DIP Joint

Since first described in 1968 by Swanson, silicone elastomer spacers have been, and are still, widely used for replacement of proximal interphalangeal (PIP) and metacarpophalangeal (MCP) joints destroyed by arthritis.[5] These implants maintain the joint space and allow motion whilst retaining stability. However, until 2011, there was little in the literature about silicone arthroplasty of the DIP joints, with the total recorded experience being only 67 distal interphalangeal replacement arthroplasties.[6,7,8,9,10,11] These papers identified this procedure as a good alternative to arthrodesis, achieving excellent pain relief and allowing stable pinch, but with the benefit of retaining 20 to 30 degrees of DIP joint movement. The complication rate leading to implant removal ranged from 1 to 10%, which is comparable to the reported complications following DIP arthrodesis. The standard technique of DIP joint replacement used in these studies involved transection of the extensor tendon, necessitating 6 to 8 weeks of postoperative joint immobilization and risking loss of some of the movement of the joint.

17.3 Own Results in the Literature

In 2011, we reported the results of a study of Swanson replacement of 131 DIP joints for painful osteoarthritis and two younger patients for ongoing joint pain after injury.[12] A total of 37 arthroplasties (28 patients) were carried out with extensor tendon division and repair, and postoperative immobilization for 8 weeks. The following 94 (60 patients) were then carried out without tendon division, allowing immediate mobilization. This group comprised 60 patients, of which 52 were female and 8 were male. Nineteen patients had two prostheses inserted at a single operation. Five patients had three prostheses at a single operation. Three patients had three prostheses inserted at two operations. One patient had five prostheses inserted at two operations. Forty prostheses were placed in the index finger, 26 in the middle finger, 15 in the ring finger, and 13 in the little finger. At assessment, after a mean period of 57 months, the mean postoperative range of movement was 39 degrees, and the mean extensor lag was 11 degrees, with a statistically significant improvement of both over the preoperative measurements in both operative groups. When compared against each other, there was no statistically significant difference between the postoperative range of movement achieved in the two groups. The severity of pain, as measured subjectively on a visual analog scale (VAS) scale, improved significantly in both groups following surgery. The overall complication rate was 7/131 (5%), with 4/131 (3%) requiring further surgery. Three joints developed cellulitis which settled with antibiotics and one developed osteomyelitis requiring removal of the implant and subsequent joint fusion. Patients were questioned about the stability of the involved joints postoperatively on each occasion on which they attended for surgical follow-up. One DIP joint had subsequent fusion because of persistent lateral instability and one had DIP joint fusion because of persistence of marked preoperative ulnar deviation. One joint had a persistent mallet-type deformity, corrected after 18 months by tendon shortening. Overall patient satisfaction with the appearance of their digit(s) postoperatively was high in both groups and all but one patient were satisfied with the cosmetic result of replacement.

17.4 Own Experience and Preferred Technique for DIP Joint Arthroplasty

Procedures involving a single joint are mostly carried out under digital ring block. Procedures involving multiple joints are carried out under multiple ring blocks, brachial

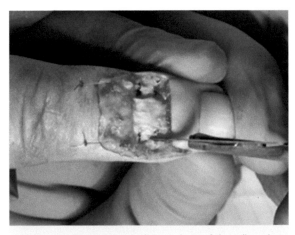

Fig. 17.1 Intraoperative view during release of the collateral ligaments from the middle phalanx, after exposure through an "H" incision.

block, or general anesthesia, according to the patient wishes. Initially, a dorsal "H-shaped" incision, creating proximal and distal flaps, was used to approach the DIP joint. More recently, the distal flap has not been raised routinely. The proximal flap is carefully elevated off the underlying extensor tendon and bone and sutured back to give good access. In those cases in which the prosthesis was inserted without extensor tendon division, the collateral ligaments were then divided from the middle phalanx proximally (▶ Fig. 17.1).

The tissues lateral to the extensor tendon were next excised. By laterally flexing the joint and retracting the extensor tendon from one side to another with a tendon hook, one is then able to remove the head of the middle phalanx with a rongeur, without damage to the extensor tendon. The intramedullary canals of the middle and distal phalanges were prepared using reamers or a burr drill. The joint was then sized for either a size 1, 0, or 00 Wright (Swanson type) silastic implants (Wright Medical Technology, Inc., Arlington, TN, USA). Finally, the distal phalangeal surface of the joint was debrided of osteophytes and the appropriate implant was inserted (▶ Fig. 17.2).

Finally, the skin was closed (▶ Fig. 17.3) and the joint placed in a small volar Zimmer splint.

17.5 Postoperative Care

All patients received a course of prophylactic oral antibiotics postoperatively for 5 days. Patients were encouraged to move the other joints of the involved finger and the remainder of the hand from the day after operation, with specific attention to the proximal interphalangeal joint of the involved finger(s) to avoid extensor tendon tethering and tightening of the dorsal capsule of this joint. Appropriate and liberal analgesia was used to allow this early active mobilization. After 2 to 4 days, patients carried out active flexion and extension exercises of the replaced DIP joint(s) of the involved finger(s) themselves five times per day.

17.6 Technique Modification

When we wrote our paper in 2011, we excised the dorsal soft tissue lateral to the extensor tendon for access to the

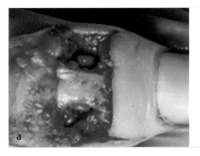
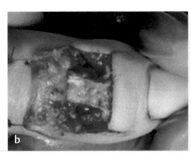

Fig. 17.2 Intraoperative view showing the resulting joint space after removal of all tissue lateral to the extensor tendon and excision of the head of the middle phalanx, **(a)** after insertion of a sizer, then **(b)** insertion of the definitive prosthesis.

17

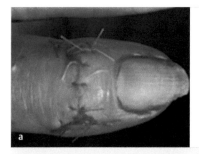 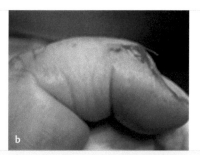 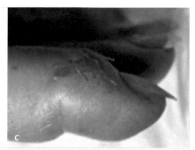

Fig. 17.3 **(a)** Intraoperative dorsal view showing the finger, after skin closure, **(b)** flexing to 40 degrees. **(c)** There remains an extensor lag of 15 degrees, which is accentuated visually to 30 degrees by dorsal bony swelling under the extensor attachment to the distal phalanx, which cannot be removed at surgery.

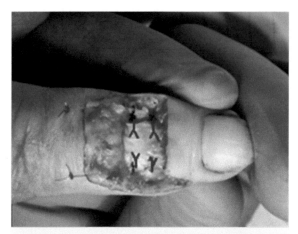

Fig. 17.4 Intraoperative view showing the new technique of retaining the tissue lateral to the extensor tendon as small laterally based flaps which are sutured back in place after insertion of the prosthesis, as a protection against prosthesis involvement in suture infection.

joint. However, soon after, we had two suture infections which went on to deep infection requiring removal of the prosthesis and we realized that, if this lateral tissue was excised, the deep part of the skin suture would be lying on the prosthesis so any infection going down the suture could infect the prosthesis. Now, on each side, the tissue between the edge of the extensor tendon and the collateral ligaments is raised as a laterally based flap based on the collateral ligament. After lifting this little flap on each side, the collateral ligament is released from the middle phalanx. After inserting the prosthesis, the flaps are sutured back in place as a barrier between the skin sutures (▶ Fig. 17.4). In addition, we now close the skin with a subcuticular suture, glue the skin, and leave the DIP joint immobile and covered by dressing for 2 weeks.

In this study, we used the Swanson prostheses manufactured by Wright Medical Technology Ltd. Usually a size 00, occasionally a size 0, rarely a size 1, prosthesis is required. Swanson prostheses made by different suppliers are not always the same size for each marked number. This has little importance when replacing larger digital

joints as each company provides a box of instruments and sizers which correspond to their own prostheses. When replacing the DIP joint, over 90 % of the prostheses used are "Wright" size 00. There may be no equivalent (sufficiently small) prosthesis in those supplied by other manufacturers, making for a dilemma after resecting the head of the middle phalanx which has no immediate solution!

Despite not showing a greater range of motion, and requiring a learning curve, albeit rapid, the extensor tendon-sparing technique has advantages of simpler postoperative management, avoiding immobilization and shortening follow-up. Consequently, we have persisted with the extensor tendon-sparing technique since 2011 and have replaced between 30 and 50 finger DIP joints and 5 and 10 thumb interphalangeal (IP) joints each year, with the number increasing slightly, year on year, to a total of 54 DIP and 15 IP joints in 2018. The complication rate remains small.

That prosthetic replacement should have stability equal to that of the original joint may be surprising, given that the lateral ligaments are divided at insertion of a Swanson prosthesis. However, two factors come into play postreplacement. The intramedullary parts of a Swanson prosthesis provide lateral stability to the replaced joint, albeit by a different process to that of intact lateral joint ligaments. As has been recognized for a long time by observation of the change from instability to stability in the fingers of patients with arthritis mutilans, passive lateral movement of the DIP joint is almost impossible when the profundus flexor tendon is activated to flex the finger. This is true both in a normal DIP joint and one which has been replaced by a Swanson prosthesis.

17.7 Thumb-IP-Joint Arthroplasty with Silicone Implant

The IP joint of the thumb is particularly subjected to radial deviating pressure on pinching. In the last 5 years, three patients have found radial deviation of the replaced IP joint on pinching to be disconcerting. We have fused one IP joint and carried out a secondary reconstruction of the ulnar collateral ligament in two patients using a 2- to 3-mm ulnar strip of the extensor tendon of the thumb, left attached distally and turned laterally and volarly across the joint to be attached to the periosteum of the middle phalanx with nonabsorbing sutures. We have also modified the surgical technique for IP joint replacement: the ulnar collateral ligament is no longer fully separated from the middle phalanx and, after inserting the prosthesis, the proximal end of this ligament is sutured to the periosteum of the middle phalanx with nonabsorbing sutures. This is also done with DIP joints of the fingers which have preoperative lateral deviation of more than 10 to 20 degrees: the contralateral collateral ligament is reattached proximally to improve the alignment of the DIP joint.

17.8 Skin Closure

The newer closure technique (▶ Fig. 17.4) has almost eliminated infection problems.

Although not a major feature of our study, and only assessed in a very rudimentary way, the appearance of these fingers is generally satisfactory to the patients. However, this may relate more to the simultaneous removal of the osteophytes around the DIP joint at surgery than to the actual joint procedure.

17.9 Discussion

Some argue that implant arthroplasty is unnecessary,[13] or should only be considered under exceptional circumstances, such as in musicians.[7,14] However, this may underestimate the functional benefits of a moving DIP joint.[15] These joints, moving through a small range of motion with speed, are integral to many daily activities. The DIP joint of the index finger and the IP joint of the thumb are particularly important for fine pinch activities. The middle finger DIP becomes involved in chuck pinch and the ring and little finger DIP joints are important for the fine control of larger objects when all five digit tips are involved in span gripping and power gripping. A surgeon raising a full-thickness graft from the forearm will use controlled movement of five finger DIP joints and both thumb IP joints to

manipulate the scalpel and forceps involved in this maneuver! We believe that more effort should be made to preserve this distal digital movement. Our 2011 study, and the cases performed routinely since, considerably extends the number of reported patients who have undergone silicone interpositional arthroplasty of the DIP joint and confirm that this procedure is an acceptable alternative to arthrodesis of this joint.

References

[1] Mantovani G, Fukushima WY, Cho AB, Aita MA, Lino W, Jr, Faria FN. Alternative to the distal interphalangeal joint arthrodesis: lateral approach and plate fixation. J Hand Surg Am. 2008; 33(1):31–34

[2] Zavitsanos G, Watkins F, Britton E, Somia N, Gupta A, Kleinert H. Distal interphalangeal joint arthrodesis using intramedullary and interosseous fixation. Hand Surg. 1999; 4(1):51–55

[3] Engel J, Tsur H, Farin I. A comparison between K-wire and compression screw fixation after arthodesis of the distal interphalangeal joint. Plast Reconstr Surg. 1977; 60(4):611–614

[4] Tomaino MM. Distal interphalangeal joint arthrodesis with screw fixation: why and how. Hand Clin. 2006; 22(2):207–210

[5] Swanson AB. Silicone rubber implants for replacement of arthritis or destroyed joints in the hand. Surg Clin North Am. 1968; 48(5):1113–1127

[6] Brown LG. Distal interphalangeal joint flexible implant arthroplasty. J Hand Surg Am. 1989; 14(4):653–656

[7] Schwartz DA, Peimer CA. Distal interphalangeal joint implant arthroplasty in a musician. J Hand Ther. 1998; 11(1):49–52

[8] Snow JW, Boyes JG, Jr, Greider JL, Jr. Implant arthroplasty of the distal interphalangeal joint of the finger for osteoarthritis. Plast Reconstr Surg. 1977; 60(4):558–560

[9] Wilgis EFS. Distal interphalangeal joint silicone interpositional arthroplasty of the hand. Clin Orthop Relat Res. 1997(342):38–41

[10] Zimmerman NB, Suhey PV, Clark GL, Wilgis EFS. Silicone interpositional arthroplasty of the distal interphalangeal joint. J Hand Surg Am. 1989; 14(5):882–887

[11] Zimmerman NB, Zimmerman SI, Wilgis EFS. Distal interphalangeal joint silicone interpositional arthroplasty: surgical technique and functional outcome. Semin Arthroplasty. 1991; 2(2):153–157

[12] Sierakowski A, Zweifel C, Sirotakova M, Sauerland S, Elliot D. Joint replacement in 131 painful osteoarthritic and post-traumatic distal interphalangeal joints. J Hand Surg Eur Vol. 2012; 37(4):304–309

[13] Rehart S, Kerschbaumer F. Endoprothetik an der Hand. Orthopade. 2003; 32(9):779–783

[14] Culver JE, Fleegler EJ. Osteoarthritis of the distal interphalangeal joint. Hand Clin. 1987; 3(3):385–403

[15] Evans RB. A study of the zone 1 flexor tendon injury and implications for treatment. J Hand Ther. 1990; 3:133–148

Section 3

Arthroplasty of the Thumb

18 Silicone Implants and Total Joint Prostheses for Osteoarthritis of the Trapeziometacarpal Joint: A Systematic Review

Nadine Hollevoet and Grey Giddins

Abstract

A systematic review about treatment of osteoarthritis of the trapeziometacarpal joint with silicone implants and total joint replacement was performed. Good subjective outcomes were reported with Swanson prostheses, but their use cannot be recommended because of the risk of dislocation, implant failure, and foreign body reaction. With some of the more recent total joint arthroplasties, good medium-term survival rates were reported and better function in comparison with trapeziectomy and tendon arthroplasty, but prospective randomized studies with strong evidence were not available.

Keywords: Trapeziometacarpal osteoarthritis, trapeziometacarpal joint replacement, thumb carpometacarpal arthroplasty, survivorship

18.1 Introduction

In 1968 Swanson published the first report of a thumb carpometacarpal (CMC) joint arthroplasty using a silicone implant.[1] In 1973 de la Caffinière reported a technique with a total joint arthroplasty.[2] Since then many different designs have been developed.

A systematic review was performed to assess the results of thumb trapeziometacarpal arthroplasty. It followed the Preferred Reporting Items for Systematic Reviews and Meta-Analyses (PRISMA) guideline but was not registered in advance as it built upon a previous review.[3]

18.2 Materials and Methods

The inclusion criteria for the systematic review were: full reports written in English or French of total joint replacement or silicone implants in patients with primary osteoarthritis of the trapeziometacarpal joint; studies reporting pain, strength, radiological changes, or failure rates as outcomes with a mean follow-up of at least 12 months; and studies with a design classification of levels I to VI, as classified by Jovell and Navarro-Rubio.[4]

The exclusion criteria were: studies with a mean follow-up of less than 12 months; reports of patients with trapeziometacarpal joint osteoarthritis that could not be separated out from cases of secondary osteoarthritis (posttraumatic, rheumatoid, gout, chondrocalcinosis, or other inflammatory conditions); studies describing only surgical techniques, case reports, short report letters, revision procedures, cadaver studies, biomechanical studies, implants other than total joint arthroplasty or silicone implants such as tendon, ceramic, pyrocarbon, or interposition arthroplasty with synthetic or biological implants; and reviews and studies in which more than one type of implants were used and results were not reported separately.

The survival rates of implants and the method to determine these were recorded. Only articles with removal or revision of the prosthesis as end point were selected to assess survival. It was noted whether a cumulative survivorship analysis was performed and with which method. Usually the product-limit method[5] or the method of Armitage[6] was used. Implants were considered to have a good result if the failure rate was lower than 1 % per year. For failure rate lower than 1 % per year, follow-up of at least 10 years should be considered before any final conclusion is made. In cases of higher failure rates, results can be reported with shorter follow-up.[7]

Assessment of the level of evidence was done according to the Jovell and Navarro-Rubio methodology[4] (▶ Table 18.1) and assessment of the methodological quality with the Coleman methodology scoring system, part A[8] (▶ Fig. 18.2).

Authors searched PubMed/Medline databases up to 31 January 2019. The following key terms were used for searching strategy: trapeziometacarpal osteoarthritis, trapeziometacarpal arthroplasty, trapeziometacarpal

Table 18.1 Classification in levels of evidence based on the type of study design (as described by Jovell and Navarro-Rubio)

Level	Strength of evidence	Type of study design
I	Good	Meta-analysis of randomized controlled trials
II	–	Large-sample randomized controlled trials (n ≥ 25)
III	Good to fair	Small-sample randomized controlled trials (n < 25)
IV	–	Nonrandomized controlled prospective trials
V	–	Nonrandomized controlled retrospective trials
VI	Fair	Cohort studies
VII	–	Case–control studies
VIII	Poor	Noncontrolled clinical series; descriptive studies
IX	–	Anecdotes or case reports

joint, trapeziometacarpal replacement, thumb CMC arthroplasty, thumb CMC joint replacement, and thumb CMC joint prosthesis. The bibliographies of all relevant papers and reviews were hand-searched.

18.3 Results

A flowchart illustrating the selection of trials included in the systematic review is shown in ▸ Fig. 18.1.

18.3.1 Silicone Implants

Reports of 12 different silicone implants were found during the search. The first four were Swanson prostheses: (1) silicone trapezium implant with convex base,[1] (2) silicone trapezium implant with concave base[9] (▸ Fig. 18.2), (3) silicone convex condylar implant,[10] (4) silicone concave condylar implant.[11] The first Swanson implants were constructed of common silicone elastomer; after 1974

high-performance elastomer was used.[11] Reports of other silicone implants found during the search include: (5) Kessler implant, a silicone implant with Dacron reinforcement. It is implanted without resection of the trapezium,[12] (6) a silicone sponge or disc for interposition in the trapeziometacarpal joint,[13] (7) the Ashworth-Blatt implant, a flat implant with a short stem that is inserted in the trapezium,[14] (8) the Niebauer arthroplasty, a Dacron-reinforced silicone trapezium implant,[15] (9) silicone implant with a tunnel in which a tendon strip can be placed to stabilize the implant,[16] (10) the Helal prosthesis, a silicone rubber ball with two stems,[17] (11) proplast silicone rubber trapezium implant without stem,[18] and (12) the tendon tie-in implant with a narrowed waist in which a tendon sling can be placed to stabilize the implant.[19]

Twenty-two articles met the inclusion criteria with seven different types of implants. Only articles of one type of Swanson prosthesis were included, i.e., the

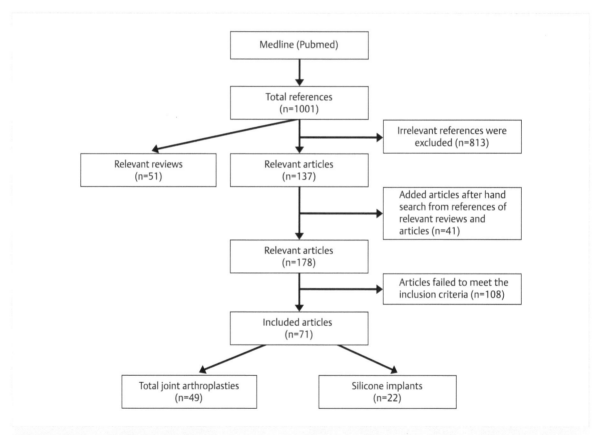

Fig. 18.1 Flowchart of the selected trials.

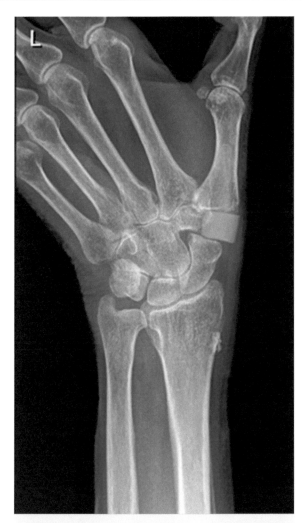

Fig. 18.2 Swanson prosthesis.

Swanson trapezium silicone prosthesis with a concave base. Articles of the condylar Eaton implant[16,20] and the proplast silicone implant[18] were excluded. Results of Swanson prostheses are reported in ► Table 18.3 and ► Table 18.4 and of other silicone implants in ► Table 18.5 and ► Table 18.6.

Of the 12 articles about the Swanson prosthesis, 7 were evidence level VI, 4 level V, and 1 level III. The mean Coleman score was 34 (range: 17–50). The most commonly reported complications were dislocation and silicone synovitis. Reported failure rates ranged between 0 and 27%. The ten articles about other types of silicone implants were all retrospective with evidence level VI and only

reported on a small number of patients. The mean Coleman score was 33 (range: 24–39). Reported complications were dislocation, foreign body reaction, and implant breakage. The highest failure rate was found with the Asworth-Blatt implant (55%).

18.3.2 Total Trapeziometacarpal Joint Implants

Results were found for 21 different total joint prostheses: Arpe prosthesis[40] (► Fig. 18.3); Braun-Cutter prosthesis[41,42,43]; Beznoska[44]; Bichat prosthesis[45]; cemented resurfacement arthroplasty[46,47,48]; de la Caffinière prosthesis[49]; Electra prosthesis[50]; Guepar I prosthesis[51,52,53]; Guepar II prosthesis[54]; Isis[55]; Ivory[56] (► Fig. 18.4); Ledoux prosthesis[57]; Maia[58,59]; Mayo Clinic prosthesis[60]; Moje Acamo[61]; Moovis[62]; Motec[63]; Nahigian prosthesis[64]; Roseland prosthesis[65] (► Fig. 18.5); Rubis II[66]; and Steffee prosthesis.[67]

Papers concerning seven of these did not fit the eligibility criteria because either they included patients with conditions other than primary osteoarthritis (Braun, Guepar I, Ledoux, Maia, Mayo Clinic, and Steffee prostheses) or the results were published in Czech (Beznoska).

Forty-nine articles of the following total joint arthroplasties were included: Arpe (8), Braun-Cutter (1), cemented resurfacement (2), de la Caffinière (8), Electra (7), Guepar II (2), Isis (1), Ivory (4), Maia (3), Moje Acamo (3), Moovis (1), Motec (2), Nahigian (1), Roseland (5) (► Fig. 18.5), and Rubis II (2). In one article results were reported of Electra and Motec prostheses.[63]

Survivorship with removal of the prosthesis as an end point was reported on ten different total joint prostheses in 21 articles (► Table 18.7). The most frequent were of the Arpe, de la Caffinière, and Electra prostheses. Results of those prostheses are presented in ► Table 18.8, ► Table 18.9, ► Table 18.10, ► Table 18.11, ► Table 18.12, and ► Table 18.13; results of other prostheses are shown in ► Table 18.14 and ► Table 18.15.

Of the 50 studies, 42 were evidence level VI, 5 level V, 2 level IV, and 1 level III. Only nine studies were prospective. Resection arthroplasty and tendon interposition and ligament reconstruction were compared with the Arpe,[87,88] de la Caffinière,[91,92] Electra,[94] Maia,[101] and Ivory prostheses.[77] Mean functional outcomes scores, visual analogue scale (VAS) for pain, and pinch grip were better, and pain relief was faster with total joint prostheses than with trapeziectomy and ligamentoplasty. The mean Coleman score was 35 (range: 19–55). The most frequent

18

Table 18.2 Coleman methodology score

		Coleman score
Study size	>60	10
	41–60	7
	20–40	4
	<20 or not stated	0
Mean duration of follow-up	>24 mo	5
	12–24 mo	2
	<12 mo, not stated or unclear	0
Number of different surgical procedures included in each reported outcome	Only one surgical procedure	10
	More than one surgical procedure, but >90% undergoing one procedure	7
	Not stated, unclear, or <90% undergoing one procedure	0
Type of study	Randomized control study	15
	Prospective cohort study	10
	Retrospective study	0
Diagnostic certainty	In all	5
	In >80%	3
	In <80%	0
Description of surgical procedure	Adequate	5
	Fair	3
	Inadequate	0
Description of postoperative rehabilitation	Well described, >80% complying	10
	Well described, 60–80% complying	5
	Protocol not reported or <60–80% complying	0

complications were loosening and dislocation. Failure rates ranged between 0 and 52%. The highest failure rates were reported for the Moje Acamo, Motec, de la Caffinière, and Electra prostheses.

18.4 Discussion

Implant survivorship of Swanson silicone implants was reported in the study by Krukhaug et al,[63] based upon the Norwegian implant registry. This study was excluded from the review as patients operated on with silicone prostheses had both osteoarthritis and rheumatoid arthritis. The 5- and 10-year survival rates were 90 and 89%, respectively; no difference in survival was found between patients with osteoarthritis and inflammatory arthritis. Despite the good survival rate and subjective outcomes and the relatively small number of patients with severe bone erosions in the included studies in this

Table 18.3 Study characteristics of the Swanson silicone trapezium implant

Authors	Patients/Implants	Mean age at surgery (yr)	Follow-up (mo) (mean)	Evidence	Coleman score	
					Separate	Total
Weilby[21]	14/14	60	6–15 (–)	VI	0,2,10,0,5,0,0	17
Amadio et al[22]	21/25	60	– (26)	V	4,5,0,0,5,5,10	29
Sollerman et al[23]	33/39	58	132–168 (144)	VI	4,5,10,0,5,5,10	39
Creighton et al[24]	124/151	62	24–128 (51)	VI	10,5,0,0,5,5,10	35
Freeman and Honner[25]	37/43	60.5 (at follow-up)	6–162 (66)	VI	7,5,10,0,5,5,10	42
Lehmann et al[26]	27	65	– (67)	V	4,5,10,0,5,5,0	30
Lovell et al[27]	52/58	–	18–90 (62) Tendon and silastic	V	7,5,10,0,5,3,5	35
Tägil and Kopylov[28]	13	62	22–66 (45)	III	0,5,10,15,5,5,10	50
van Cappelle et al[29]	35/45	61	90–282 (164)	VI	7,5,0,0,5,5,10	29
MacDermid et al[30]	25/30	64	36–120 (54)	VI	4,5,10,0,5,5,10	39
Taylor et al[31]	22	66	≥12 (–)	V	4,2,10,0,5,0,0	21
Burke et al[32]	58/69	62	9–228 (92)	VI	10,5,10,0,5,5,10	45

review, the use of a silicone implant cannot be recommended. The implant often fails with dislocation or fracture but is not changed as the patient is satisfied. The risk of silicone synovitis can be avoided with alternative treatment methods not least trapeziectomy with or without some form of suspension procedure.

Survival rates of the Arpe, Ivory, and Maia implants were promising at 5 years (≥95%) in some studies,[56,69,70,79] but it is not certain if they remain so high at 10 years. The 5-year survival rate of the Ivory was initially 95%[56] but at 10 years it decreased to 85%.[107] The paper by Vissers et al[107] was not included in the review because

18

Table 18.4 Details of outcome measurements of the Swanson silicone trapezium implant

Authors	Pain	Mean grip strength (kg)	Mean key pinch strength (kg)	Mean tip pinch strength (kg)	Radiographic findings	Failure rate	Predominant complication
Weilby[21]	5/14 had pain	–	–	–	2 dislocation 1 subluxation	14%	Dislocation 2/14
Amadio et al[22]	2/25 still pain	17.9/ silastic/ trapeziectomy	5/4.6 silastic/ trapeziectomy	–	3 subluxation 1 malposition	0%	Subluxation
Sollerman et al[23]	26/39 no pain	6.2/6.2 N/cm² operated/ contralateral hand	2.3/4.1 preop/postop	4.0/4.4 N/cm² operated/contra-lateral hand	56% dislocation or subluxation 51% cyst formation	0%	Dislocation
Creighton et al[24]	85% less pain than preop	12 no difference with preop	3.5 no difference with preop		56% scaphoid cysts (85/151) 74% metacarpal lucencies	1.6% 2/124	Pancarpal cysts 3/124
Freeman and Honner[25]	1.7 (on a scale of 1 to 6)	102% of other side	71% of other side	77% of other side	79% stable 23% wear 53% lucencies	8%	Synovitis 3/37
Lehmann et al[26]	8.0/8.2 (VAS) silastic/tendon	–	4.8/3.6 silastic/tendon	–	Proximalization first metacarpal less with silastic than with tendon	–	–
Lovell et al[27]	78/76 on a scale 0–100, 100: no pain silastic/tendon	–	–	–	4 subluxation 1 stem fracture 1 dislocation	14%	Subluxation 4/58
Tägil and Kopylov[28]	9/14 (VAS 0–100) silastic/tendon	0.56/0.54 kp/ cm² silastic/tendon	0.34/0.35 kp/cm² silastic/tendon		2 dislocations dynamic subluxation Bone cysts	0%	Subluxation 5/13
van Cap-pelle et al[29]	9 (VAS) 10 meant no pain	–	–	–	50% dislocation or subluxation 16% osteolysis	27%	Dislocation (40%)
MacDer-mid et al[30]	5.7/10 = average amount of improvement in pain	18.2/22.3 operated/ nonoperated	4.7/6.7 operated/ nonoperated	3.3/4.5 operated/ nonoperated	90% had osteol-ysis (1 pancarpal) 10% dislocation	20% 6/30	Silicone synovitis (90%)
Taylor et al[31]	18 on a scale of 0 to 100 0 no pain	–	11	7	1 dislocation	9% 2/22	Dislocation 1/22
Burke et al[32]	34 on a scale of 0 to 100 0 no pain	–	–	–	–	1.5% 1/69	Infection 1

Table 18.5 Study characteristics of other silicone implants

Implant	Authors	Patients/Implants	Mean age at surgery (yr)	Follow-up (mo) (mean)	Evidence	Coleman score	
						Separate	Total
Ashworth-Blatt	Ashworth et al[14]	37	56	1–75 (34)	VI	4,5,10,0,5,5,10	39
	Karlsson et al[33]	19/20	56	36–96 (54)	VI	4,5,10,0,5,0,0	24
	Oka and Ikeda[34]	16/16	60	12–144 (57)	VI	0,5,10,0,5,5,5	30
	Minami et al[35]	10/12	66	120–252 (180)	VI	0,5,10,0,5,5,10	35
Helal	O'Leary et al[36]	23/27	63	12–138 (59)	VI	4,5,10,0,5,5,10	39
Kessler	Kessler[37]	17/18	Range: 44–66	At least 24 mo	VI	0,5,10,0,5,5,5	30
Niebauwer	Ferlic et al[38]	11	54	12–36 (20)	VI	0,2,10,0,5,5,10	32
	Adams et al[39]	18/22	60	6–68 (28.8)	VI	4,5,10,0,5,5,10	39
Silicone sponge	Dickson[13]	12/16	–	12–60 (38)	VI	0,2,10,0,5,5,10	32
Tendon tie-in	Avisar et al[19]	22/28	66	12–26 (18)	VI	4,2,10,0,0,5,10	31

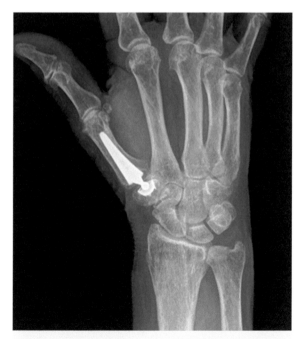

Fig. 18.3 Arpe prosthesis.

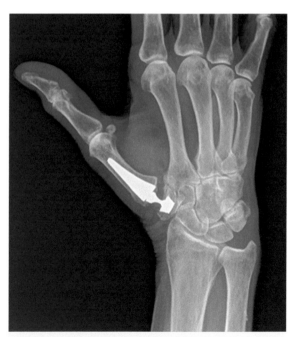

Fig. 18.4 Ivory prosthesis.

Table 18.6 Details of outcome measurements of other silicone implants

Implant	Authors	Pain	Mean grip strength (kg)	Mean key pinch strength (kg)	Mean tip pinch strength (kg)	Radiographic findings	Failure rate	Predominant complication
Ashworth-Blatt	Ashworth et al[14]	3/37 no pain	–	–	–	–	3%	Implant fracture 1/37
	Karlsson et al[33]	–	0.46/0.24 kp/cm² operated/ nonoperated	191/152 Units operated/ nonoperated	–	5 subluxation 7 dislocation In all carpal cysts	55%	Foreign body reaction
	Oka and Ikeda[34]	75% pain-free	7 out of 12 improved postop	–	–	5 brim rupture of implant 1 implant breakage	6%	Partial rupture 5/16
	Minami et al[35]	17% pain-free 58% severe pain	12/9.5 preop/ postop	3.2	3.2	4 silicone synovitis 5 implant fracture 2 dislocations	17%	Implant breakage 5/12
Helal	O'Leary et al[36]	26% signifi-cant postop pain	19	5	4	no osteolysis no dislocation	3.7%	Pain
Kessler	Kessler[37]	61% pain-free	–	–	–	1 dislocation	5.5%	Dislocation
Niebauer	Ferlic et al[38]	6 moderate and 5 marked pain relief	87% of opposite hand	85% of oppo-site hand	79% of opposite hand	No dislocation No bone erosion	0%	–
	Adams et al[39]	14% no improvement	16/20 operated/ nonoperated	4.3/6 operated/ nonoperated	–	2/22 instability	9%	Dislocation
Silicone sponge	Dickson[13]	94% no pain	–	–	–	–	6%	Insufficient removal of osteophyte 1
Tendon tie-in	Avisar et al[19]	7.4/1.2 preop/postop p<0.05	11/11 operated/ nonoperated	5.5/6 operated/ nonoperated	–	2 dislocations	7%	Dislocation 2/28

it included a case with posttraumatic osteoarthritis. The best 10-year survival rate (91%) was reported with the Roseland prosthesis.[81] A good survival rate (74% at 26 years) was also reported with the de la Caffinière pros-thesis,[76] but this was not confirmed by other studies in which higher failure rates were reported.[73,74]

In comparison with our previous review of total joint implants,[3] the level of evidence and the quality of more recent articles have improved. Better functional outcome scores were reported with the Arpe[87] and Ivory prosthe-ses[77,100] than with trapeziectomy and tendon arthro-plasty. Better strength was noted with the Arpe,[88] Ivory,[77] and Maia prostheses.[101] Faster recovery and pain relief were reported with the Electra prosthesis, but follow-up

was not more than 1 year.[94] The risk of dislocation may have decreased with the newer type of implants with dual mobility, but follow-up of these implants is still rela-tively short.

Patients should be informed that the risk of revision is higher if a total joint arthroplasty is chosen instead of a trapeziectomy with or without a suspension procedure such as tendon interposition and ligament reconstruc-tion. There is some evidence that function may be better with some types of total joint prostheses, but the ques-tion remains how long this will last. Some implants (Elec-tra, Moje Acamo, Motec) have been reported to have high failure rates; the use of these implants cannot be recommended.

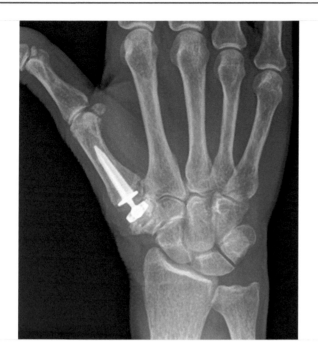

Fig. 18.5 Roseland prosthesis.

Table 18.7 Survivorship of total joint implants for the trapeziometacarpal joint

Implant	Authors	N	% men	% lost	Survival	Cumulative survival analysis
Arpe	Apard and Saint-Cast[68]	43	6	26	85 % at 5 yr 79 % at 11 yr	Armitage
	der Eecken et al[69]	49	18	12	97 % at 5 yr	None
	Cootjans et al[70]	166	13	4	96 % at 6.5 yr	Kaplan Meier
	Craig et al	110	39	24.5	95 % at 2 yr	None
Cemented surface replacement	Pendse et al[71]	62	34	0	91 % at 3 yr	Kaplan Meier
	Ten Brinke et al[72]	10	10	0	80 % at 5 yr	None
de la Caffinière	Wachtl et al[73]	43	n/a	19	66 % at 5 yr	Armitage
	Van Cappelle et al[74]	77	14	0	72 % at 16 yr	Armitage
	Chakrabarti et al[75]	93	12	22	89 % at 16 yr	Armitage
	Johnston et al[76]	93	12	47	74 % at 26 yr	Kaplan Meier
Electra	Krukhaug et al[63]	29	28	n/a	90 % at 5 yr	Kaplan Meier
Ivory	Goubau et al[56]	24	5	8	95 % at 5 yr	None
	Cebrian-Gomez et al[77]	84	8	0	96 % at 5 yr	Kaplan Meier
Maia	Toffoli and Teissier[78]	116	28	31	93 % at 5 yr	Kaplan Meier
	Caekebeke and Duerinckx[79]	50	46	0	96 % a 5 yr	Kaplan Meier
Moje Acamo	Hansen and Vainorius[61]	9	33	0	66 % at 1 yr	None
Motec	Krukhaug et al[63]	53	40	-	91 % at 5 yr	Kaplan Meier
	Thilleman et al[80]	42	19	0	58 % at 2 yr	Kaplan Meier
Roseland	Semere et al[81]	64	6	24	91 % at 10 yr	None
Rubis II	Maes et al[82]	118	6	14	93 % at 5 yr 90 % at 12 yr	Kaplan Meier
	Dehl et al[83]	115	7	45	89 % at 10 yr	Kaplan Meier

18

Table 18.8 Study characteristics of the Arpe prosthesis

Authors	Patients/ Implants	Mean age at surgery (yr)	Follow-up (mo) (mean)	Evidence	Coleman score	
					Separate	Total
Brutus and Kinnen[84]	52/63	55	5–40 (14.8)	VI	10,2,10,0,3,5,5	35
Jacoulet[85]	29/37	67	– (36)	VI	4,5,10,0,3,5,10	37
Apard and Saint-Cast[68]	25/32	59	60–138 (86)	VI	7,5,10,0,0,5,5	32
der Eecken et al[69]	41/49	55	36–132 (72)	VI	7,5,10,0,3,5,5	35
Martin-Ferrero[86]	60/65	58	120–150 (127.2)	VI	10,5,10,10,3,5,0	43
Cootjans et al[70]	156/166	58	– (80)	VI	10,5,10,10,5,5,10	55
Craik et al[87]	83/83	69	– (24)	V	10,2,10,0,5,5,10	42
Robles-Molina et al[88]	31/31	56	– (56)	V	4,5,10,0,5,5,10	39

Table 18.9 Details of outcome measurements of the Arpe prosthesis

Authors	Pain	Mean grip strength (kg)	Mean key pinch strength (kg)	Mean tip pinch strength (kg)	Radiographic findings	Failure rate	Predominant complication
Brutus and Kinnen[84]	0.1 on a scale 0–4.	–	6.6 (98.5 % of opposite side)	–	3/63 cup loosening; 1/63 stem loosening	5 % (3/63)	Dislocation 6/63
Jacoulet[85]	All pain-free	23	4	–	1/37 cup loosening	8 % (3/37)	Dislocation 2/37
Apard and Saint-Cast[68]	5/32 pain with prolonged use; 3/32 pain in cold	20	5.7	–	2/32 dislocation, 5/32 loosening	22 % (7/ 32)	Loosening
der Eecken et al[69]	1 (VAS) postop	–	–	–	1/43 cup loosening; 1/43 cup perforation, 1/43 polyethylene wear	9 % (4/43)	Dislocation 2/43
Martin-Ferrero[86]	7.4/1.1 (VAS) preop/postop p < 0.001	–	4.3/5.6 preop/postop p = 0.005	–	14 % minor loosening; 8 % failed	5 % (3/65)	Loosening
Cootjans et al[70]	Mean VAS 0 (range: 0–9)	19/25 preop/postop	4/5 preop/postop	–	1/166 cup loosening 1/166 cup subsidence	4 % 6/166	Dislocation 8/166
Craik et al[87]	–	–	–	–	1 fracture, 1 heterotopic ossification	5 % (4/83)	Dislocation 8/83
Robles-Molina et al[88]	VAS 1.3/1.4 Arpe/ tendon	–	11.8/8.4 lb Arpe/tendon p < 0.001	–	–	7 % (3/31)	Dislocation 3/31

Table 18.10 Study characteristics of the de la Caffinière prosthesis

Authors	Patients/Implants	Mean age at surgery	Follow-up (mo) (mean)	Evidence	Coleman score	
					Separate	Total
de la Caffinière[89]	13/13	–	– (144)	VI	0,5,10,0,5,0,0,	20
Nicholas and Calderwood[90]	17/20	57	8–120 (64.2)	VI	4,5,10,0,5,0,0	24
Chakrabarti et al[75]	71/93	57	72–192 (132)	VI	10,5,10,0, 0,5,0	30
Wachtl et al[73]	– /43	–	45–81 (64)	VI	7,5,10,0,3,5,5	35
van Cappelle et al[74]	63/77	62	24–192 (102)	VI	10,5,10,0,5,0,0	30
De Smet et al[91]	40/43	54	15–69 (26)	VI	7,5,10,0,5,5,0	32
De Smet et al[92]	27	54	6–52 (25)	V	4,5,10,0,5,0,0	24
Johnston et al[76]	26/39	57	192–312 (228)	VI	4,5,10,0,0,0,0	19

Table 18.11 Details of outcome measurements using de la Caffinière prosthesis

Authors	Pain	Mean grip strength (kg force)	Mean key pinch strength (kg force)	Mean tip pinch strength (kg force)	Radiographic findings	Failure rate	Predominant complication
de la Caffinière[89]	9/13 without pain	–	–	–	4 early loosening 4 gradual loosening	31%	Loosening
Nicholas and Calderwood[90]	80% pain-free	–	–	–	1/20 dislocation; 1/20 trapezial collaps; 1/20 radiolucent lines	0%	Pain
Chakrabarti et al[75]	93% good pain relief (VAS)	22/21 operated/ nonoperated	–	–	10/93 loosening (7 cups, 3 stems)	12% (11/93)	Loosening
Wachtl et al[73]	44% no pain 48% pain with effort 4% pain at rest	28/27.6 operated/ nonoperated	7.5/8 operated/ nonoperated	3.9/3.8 operated/ nonoperated	1/43 dislocation; 9/43 loosening	23% (10/43)	Loosening
van Cappelle et al[74]	75.4% good pain relief (VAS)	–	–	–	13/77 loosening; 15/77 severe loosening with need for revision	21% (16/77)	Loosening
De Smet et al[91]	70% good pain relief (VAS)	17.6/23.8 preop/postop p<0.05	5.32/5.97 preop/postop p<0.01	–	19/43 loosening; 4/43 cup fracture; 1/43 cortex perforation	2% (1/43)	Loosening
De Smet et al[92]	–	–	6.1/5.3 prosthesis versus tendon p > 0.05	–	17/27 loosening	–	–
Johnston et al[76]	27 (VAS)	15.7/17.8 operated/ nonoperated	–	2.9/3.7 operated/ nonoperated	14/39 loosening (11 cups, 3 stems)	26%	Loosening

18

Table 18.12 Study characteristics the Electra prosthesis

Authors	Patients/Implants	Mean age at surgery in yr	Follow-up (mo) (mean)	Evidence	Coleman score	
					Separate	Total
Regnard[50]	100/100	59	36–78 (54)	VI	10,5,10,10,5,5,0	45
Hansen and Snerum[93]	16/17	54	22–52 (35)	VI	0,5,10,0,5,5,10	35
Ulrich-Vinther et al[94]	36/36	58	12	IV	10,2,0,15,5,5,0	37
Hernández-Cortés et al[95]	19/19	57	24–36 (29)	VI	0,2,10,10,5,5,0	32
Hansen and Stilling[96]	11/11	60	24	III	0,2,10,15,5,5,10	47
Krukhaug et al[63]	– /29	62	– (24)	VI	4,2,10,0,5,0,0	21
Chug et al[97]	14/16	70	12–38 (26)	VI	0,5,10,0,5,3,10	23

Table 18.13 Details of outcome measurements the Electra prosthesis

Authors	Pain	Mean grip strength (kg)	Mean key pinch strength (kg)	Mean tip pinch strength (kg)	Radiographic findings	Failure rate	Predominant complication
Regnard[50]	81 % pain-free	28	6	–	15/100 loosening; 7/100 dislocation	17 % (17/100)	Loosening
Hansen and Snerum[93]	–	–	–	–	5/17 cup loosening; 1/17 dislocation	35 % (6/17)	Loosening
Ulrich-Vinther et al[94]	3.8/0.5 (VAS) preop /postop p < 0.001	10.5/25.6 preop / postop p < 0.05	5.0/5.6 preop/postop p < 0.05	4.0/5.3 preop/postop p < 0.05	2/19 osteolysis around cup	3 % (1/36)	Tendon problems
Hernández-Cortés et al[95]	8.4/4.6 (VAS) preop/postop p < 0.001	–	3.1/2.2 preop/postop	–	10/19 osteolysis; 1/19 periprosthetic fracture	16 % (3/19)	Cup loosening
Hansen and Stilling[96]	No significant differences to DLC cup (VAS)	No significant difference to DLC cup	–	–	0.8-mm mean implant migration	9 % (1/11)	Cup loosening
Krukhaug et al[63]	–	–	–	–	1/29 loosening; 1/29 dislocation; 1/29 instability	10 % (5-yr failure rate)	Dislocation and pain
Chug et al[97]	34.2/5.4 preop/postop PRWE (p < 0.01)	27/28 operated/nonoperated	3.6/3.9 operated/nonoperated	4/4.3 operated/nonoperated	1/16 cup loosening	6 % (1/16)	Intraoperative trapezium fracture

Table 18.14 Study characteristics of total arthroplasty using other prostheses

Implant	Authors	Patients/ Implants	Mean age at surgery (yr)	Follow-up (mo) (mean)	Evidence	Coleman score Separate	Total
Braun-Cutter	Badia and Sambandam[41]	25/26	71	26–68 (59)	VI	4,5,10,10,5,5,0	39
Cemented resurfacement arthroplasty	Pendse et al[71]	50/62	64.5	24–84 (36)	VI	10,5,10,0,3,5,10	43
	Ten Brinke et al[72]	10/10	n/a	60	VI	0,5,10,10,5,0,0	30
Guepar II	Masmejean et al[54]	60/64	58	12–84 (29)	VI	10,5,10,0,3,5,5	38
	Lemoine et al[98]	68/84	61	12–115 (50)	VI	10,5,10,0,3,0,0	28
Isis	Seng et al[55]	26/30	n/a	18–47 (30)	VI	4,5,7,0,3,10,5	34
Ivory	Goubau et al[56]	22/22	66	60–77 (67)	VI	4,5,10,10,5,5,10	49
	Spaans et al[99]	20/20	60	26–52 (37)	VI	4,5,10,0,3,5,10	37
	Erne et al[100]	39/39	56	12–72 (42)	V	4,5,10,0,5,5,10	39
	Cebrian-Gomez et al[77]	84/84	60	24–60 (48)	IV	10,5,10,10,5,5,10	55
Maia	Toffoli and Teissier[78]	80/96	68	60–102 (76)	VI	10,5,10,0,5,5,10	45
	Degeorge et al[101]	41/41	63	6–36 (20)	V	7,2,10,0,5,3,5	32
	Caekebeke and Duerinckx[79]	35/50	57	56–71 (65)	VI	7,5,10,0,5,5,10	42
Moje Acamo	Hansen and Vainorius[61]	9/9	58	12 (12)	VI	0,2,10,0,5,5,0	22
	Kaszap et al[102]	12/12	64	– (50)	VI	0,5,10,0,5,5,0	25
	Kollig et al[103]	28/29	63	9–62 (33)	VI	4,5,10,0,5,5,10	39
Moovis	Dreant and Poumellec[62]	25/28	63	– (27.5)	VI	4,5,10,0,5,5,10	39
Motec	Krukhaug et al[63]	– /53	63	– (22.8)	VI	4,2,10,0,5,0,0	21
	Thillemann et al[80]	40 /42	59	14–46 (27)	VI	7,5,10,0,5,5,10	42
Nahigian prosthesis	Hannula and Nahigian[64]	30/34	58	15–86 (47)	VI	4,5,10,0,3,3,0	25

(Continued)

18

Table 18.14 (*Continued*) Study characteristics of total arthroplasty using other prostheses

Implant	Authors	Patients/ Implants	Mean age at surgery (yr)	Follow-up (mo) (mean)	Evidence	Coleman score	
						Separate	Total
Roseland	Schuhl[104]	43/45	59	1–50 (14)	VI	7,2,0,0,3,3,5	20
	Moutet et al[65]	24/27	62	24–61 (38)	VI	4,2,10,0,3,5,10	34
	Zollinger et al[105]	27/32	n/a	7–66 (39)	VI	4,5,10,0,5,0,10	34
	Guardia et al[106]	68/79	61	– (44)	VI	10,5,10,0,3,5,5	38
	Semere et al[81]	51/64	58	≥ 120 (150)	VI	10,5,10,0,0,5,10	40
Rubis II	Maes et al[82]	106/118	62	– (88)	VI	10,5,10,0,0,3,5	33
	Dehl et al[83]	95/115	61	– (126)	VI	10,5,10,0,5,5,10	45

Table 18.15 Details of outcome measurements of other prostheses

Implant	Authors	Pain	Mean grip strength (kg)	Mean key pinch strength (kg)	Mean tip pinch strength (kg)	Radiographic findings	Failure rate	Predominant complication
Braun-Cutter	Badia and Sambandam[41]	24/26 complete pain relief	–	3.5/5.5 preop/ postop	–	No loosening or subsidence	4 % (1/26)	Posttraumatic dislocation 1/26
Cemented resurfacement arthroplasty	Pendse et al[71]	1.29 (VAS)	19.6	–	4	11/62 trapezial loosening 1/62 metacarpal loosening	11 % (7/62)	Loosening
	Ten Brinke et al[72]	–	–	–	–	–	20 % 2/10	–
Guepar II	Masmejean et al[54]	78 % (50/64) pain-free (Alnot and Muller's classification)	19 79 % of opposite side	6 94 % of opposite side	–	6/64 radiolucent lines 1/64 metacarpal sinking	2 % (1/64)	Loosening
	Lemoine et al[98]	3.5/0.7 (Alnot and Muller's classification) p < 0.0001	20.8/20.4 operated/ nonoperated	4/4.2 operated/ nonoperated	–	33 % lucent lines; 3 % cup loosening; 3 % stem loosening	1 % (1/84)	Pain
Isis	Seng et al[55]	8.1/3.4 (VAS) preop/postop	17 75 % of opposite side	5 75 % of opposite side	3 73 % of opposite side	20 % radiolucent lines; 10 % loosening	3 % (1/30)	Loosening

(*Continued*)

Table 18.15 (*Continued*) Details of outcome measurements of other prostheses

Implant	Authors	Pain	Mean grip strength (kg)	Mean key pinch strength (kg)	Mean tip pinch strength (kg)	Radiographic findings	Failure rate	Predominant complication
Ivory	Goubau et al[56]	8.1/1.2 (VAS) preop/postop p < 0.0001	17.2/22.5 preop/postop p < 0.001	4.5/5.1 preop/postop p = 0.18	–	1/22 cup instability; 1/22 osteolysis	5 % (1/22)	Cup instability 1/22
	Spaans et al[99]	1.9 (VAS)	23.7/26.1 operated/nonoperated	4.5/4.5 operated/nonoperated	2.4/2.6 operated/nonoperated	2/20 minor osteolysis cup; 1/20 trapezium collaps	10 % (2/20)	Dislocation 2/20
	Erne et al[100]	0.5/1.0 Ivory/tendon p > 0.05		1.0/0.8 bar Ivory/tendon p > 0.05		2 breakage proximal component, 1 loosening	8 % (3/39)	Breakage proximal component
	Cebrian-Gomez et al[77]	0.6/1.7 (VAS) Ivory / tendon P = 0.001	20/19 Ivory /tendon	2.3/1.7 Ivory/tendon P = 0.014	–	2 dislocation 2 cup loosening	3.5 %	Dislocation 2/84
Maia	Toffoli and Teissier[78]	7.1/1.2 (VAS) preop/postop p < 0.05	13.3/23.4 preop/postop P < 0.05	4.3/5.8 preop/postop not significant		4 cup subsidence, 16 heterotopic ossification	5 %	Cup loosening 5/96
	Degeorge et al[101]	–	–	3.9/3.1 Maia/LRTI p = 0.003	–	–	–	–
	Caekebeke and Duerinckx[79]	Mean VAS at rest 0 and 1 with loading	29/27 operated/nonoperated hand	7/7 operated/nonoperated hand	–	1 polyethylene wear, 1 intra-articular bone growth	4 %	Traumatic trapezial fractures 2/50
Moje Acamo	Hansen and Vainorius[61]	–	–	–	–	8/9 osteolysis	33 % (3/9)	Osteolysis around the implant
	Kaszap et al[102]	92 % pain	–	–	–	10/12 implant migration; 11/12 implant tilting; 9/12 radiolucent lines	42 % (5/12)	Implant migration or loosening
	Kollig et al[103]	1.9 (VAS at 33 mo)				At 6 mo 48 % radiolucent lines	52 %	Loosening
Moovis	Dreant and Poumellec[62]	8/1 (VAS) preop/postop	28	7.5	4.5	1 osteolytic trapezial lesion	4 %	Loosening 1/28

(*Continued*)

18

Table 18.15 (*Continued*) Details of outcome measurements of other prostheses

Implant	Authors	Pain	Mean grip strength (kg)	Mean key pinch strength (kg)	Mean tip pinch strength (kg)	Radio-graphic findings	Failure rate	Predominant complication
Motec	Krukhaug et al[63]	–	–	–	–	3/53 loosening	9 % at 5 yr	Dislocation and pain
	Thilleman et al[80]	1/4 with activity/at rest (NRS)	–	–	–	9/42 cup loosening 3/42 dislocation	42 % at 2 yr	Loosening
Nahigian prosthesis	Hannula and Nahigian[64]	23 % excellent results, 51 % good results	36.2/43.4 preop/postop	3.6/6.2 preop/postop p < 0.001	n/a	13/23 radio-lucent lines	13 % (5/39)	Loosening
Roseland	Schuhl[104]	35 % pain-free; 39 % infre-quent pain	–	–	–	8/45 cup loosening; 2/45 stem loosening; 1/45 dislocation	18 % (8/45)	loosening
	Moutet et al[65]	67 % pain-free	89 % of the other side	95 % of the other side	–	1/27 stem loosening; 1/27 trape-zial fracture	0 %	Trapezial fracture and loosening
	Zollinger et al[105]	7.4/1.2 (VAS) preop/postop p = 0.000	–	–	–	2/32 dislocation	9 % (3/32)	Dislocation
	Guardia et al[106]	70 % satisfac-tory results	–	–	–	2/79 disloca-tion; 1/79 trapezium fracture	4 % (3/79)	Dislocation
	Semere et al[81]	41 % pain-free; 50 % occasional pain	22	6	4.5	33/47 cup subsidence; 31/47 stem subsidence	9 % (6/64)	Loosening
Rubis II	Maes et al[82]	77 % pain-free; 33 % moder-ate pain	–	–	100 % of opposite side	5 % osteoly-sis base stem; 9 % osteolysis around stem and cup	8 % (9/118)	Dislocation 8 %
	Dehl et al[83]	Mean VAS at rest 1; during activities 5	92 % of the other side	98 % of the other side	92 % of the other side	Peripros-thetic ossifi-cation: 27 %; radiolucent lines: 13 %	9.5 % (11/115)	Dislocation 13 %

References

[1] Swanson AB. Silicone rubber implants for replacement of arthritis or destroyed joints in the hand. Surg Clin North Am. 1968; 48 (5):1113–1127

[2] de la Caffinière JY. Total trapezo-metacarpal prosthesis. Rev Chir Orthop Repar Appar Mot. 1974; 60(4):299–308

[3] Huang K, Hollevoet N, Giddins G. Thumb carpometacarpal joint total arthroplasty: a systematic review. J Hand Surg Eur Vol. 2015; 40 (4):338–350

[4] Jovell AJ, Navarro-Rubio MD. Evaluation of scientific evidence. Med Clin (Barc). 1995; 105(19):740–743

[5] Kaplan EL, Meier P. Nonparametric estimation from incomplete observations. J Am Stat Assoc. 1958; 53:457–481, 425

[6] Armitage P. Statistical methods in medical research. Oxford: Blackwell; 1971:408–414

[7] Murray DW, Carr AJ. Bulstrode C: survival analysis of joint replacements. J Bone Joint Surg Br. 1993; 75:697–704

[8] Tallon C, Coleman BD, Khan KM, Maffulli N. Outcome of surgery for chronic Achilles tendinopathy: a critical review. Am J Sports Med. 2001; 29(3):315–320

[9] Swanson AB. Disabling arthritis at the base of the thumb: treatment by resection of the trapezium and flexible (silicone) implant arthroplasty. J Bone Joint Surg Am. 1972; 54(3):456–471

[10] Swanson AB, deGoot Swanson G, Watermeier JJ. Trapezium implant arthroplasty: long-term evaluation of 150 cases. J Hand Surg Am. 1981; 6(2):125–141

[11] Swanson AB, de Groot Swanson G. Reconstruction of the thumb basal joints: development and current status of implant techniques. Clin Orthop Relat Res. 1987(220):68–85

[12] Kessler I, Axer A. Arthroplasty of the first carpometacarpal joint with a silicone implant. Plast Reconstr Surg. 1971; 47(3):252–257

[13] Dickson RA. Arthritis of the carpometacarpal joint of the thumb: treatment by silicone sponge interposition arthroplasty. An experimental and clinical study. Hand. 1976; 8(3):197–208

[14] Ashworth CR, Blatt G, Chuinard RG, Stark HH. Silicone-rubber interposition arthroplasty of the carpometacarpal joint of the thumb. J Hand Surg Am. 1977; 2(5):345–357

[15] Poppen NK, Niebauer JJ. "Tie-in" trapezium prosthesis: long-term results. J Hand Surg Am. 1978; 3(5):445–450

[16] Eaton RG. Replacement of the trapezium for arthritis of the basal articulations: a new technique with stabilization by tenodesis. J Bone Joint Surg Am. 1979; 61(1):76–82

[17] Grange WJ, Helal B. Replacement of the trapezium with a silicone rubber ball spacer. Hand. 1983; 15(1):53–56

[18] Kessler FB, Epstein MJ, Culver JE, Jr, Prewitt J, Homsy CA. Proplast stabilized stemless trapezium implant. J Hand Surg Am. 1984; 9 (2):227–231

[19] Avisar E, Elvey M, Tzang C, Sorene E. Trapeziectomy with a tendon tie-in implant for osteoarthritis of the trapeziometacarpal joint. J Hand Surg Am. 2015; 40(7):1292–1297

[20] Ho PK, Jacobs JL, Clark GL. Trapezium implant arthroplasty: evaluation of a semiconstrained implant. J Hand Surg Am. 1985; 10 (5):654–660

[21] Weilby A. Surgical treatment of osteoarthritis of the carpo-metacarpal joint of the thumb: indications for arthrodesis, excision of the trapezium, and alloplasty. Scand J Plast Reconstr Surg. 1971; 5 (2):136–141

[22] Amadio PC, Millender LH, Smith RJ. Silicone spacer or tendon spacer for trapezium resection arthroplasty: comparison of results. J Hand Surg Am. 1982; 7(3):237–244

[23] Sollerman C, Herrlin K, Abrahamsson SO, Lindholm A. Silastic replacement of the trapezium for arthrosis: a twelve year follow-up study. J Hand Surg [Br]. 1988; 13(4):426–429

[24] Creighton JJ, Jr, Steichen JB, Strickland JW. Long-term evaluation of silastic trapezial arthroplasty in patients with osteoarthritis. J Hand Surg Am. 1991; 16(3):510–519

[25] Freeman GR, Honner R. Silastic replacement of the trapezium. J Hand Surg [Br]. 1992; 17(4):458–462

[26] Lehmann O, Herren DB, Simmen BR. Comparison of tendon suspension-interposition and silicon spacers in the treatment of degenerative osteoarthritis of the base of the thumb. Ann Chir Main Memb Super. 1998; 17(1):25–30

[27] Lovell ME, Nuttall D, Trail IA, Stilwell J, Stanley JK. A patient-reported comparison of trapeziectomy with Swanson Silastic implant or sling ligament reconstruction. J Hand Surg [Br]. 1999; 24(4):453–455

[28] Tägil M, Kopylov P. Swanson versus APL arthroplasty in the treatment of osteoarthritis of the trapeziometacarpal joint: a prospective and randomized study in 26 patients. J Hand Surg [Br]. 2002; 27 (5):452–456

[29] van Cappelle HG, Deutman R, van Horn JR. Use of the Swanson silicone trapezium implant for treatment of primary osteoarthritis: long-term results. J Bone Joint Surg Am. 2001; 83(7):999–1004

[30] MacDermid JC, Roth JH, Rampersaud YR, Bain GI. Trapezial arthroplasty with silicone rubber implantation for advanced osteoarthritis of the trapeziometacarpal joint of the thumb. Can J Surg. 2003; 46 (2):103–110

[31] Taylor EJ, Desari K, D'Arcy JC, Bonnici AV. A comparison of fusion, trapeziectomy and silastic replacement for the treatment of osteoarthritis of the trapeziometacarpal joint. J Hand Surg [Br]. 2005; 30 (1):45–49

[32] Burke NG, Walsh J, Moran CJ, Cousins G, Molony D, Kelly EP. Patient-reported outcomes after silastic replacement of the trapezium for osteoarthritis. J Hand Surg Eur Vol. 2012; 37(3):263–268

[33] Karlsson MK, Necking LE, Redlund-Johnell I. Foreign body reaction after modified silicone rubber arthroplasty of the first carpometacarpal joint. Scand J Plast Reconstr Surg Hand Surg. 1992; 26 (1):101–103

[34] Oka Y, Ikeda M. Silastic interposition arthroplasty for osteoarthrosis of the carpometacarpal joint of the thumb. Tokai J Exp Clin Med. 2000; 25(1):15–21

[35] Minami A, Iwasaki N, Kutsumi K, Suenaga N, Yasuda K. A long-term follow-up of silicone-rubber interposition arthroplasty for osteoarthritis of the thumb carpometacarpal joint. Hand Surg. 2005; 10 (1):77–82

[36] O'Leary ST, Grobbelaar AO, Goldsmith N, Smith PJ, Harrison DH. Silicone arthroplasty for trapeziometacarpal arthritis. J Hand Surg [Br]. 2002; 27(5):457–461

[37] Kessler I. Silicone arthroplasty of the trapezio-metacarpal joint. J Bone Joint Surg Br. 1973; 55(2):285–291

[38] Ferlic DC, Busbee GA, Clayton ML. Degenerative arthritis of the carpometacarpal joint of the thumb: a clinical follow-up of eleven Niebauer prostheses. J Hand Surg Am. 1977; 2(3):212–215

[39] Adams BD, Unsell RS, McLaughlin P. Niebauer trapeziometacarpal arthroplasty. J Hand Surg Am. 1990; 15(3):487–492

[40] Isselin J. ARPE prosthesis: preliminary results. Chir Main. 2001; 20 (1):89–92

[41] Badia A, Sambandam SN. Total joint arthroplasty in the treatment of advanced stages of thumb carpometacarpal joint osteoarthritis. J Hand Surg Am. 2006; 31(10):1605–1614

[42] Braun RM. Total joint replacement at the base of the thumb: preliminary report. J Hand Surg Am. 1982; 7(3):245–251

[43] Braun RM. Total joint arthroplasty at the carpometacarpal joint of the thumb. Clin Orthop Relat Res. 1985(195):161–167

[44] Jurča J, Němejc M, Havlas V. Surgical treatment for advanced rhizarthrosis. comparison of results of the Burton-Pellegrini technique and trapeziometacarpal joint arthroplasty. Acta Chir Orthop Traumatol Cech. 2016; 83(1):27–31

[45] Alnot JY. Trapezo-metacarpal prosthesis (author's trans.). Ann Radiol (Paris). 1982; 25(4):294–296

[46] Pérez-Ubeda MJ, García-López A, Marco Martinez F, Junyent Vilanova E, Molina Martos M, López-Duran Stern L. Results of the cemented SR trapeziometacarpal prosthesis in the treatment of thumb carpometacarpal osteoarthritis. J Hand Surg Am. 2003; 28 (6):917–925

18

18

[47] Uchiyama S, Cooney WP, Niebur G, An KN, Linscheid RL. Biomechanical analysis of the trapeziometacarpal joint after surface replacement arthroplasty. J Hand Surg Am. 1999; 24(3):483–490

[48] van Rijn J, Gosens T. A cemented surface replacement prosthesis in the basal thumb joint. J Hand Surg Am. 2010; 35(4):572–579

[49] de la Caffiniere JY, Aucouturier P. Trapezio-metacarpal arthroplasty by total prosthesis. Hand. 1979; 11(1):41–46

[50] Regnard PJ. Electra trapezio metacarpal prosthesis: results of the first 100 cases. J Hand Surg [Br]. 2006; 31(6):621–628

[51] Alnot JY, Beal D, Oberlin C, Salon A. Guepar total trapeziometacarpal prosthesis in the treatment of arthritis of the thumb: 36 case reports. Ann Chir Main Memb Super. 1993; 12(2):93–104

[52] Alnot JY, Muller GP. A retrospective review of 115 cases of surgically-treated trapeziometacarpal osteoarthritis. Rev Rhum Engl Ed. 1998; 65(2):95–108

[53] Alnot JY, Saint Laurent Y. Total trapeziometacarpal arthroplasty: report on seventeen cases of de generative arthritis of the trapeziometacarpal joint. Ann Chir Main. 1985; 4(1):11–21

[54] Masmejean E, Alnot JY, Chantelot C, Beccari R. Guepar anatomical trapeziometacarpal prosthesis. Chir Main. 2003; 22(1):30–36

[55] Seng VS, Chantelot C. Isis(®) trapeziometacarpal prosthesis in basal thumb osteoarthritis: 30 months follow-up in 30 cases. Chir Main. 2013; 32(1):8–16

[56] Goubau JF, Goorens CK, Van Hoonacker P, Berghs B, Kerckhove D, Scheerlinck T. Clinical and radiological outcomes of the Ivory arthroplasty for trapeziometacarpal joint osteoarthritis with a minimum of 5 years of follow-up: a prospective single-centre cohort study. J Hand Surg Eur Vol. 2013; 38(8):866–874

[57] Ledoux P. Failure of total uncemented trapeziometacarpal prosthesis: a multicenter study. Ann Chir Main Memb Super. 1997; 16(3):215–221

[58] Bricout M, Rezzouk J. Complications and failures of the trapeziometacarpal Maia® prosthesis: a series of 156 cases. Hand Surg Rehabil. 2016; 35(3):190–198

[59] Jager T, Barbary S, Dap F, Dautel G. Evaluation of postoperative pain and early functional results in the treatment of carpometacarpal joint arthritis: comparative prospective study of trapeziectomy vs. MAIA(®) prosthesis in 74 female patients. Chir Main. 2013; 32(2):55–62

[60] Cooney WP, Linscheid RL, Askew LJ. Total arthroplasty of the thumb trapeziometacarpal joint. Clin Orthop Relat Res. 1987(220):35–45

[61] Hansen TB, Vainorius D. High loosening rate of the Moje Acamo prosthesis for treating osteoarthritis of the trapeziometacarpal joint. J Hand Surg Eur Vol. 2008; 33(5):571–574

[62] Dreant N, Poumellec MA. Total thumb carpometacarpal joint arthroplasty: a retrospective functional study of 28 Moovis prostheses. Hand (N Y). 2019; 14(1):59–65

[63] Krukhaug Y, Lie SA, Havelin LI, Furnes O, Hove LM, Hallan G. The results of 479 thumb carpometacarpal joint replacements reported in the Norwegian Arthroplasty Register. J Hand Surg Eur Vol. 2014; 39(8):819–825

[64] Hannula TT, Nahigian SH. A preliminary report: cementless trapeziometacarpal arthroplasty. J Hand Surg Am. 1999; 24(1):92–101

[65] Moutet F, Lebrun C, Massart P, Sartorius C. The Roseland prosthesis. Chir Main. 2001; 20(1):79–84

[66] Dunaud JL, Moughabghab M, Benaïssa S, Vimont E, Degandt A. Rubis 2 trapezometacarpal prosthesis: concept, operative technique. Chir Main. 2001; 20(1):85–88

[67] Ferrari B, Steffee AD. Trapeziometacarpal total joint replacement using the Steffee prosthesis. J Bone Joint Surg Am. 1986; 68(8):1177–1184

[68] Apard T, Saint-Cast Y. Results of a 5 years follow-up of Arpe prosthesis for the basal thumb osteoarthritis. Chir Main. 2007; 26(2):88–94

[69] Eecken SV, Vanhove W, Hollevoet N. Trapeziometacarpal joint replacement with the Arpe prosthesis. Acta Orthop Belg. 2012; 78(6):724–729

[70] Cootjans K, Vanhaecke J, Dezillie M, Barth J, Pottel H, Stockmans F. Joint survival analysis and clinical outcome of total joint arthroplasties with the ARPE implant in the treatment of trapeziometacarpal

osteoarthritis with a minimal follow-up of 5 years. J Hand Surg Am. 2017; 42(8):630–638

[71] Pendse A, Nisar A, Shah SZ, Bhosale A, Freeman JV, Chakrabarti I. Surface replacement trapeziometacarpal joint arthroplasty: early results. J Hand Surg Eur Vol. 2009; 34(6):748–757

[72] Ten Brinke B, Mathijssen NMC, Blom I, Deijkers RLM, Ooms EM, Kraan GA. Model-based roentgen stereophotogrammetric analysis of the surface replacement trapeziometacarpal total joint arthroplasty. J Hand Surg Eur Vol. 2016; 41(9):925–929

[73] Wachtl SW, Guggenheim PR, Sennwald GR. Cemented and noncemented replacements of the trapeziometacarpal joint. J Bone Joint Surg Br. 1998; 80(1):121–125

[74] van Cappelle HG, Elzenga P, van Horn JR. Long-term results and loosening analysis of de la Caffinière replacements of the trapeziometacarpal joint. J Hand Surg Am. 1999; 24(3):476–482

[75] Chakrabarti AJ, Robinson AHN, Gallagher P. De la Caffinière thumb carpometacarpal replacements. 93 cases at 6 to 16 years follow-up. J Hand Surg [Br]. 1997; 22(6):695–698

[76] Johnston P, Getgood A, Larson D, Chojnowski AJ, Chakrabarti AJ, Chapman PG. De la Caffinière thumb trapeziometacarpal joint arthroplasty: 16–26 year follow-up. J Hand Surg Eur Vol. 2012; 37(7):621–624

[77] Cebrian-Gomez R, Lizaur-Utrilla A, Sebastia-Forcada E, Lopez-Prats FA. Outcomes of cementless joint prosthesis versus tendon interposition for trapeziometacarpal osteoarthritis: a prospective study. J Hand Surg Eur Vol. 2019; 44(2):151–158

[78] Toffoli A, Teissier J. Maïa trapeziometacarpal joint arthroplasty: clinical and radiological outcomes of 80 patients with more than 6 years of follow-up. J Hand Surg Am. 2017; 42(10):838.e1–838.e8

[79] Caekebeke P, Duerinckx J. Can surgical guidelines minimize complications after Maïa® trapeziometacarpal joint arthroplasty with unconstrained cups? J Hand Surg Eur Vol. 2018; 43(4):420–425

[80] Thillemann JK, Thillemann TM, Munk B, Krøner K. High revision rates with the metal-on-metal Motec carpometacarpal joint prosthesis. J Hand Surg Eur Vol. 2016; 41(3):322–327

[81] Semere A, Vuillerme N, Corcella D, Forli A, Moutet F. Results with the Roseland(®) HAC trapeziometacarpal prosthesis after more than 10 years. Chir Main. 2015; 34(2):59–66

[82] Maes C, Dunaud JL, Moughabghab M, Benaissa S, Henry L, Guériat F. Results of the treatment of basal thumb osteoarthritis by Rubis II prosthesis after more than 5 years: a retrospective study of 118 cases. Chir Main. 2010; 29(6):360–365

[83] Dehl M, Chelli M, Lippmann S, Benaissa S, Rotari V, Moughabghab M. Results of 115 Rubis II reverse thumb carpometacarpal joint prostheses with a mean follow-up of 10 years. J Hand Surg Eur Vol. 2017; 42(6):592–598

[84] Brutus JP, Kinnen L. Total carpometacarpal joint replacement surgery using the ARPE implant for primary osteoarthritis of the thumb: our short-term. Chir Main. 2004; 23:224–228

[85] Jacoulet P. Results of the ARPE trapezometacarpal prosthesis: a retrospective study of 37 cases. Chir Main. 2005; 24(1):24–28

[86] Martin-Ferrero M. Ten-year long-term results of total joint arthroplasties with ARPE® implant in the treatment of trapeziometacarpal osteoarthritis. J Hand Surg Eur Vol. 2014; 39(8):826–832

[87] Craik JD, Glasgow S, Andren J, et al. Early results of the ARPE arthroplasty versus trapeziectomy for the treatment of thumb carpometacarpal joint osteoarthritis. J Hand Surg Asian Pac Vol. 2017; 22(4):472–478

[88] Robles-Molina MJ, López-Caba F, Gómez-Sánchez RC, Cárdenas-Grande E, Pajares-López M, Hernández-Cortés P. Trapeziectomy with ligament reconstruction and tendon interposition versus a trapeziometacarpal prosthesis for the treatment of thumb basal joint osteoarthritis. Orthopedics. 2017; 40(4):e681–e686

[89] De la Caffinière JY. Long term results of the total prosthesis of the trapezio-metacarpal joint in osteo-arthritis of the thumb. Rev Chir Orthop Repar Appar Mot. 1991; 77:312–321

[90] Nicholas RM, Calderwood JW. De la Caffinière arthroplasty for basal thumb joint osteoarthritis. J Bone Joint Surg Br. 1992; 74(2):309–312

[91] De Smet L, Sioen W, Spaepen D. Changes in key pinch strength after excision of the trapezium and total joint arthroplasty. J Hand Surg [Br]. 2004; 29(1):40–41

[92] De Smet L, Sioen W, Spaepen D, Van Ransbeeck H. Total joint arthroplasty for osteoarthritis of the thumb basal joint. Acta Orthop Belg. 2004; 70(1):19–24

[93] Hansen TB, Snerum L. Elektra trapeziometacarpal prosthesis for treatment of osteoarthrosis of the basal joint of the thumb. Scand J Plast Reconstr Surg Hand Surg. 2008; 42(6):316–319

[94] Ulrich-Vinther M, Puggaard H, Lange B. Prospective 1-year follow-up study comparing joint prosthesis with tendon interposition arthroplasty in treatment of trapeziometacarpal osteoarthritis. J Hand Surg Am. 2008; 33(8):1369–1377

[95] Hernández-Cortés P, Pajares-López M, Robles-Molina MJ, Gómez-Sánchez R, Toledo-Romero MA, De Torres-Urrea J. Two-year outcomes of Elektra prosthesis for trapeziometacarpal osteoarthritis: a longitudinal cohort study. J Hand Surg Eur Vol. 2012; 37(2):130–137

[96] Hansen TB, Stilling M. Equally good fixation of cemented and uncemented cups in total trapeziometacarpal joint prostheses. A randomized clinical RSA study with 2-year follow-up. Acta Orthop. 2013; 84(1):98–105

[97] Chug M, Williams N, Benn D, Brindley S. Outcome of uncemented trapeziometacarpal prosthesis. Indian J Orthop. 2014; 48(4):394–398

[98] Lemoine S, Wavreille G, Alnot JY, Fontaine C, Chantelot C, groupe GUEPAR. Second generation GUEPAR total arthroplasty of the thumb basal joint: 50 months follow-up in 84 cases. Orthop Traumatol Surg Res. 2009; 95(1):63–69

[99] Spaans AJ, van Minnen LP, Weijns ME, Braakenburg A, van der Molen AB. Retrospective study of a series of 20 Ivory prostheses in the treatment of trapeziometacarpal osteoarthritis. J Wrist Surg. 2016; 5(2):131–136

[100] Erne H, Scheiber C, Schmauss D, et al. Total endoprothesis versus Lundborg's resection arthroplasty for the treatment of trapeziometacarpal joint osteoarthritis. Plast Reconstr Surg Glob Open. 2018; 6(4):e1737

[101] Degeorge B, Dagneaux L, Andrin J, Lazerges C, Coulet B, Chammas M. Do trapeziometacarpal prosthesis provide better metacarpophalangeal stability than trapeziectomy and ligamentoplasty? Orthop Traumatol Surg Res. 2018; 104(7):1095–1100

[102] Kaszap B, Daecke W, Jung M. High frequency failure of the Moje thumb carpometacarpal joint arthroplasty. J Hand Surg Eur Vol. 2012; 37(7):610–616

[103] Kollig E, Weber W, Bieler D, Franke A. Failure of an uncemented thumb carpometacarpal joint ceramic prosthesis. J Hand Surg Eur Vol. 2017; 42(6):599–604

[104] Schuhl JF. The Roseland prosthesis in the treatment of osteoarthritis: a five years experience with the same surgeon. Chir Main. 2001; 20(1):75–78

[105] Zollinger PE, Ellis ML, Unal H, Tuinebreijer WE. Clinical outcome of cementless semi-constrained trapeziometacarpal arthroplasty, and possible effect of vitamin C on the occurrence of complex regional pain syndrome. Acta Orthop Belg. 2008; 74(3):317–322

[106] Guardia C, Moutet F, Corcella D, Forli A, Pradel P. Roseland® prosthesis: quality of life's studies about 68 patients with a mean followed-up of 43.8 months. Chir Main. 2010; 29(5):301–306

[107] Vissers G, Goorens CK, Vanmierlo B, et al. Ivory arthroplasty for trapeziometacarpal osteoarthritis: 10-year follow-up. J Hand Surg Eur Vol. 2018; 44(2):138–145

18

19 Pi² and Nugrip Pyrocarbon Arthroplasties of the Thumb CMC Joint

Ludovic Ardouin

Abstract

Pi² and Nugrip are pyrocarbon implants for thumb basal joint osteoarthritis after trapeziectomy. Pi² implant is a free spacer whereas the Nugrip is an hemiprosthesis. The author reports the results in the literature of both implants and describes Pi² pyrocarbon implant technique for primary thumb basal joint osteoarthritis. The key points of the Pi² procedure are: preservation of the soft tissue environment during the trapeziectomy, partial trapezoidectomy to medialize the implant, and careful capsuloplasty and ligamentoplasty to stabilize the implant.

Keywords: Pyrocarbon, thumb basal joint, osteoarthritis, arthroplasty, CMC implant, trapeziectomy

19.1 Introduction

Today's bioindustrial proficiency in pyrocarbon technology has led to its use in the field of orthopedics, most particularly in hand and wrist surgery with the development of joint prostheses or hemiprostheses and new implants.[1,2,3]

19.2 Characteristic of Implants

19.2.1 Pi²

Whright Pi² implant is a free spacer because there is no bone or ligament fixation (▸ Fig. 19.1). It can therefore be mobile, and its shape allows it to adapt its position to thumb movements. Implant stability is based to a large extent on the soft tissues, which prevent it from coming out of its trapezium fossa. The implant is oval with two axes. When the implant is positioned, its largest axis is perpendicular to the thumb column. The implant comes in two sizes (thickness by length): 9 × 13 mm and 9 × 15 mm. The 9-mm thickness was chosen to be slightly smaller than the trapezium height, which is on average 11 mm. The implant thus maintains a certain height in its trapezium compartment without being subjected to or subjecting the scaphoid or the metacarpal base to excessive stresses that could result in bone resorption.

19.2.2 Nugrip

Ascension NuGrip™ CMC Implant is not a free spacer but a pyrocarbon hemiprosthesis. This is the second-generation PyroHemiSpher implant that has been specifically designed for the treatment of osteoarthritis in the thumb carpometacarpal joint (▸ Fig. 19.2).

19.3 Results in the Literature

19.3.1 Pi²

This ellipsoidal free implant was originally intended for total TMC implant failures before being routinely used as a trapezium spacer for primary treatment of TMC

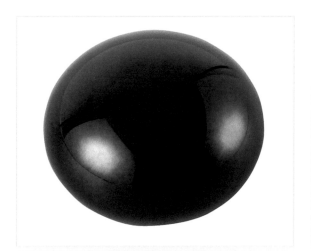

Fig. 19.1 Pi² implant.

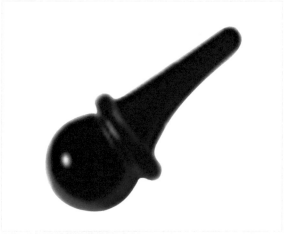

Fig. 19.2 Nugrip hemiprosthesis.

osteoarthritis.[4] The Pi^2 implant has been afterward our technique of choice for treating TMC osteoarthritis. In a short-term prospective and comparative study, Alligand-Perrin et al[5] found earlier functional recovery and better overall patient satisfaction with the Pi^2 implant than with trapeziectomy stabilization. The Ardouin and Bellemère study at 5-year follow-up[6] was supplemented by that of Agout et al[7] at a minimum of 10-year follow-up. Of the 29 implants reviewed, 96.6% of patients were satisfied or very satisfied, pain measured 1.6/10, and the QuickDASH was 19.9%, while grip strength was 24 kg and key pinch was 5.9 kg.[7] The preoperative metacarpophalangeal (MCP) hyperextension did not get worse and the thumb column's mobility increased.[7] No implants were revised.[7] Radiologically, 4.2% of the implants were dislocated, 48.2% (29% at 5-year follow-up) had signs of bone remodeling, mainly of the scaphoid distal pole, averaging 11.2% (8.5% at 5-year follow-up) of its height, without functional repercussions.[7] These good results are unusual. Many authors[8,9,10,11,12] found an early implant dislocation rate between 12.5 and 33% and a revision rate between 4 and 33%. However, the implantation method in these studies differed from ours, either in the approach or the stabilization technique (when performed). This underlines the demanding and precise nature of this procedure, mastery of which may require a lengthy learning curve.

19.3.2 Nugrip

In a recent publication comparing the results of 47 pyrocarbon hemiarthroplasties (24 Nugrip and 23 PyroHemiSpher) with those of 40 trapeziectomies performed using Thompson technique, there was no significant difference in pain, strength, mobility, and QuickDASH scores at an average follow-up of more than 24 months.[13] PyroHemiSpher implants have a significantly better functional thumb score (Nelson score) but higher complication, revision, and failure rates. Scaphotrapeziotrapezoid (STT) osteoarthritis (OA) decompensation occurred in 23% of cases and there was a 30% revision rate mainly due to STT OA; 17% were failures revised by trapeziectomy. Radiologically, 23% of cases had signs of implant instability and 32% had radiolucent lines up to 0.5 mm thick around the stem.

19.4 Indications/Contraindications

19.4.1 Indications

Indications are basal joint osteoarthritis in patients with primarily Eaton stage III–IV arthritic changes. It can be used in stage II osteoarthritis, but as this technique involves total trapeziectomy, the scaphotrapezial joint will also be removed.

19.4.2 Contraindications

We do not have any contraindications unless hyperextension of the MCP joint is treated when preoperatively hyperextension in the MP joint is 40 degrees or more.

19.5 Pi^2 Implant: Author's Own Experience and Preferred Technique

This procedure does not simply remove the trapezium and replace it with an implant. The technique requires several surgical stages whose sequence and execution must be scrupulously respected.[14] The intervention takes place under locoregional anesthesia with a pneumatic tourniquet at the root of the arm.

19.5.1 Anteroexternal Approach

We use a modified anterior Gedda-Moberg approach (► Fig. 19.3), i.e., slightly medial and centered in a V on the trapezium tubercle. It provides easy access to the abductor pollicis longus (APL) tendon as well as to the flexor carpi radialis (FCR) tendon, which will be used to stabilize the implant. The fascia of the external thenar muscles is detached on its external edge, so that the muscles can be retracted internally, and the trapeziometacarpal joint can be approached as well as the trapezium tubercle. There often is an accessory tendon of the APL, highly variable in size, which is frequently inserted on the thenar muscle fascia or more rarely on the trapezium. This accessory tendon can be left in place or resected.

19.5.2 Nontraumatic Trapeziectomy

Before proceeding to the trapeziectomy, it is important to identify the FCR tendon immediately above the trapezium tubercle. This tendon should be preserved for the duration of the trapeziectomy. This should be done as gently

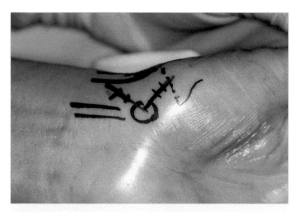

Fig. 19.3 Modified anterior Gedda-type approach.

as possible by disinsertion of the soft peritrapezial tissues at the bone level using a no. 15 blade or a fine periosteal elevator. We use a "corkscrew" screwed into the trapezium and handled like a joystick to expose each facet of the trapezium as much as possible and release them from the surrounding soft tissue (▶ Fig. 19.4). This allows the trapezium to be extracted in the majority of cases in a single piece. The corkscrew is never used as an extractor, which would tear and weaken soft tissue environment. The internal osteophyte of the trapezium, often fractured during trapeziectomy, is removed with the same care as the trapezium.

19.5.3 Partial Trapezoidectomy

A partial trapezoidectomy (approximately one-third of the trapezoid volume) is necessary to slightly medialize the implant in relation to the thumb axis and to treat scaphotrapezoid osteoarthritis if need be (▶ Fig. 19.5). This is done either with a 5-mm curved Lambotte osteotome or gouge forceps. Only the trapezium and scaphoid facets of the trapezoid are resected so that the remaining bone is

at the level of the second metacarpal joint surface, taking care, however, not to go beyond this point.

19.5.4 Placing a Trial Implant and the Final Implant

The 9 × 13 trial implant size is used most frequently. It allows checking whether the implant is properly medialized. Circumduction, opposition, and adduction movements as well as axial compression at the thumb will tend to posteriorly dislocate the implant into the dorsal capsule-ligament redundancy, and anteriorly by the opening. This instability will be treated with capsuloplasty and ligament reconstruction. The final implant is then placed.

19.5.5 Capsuloplasty and Ligament Reconstruction

Capsuloplasty can remove the dorsal capsular redundancy, which varies from case to case. A kinking of the tissues with two cross-stitches of 3/0 or a reinsertion-retension at the scaphoid or the metacarpal (▶ Fig. 19.6) is performed. This kinking must be adjusted so as to prevent dorsal luxation of the implant and to avoid an overload between the scaphoid and the metacarpal base.

The ligamentoplasty is made using two tendon strips resected 2 to 3 cm proximally from their distal insertion. One is harvested from the APL and the other from the FCR (▶ Fig. 19.7). The size of each strip is approximately half of the harvested tendon. The FCR strip is attached to the dorsal capsule and the APL strip to the remnants of palmar capsule and ligament. Then the two strips are attached together by crossing each other so the implant is covered, thus stabilizing it with a ligament barrier.

Poorly performed capsuloplasty creates a bulge in the radial fossa by dorsal dislocation of the implant. Poor ligamentoplasty causes subluxation or dislocation of the implant in the thenar muscles. However, capsuloplasty or

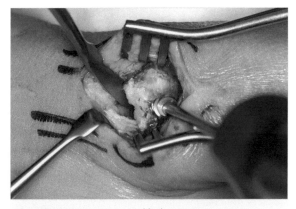

Fig. 19.4 Nontraumatic monoblock trapeziectomy using a corkscrew.

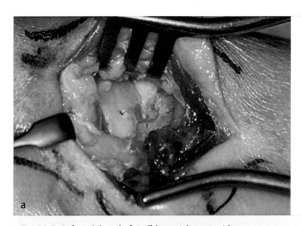
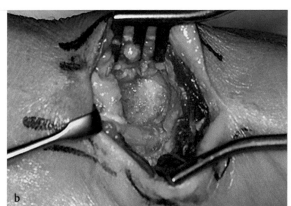

Fig. 19.5 Before (a) and after (b) partial trapezoidectomy.

ligament reconstruction should never constrain the implant: it should remain relatively free in its movements.

All the steps are summarized in ▶ Fig. 19.8.

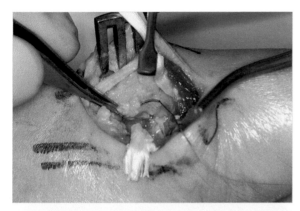

Fig. 19.6 Capsuloplasty. Note the dorsal capsule redundancy.

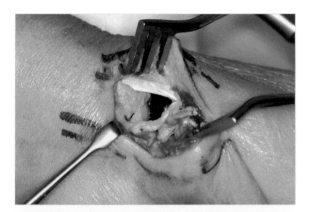

Fig. 19.7 Capsuloplasty and ligament reconstruction. The two-tendon strips harvested from the abductor pollicis longus and the flexor carpi radialis.

19.5.6 Closure and X-Rays

The external thenar muscles are repositioned with regard to the ligament reconstruction and their fascia reattached. No drainage is necessary. The skin is closed using resorbable intradermic suture. The implant position is verified scopically (▶ Fig. 19.9).

19.5.7 Postoperative Care and Rehabilitation

A removable splint is worn continually for the first 2 weeks postoperative. After removal of the bandage on the 15th day, self-rehabilitation is begun aiming to restore range of motion of the thumb. The splint is worn at night and episodically as needed during the day until the fourth week.

19.5.8 Possible Complementary Procedures

Treatment of Associated Carpal Tunnel Syndrome

The flexor retinaculum via its external edge can be opened by the same approach and released from its attachments to the trapezium, trapezoid, and scaphoid.[6] The FCR opened sheath reveals the flexor pollicis longus.

Treatment of MP Joint Hyperextension

When preoperatively hyperextension in the MP joint is 40 degrees or more and is partially corrected by the Pi^2, we correct the residual hyperextension during the same procedure. We first perform an anterior sesamoidesis and capsulodesis with an oblique incision centered on the MP joint. The neck of the metacarpal is approached between

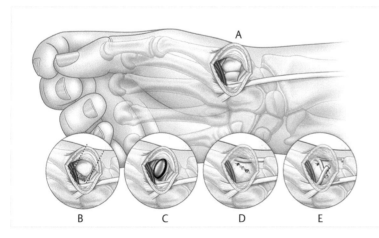

Fig. 19.8 Summary of the procedure. (A) Monoblock trapeziectomy. (B) Partial trapezoidectomy. (C) Placing the final implant. (D) Capsuloplasty. (E) Ligament reconstruction.

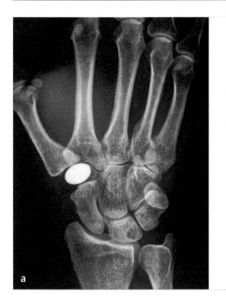

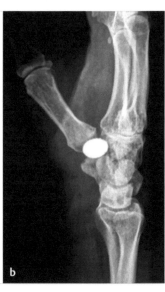

Fig. 19.9 X-ray of Pi² implant in place: **(a)** anteroposterior and **(b)** lateral. The implant is slightly medialized in relation to the thumb column axis.

19

the thenar muscles and roughened with a curette. An intraosseous minianchor is pinned in the bone which fastens the anterior capsule and the external sesamoid, with the MP joint slightly flexed. The second step is the tenodesis of the extensor pollicis brevis, which is done either by extending the opening dorsally or by a new incision on the dorsal surface of the metacarpal neck, which is then roughened. A second anchor provides fixation of the extensor pollicis brevis in slight tension to the metacarpal neck.

References

[1] Cook SD, Beckenbaugh RD, Redondo J, Popich LS, Klawitter JJ, Linscheid RL. Long-term follow-up of pyrolytic carbon metacarpophalangeal implants. J Bone Joint Surg Am. 1999; 81(5):635–648

[2] Péquignot JP, Lussiez B, Allieu Y. Implant adaptatif du scaphoïde proximal. Chir Main. 2000; 19(5):276–285

[3] Bellemère P. Pyrocarbon implants for the hand and wrist. Hand Surg Rehabil. 2018; 37(3):129–154

[4] Péquignot JP, Belleme're P, Berthe A. Les reprises de prothe' ses trape´zo- me´ tacarpiennes par implant mobile en pyrocarbone: PI2. Etude d'une série rétrospective de 30 cas avec un recul moyen de 5,5 ans (4 à` 7 ans). Chir Main. 2011; 30:S117–S122

[5] Alligand-Perrin P, Bellemère P, Gaisne E, et al. Pyrocarbon Pi2 interposition arthroplasty versus trapeziectomy-ligament reconstruction-suspension in the treatment of trapeziometacarpal osteoarthritis: preliminary comparative study of two series over one year. Rev Chir Orthop Repar Appar Mot. 2010; 96S:S66–S71

[6] Ardouin L, Bellemère P. A 5-year prospective outcome study of Pi2 pyrocarbon arthroplasty for the treatment of thumb carpometacarpal joint osteoarthritis. Chir Main. 2011; 30:S17–S23

[7] Agout C, Ardouin L, Bellemère P. A ten-year prospective outcome study of Pi2 pyrocarbon spacer arthroplasty in carpometacarpal joint osteoarthritis. Hand Surg Rehabil. 2016; 35(4):255–261

[8] Colegate-Stone TJ, Garg S, Subramanian A, Mani GV. Outcome analysis of trapezectomy with and without pyrocarbon interposition to treat primary arthrosis of the trapeziometacarpal joint. Hand Surg. 2011; 16(1):49–54

[9] Maru M, Jettoo P, Tourret L, Jones M, Irwin L. Thumb carpometacarpal osteoarthritis: trapeziectomy versus pyrocarbon interposition implant (Pi2) arthroplasty. J Hand Surg Eur Vol. 2012; 37(7):617–620

[10] Cheval D, Sauleau V, Moineau G, Le Jacques B, Le Nen D. Total trapeziectomy and suspension ligamentoplasty: is there any interest to interpose a pyrocarbon Pi2® implant? Chir Main. 2013; 32(3):169–175

[11] Szalay G, Meyer C, Scheufens T, Schnettler R, Christ R, Schleicher I. Pyrocarbon spacer as a trapezium replacement for arthritis of the trapeziometacarpal joint; a follow-up study of 60 cases. Acta Orthop Belg. 2013; 79(6):648–654

[12] van Aaken J, Holzer N, Wehrli L, Delaquaize F, Gonzalez IA, Beaulieu JY. Unacceptable failure of the PI2® implant. J Hand Surg Eur Vol. 2016; 41(9):917–922

[13] Vitale MA, Hsu CC, Rizzo M, Moran SL. Pyrolytic carbon arthroplasty versus suspensionplasty for trapezial-metacarpal arthritis. J Wrist Surg. 2017; 6(2):134–143

[14] Bellemère P, Ardouin L. Pi2 spacer pyrocarbon arthroplasty technique for thumb basal joint osteoarthritis. Tech Hand Up Extrem Surg. 2011; 15(4):247–252

20 Pyrocardan and Pyrodisk Arthroplasties of the Thumb CMC Joint

Philippe Bellemère

Abstract

Pyrocardan and Pyrodisk implants are made of pyrocarbon and used as interposition arthroplasty for the treatment of the thumb CMC joint osteoarthritis. The aim of interposition implants is to preserve the thumb length to allow normal thumb motion and function.

Pyrodisk is a biconvex disk with a central hole used for a ligamentoplasty to stabilize the implant and the base of the metacarpal. It may be used after partial or total trapeziectomy in any stage of osteoarthritis. Pyrocardan implant is biconcave and rectangular-shaped. It is thinner than Pyrodisk. It is used as an interfacing arthroplasty between the trapezoid and the metacarpal in early stages of osteoarthritis (Eaton's stage 1, 2 and early stage 3). Its implantation preserves capsuloligamentous soft tissues of the joint and therefore no ligamentoplasty is required.

Mid- to long-term outcomes of these two implants have been reported. They show marked improvement on pain, strength, and function. Recovery seems quicker compared to trapeziectomy. With the follow-up bone tolerance is good and clinical outcomes remain stable or tend to progress. Complication rates are low and survival rates are 94% at 8 years for Pyrodisk and 96.2% at 5.5 years for Pyrocardan. Due to Pyrocarbon material these interposition arthroplasties are well tolerated and have eliminated the problems encountered with silicone implants or metallic and polyethylene total prosthesis used in CMC joint.

Keywords: pyrocarbon, CMC joint, implant, arthroplasty, interposition, arthritis, Pyrocardan, Pyrodisk

20.1 Introduction

Because of the remarkable mechanical properties of the pyrocarbon (elasticity, density, roughness, hardness, and resistance to wear durability) and its biocompatibility, pyrocarbon implants have been proposed as an alternative to silicon and other synthetic implants. They have been used in hand since the 1980s and later in wrist.[1]

For the treatment of basal thumb osteoarthritis (OA), two categories of pyrocarbon implants are available:
1. Hemiarthroplasty implants: They replace the metacarpal surface and are stabilized by an intramedullary metacarpal stem: PyroHemiSpher, CMI, Nugrip (see Chapter 19), and Saddle implants.
2. Interposition implants: They are placed between two articulating surfaces either after total or partial trapeziectomy for the Pi[2] (see Chapter 19) and Pyrodisk

implants, or in the trapeziometacarpal (TMC) joint for the Pyrocardan implant. Pyrodisk implant has been used since 2005[2] and Pyrocardan since 2009.[3]

The aim of interposition implants is to preserve the thumb length to allow normal thumb motion and function.

20.2 Pyrodisk

20.2.1 Characteristics of the Implant

Pyrodisk implant (Integra Life Sciences, Plainsboro, NJ, USA) (► Fig. 20.1) is a nonanatomical interposition shaped as a biconvex disk with a central hole to allow stabilization with an autograft tendon, transferred and passed through the trapezium, the implant, and the thumb metacarpal. Six available sizes exist with various combinations of diameters (14 mm, 16 mm, 18 mm) and heights (5.5 mm, 7 mm, 8 mm, 9 mm).

20.2.2 Indications

Pyrodisk implant may be indicated for the treatment of any stages of OA. In the early stages (Eaton's stage 1, 2, and 3), Pyrodisk implant is originally used after partial trapeziectomy. The implant is positioned between the metacarpal and the remaining trapezium (► Fig. 20.2). More severe stages of OA may require total trapeziectomy with interposition of Pyrodisk articulated between the metacarpal and the scaphoid (► Fig. 20.3).

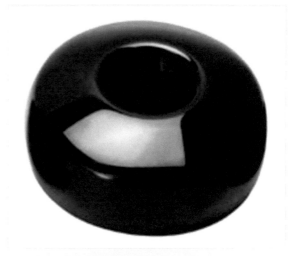

Fig. 20.1 Pyrodisk implant.

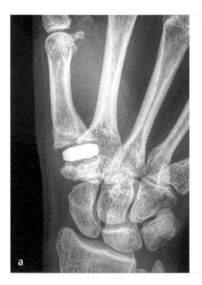
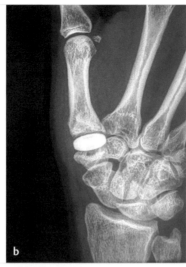

Fig. 20.2 Partial trapeziectomy with Pyrodisk implant. **(a)** Lateral view. **(b)** Frontal view.

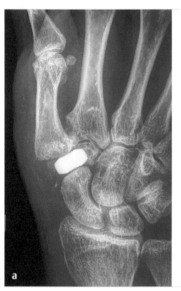
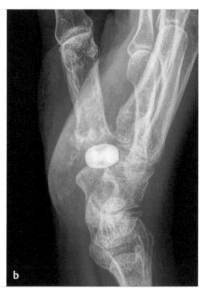

Fig. 20.3 Total trapeziectomy with Pyrodisk implant. **(a)** Lateral view. **(b)** Frontal view.

20.2.3 Surgical Technique

The approach is dorsal over the trapezium. Two to 3 mm of bone is removed with an oscillating saw from the metacarpal base perpendicular from its long axis. The trapezial surface is flattened with the saw with a cut parallel to the metacarpal cut. A reamer is used to dig a small concavity on the trapezium and metacarpal surfaces. In each bone a 3.2-mm drill hole is created obliquely toward the center of the TMC joint in the middle of the cavities starting for the trapezium from the center of the scaphotrapezial joint and for the metacarpal from its dorsal radial aspect. The proper implant diameter is determined by selecting the size that provides the best fit to the diameter of the thumb metacarpal base without overhang. If the best size falls between two available sizes, then the smaller size is chosen. The goal is to achieve a gentle rocking motion of the biconvex disk on the concave surfaces of both the thumb metacarpal base and the trapezium.

Intraoperative fluoroscopy confirms proper sizing.

One of the bundles of the abductor pollicis longus tendon or half of the flexor carpi radialis (FCR) tendon[4] is used as a stabilizer tendon. The distal stump of the distally based tendon is passed through the trapezium, into the resected joint through the selected Pyrodisk implant and into the thumb metacarpal base to exit dorsally through the prepared passage. Gentle traction is applied to the tendon prior to closure to enhance stability. The remaining tendon then is folded back and incorporated into a secure capsular closure.

After surgery, the wrist and thumb are immobilized in a thumb spica plaster orthosis for 3 weeks. A removable orthosis is used during the next 8 to 9 weeks during which the patient performs active range of motion exercises and uses the hand for daily activities. After 11 to 12 weeks, unrestricted activities are allowed.

20.2.4 Results in the Literature

A retrospective series by Barrera-Ochoa et al[2] included 19 patients reviewed at a minimum 5-year follow-up. Eighty-nine percent of patients were satisfied or very satisfied, pain measured 1.7 (visual analog scale [VAS]), Quick-DASH scored 20.2, mobility was not significantly improved, and grip strength (20 kg) increased significantly. The failure rate was 10.5%, associated with painful instabilities, revised by trapeziectomy after 1 year. Long-term outcomes of reported similar results with a survival rate of 94% at 8 years.[5]

The series by Mariconda et al[6] included 27 patients reviewed at an average follow-up of 37 months. It showed better results on pain and Quick-DASH score. Ninety-six percent of patients were satisfied or very satisfied. There were no complications or revisions. Radiologically, one implant was dislocated and no bone subsidence was noted.

In indications of perfectly centered rhizarthrosis, Odella et al[7] generally obtained good pain results with Pyrodisk. However their results on strength (a 20% loss) were in contradiction with those of Barrera-Ochoa et al (a 26% gain).[2] They also reported a failure rate of 3% and 3% implant dislocation.

A recent retrospective comparative series[2] of ligament reconstruction and tendon interposition (LRTI) (19 cases) versus Pyrodisk (20 cases) showed a significant better key pinch strength (1.8 kg higher) with the Pyrodisk after a minimum follow-up of 2 years. No differences were found in other functional criteria or in complication rates.

20.2.5 Author's Experience

The Pyrodisk implant can also be used after total trapeziectomy (▶ Fig. 20.4), as proposed by Vitale et al[8] and Chaise.[9] Like the Pi[2] implantation (see Chapter 19), a partial trapezoidectomy is required to medialize the implant and for the treatment of an associated scapho-trapezoid OA (▶ Fig. 20.4). To stabilize the implant a strip of the FCR tendon,[8] or a ligamentoplasty with a thread of Goretex CV/0[9] may be used. This latter implant stabilization technique is simpler and less invasive than that used for the Pi[2] implant (see Chapter 19). However, in our experience of more than 80 implants, the failure rate (revised by implant) for chronic pain enduring beyond 1 year was 6% and we found that the overall clinical results, especially regarding pain, seemed inferior to those of the Pi[2] implant. Since the Pyrodisk implant is more constrained than the Pi[2], pain originating in the bone may be associated with excessive stress peaks. Failure to stabilize the implant and the base of the metacarpal with the follow-up may occur with the follow-up as shown in some cases of our series (▶ Fig. 20.5). It may be due to frictional wear of the ligamentoplasty in the articulating surfaces and can be facilitated by the biconvex shape of the implant.

20

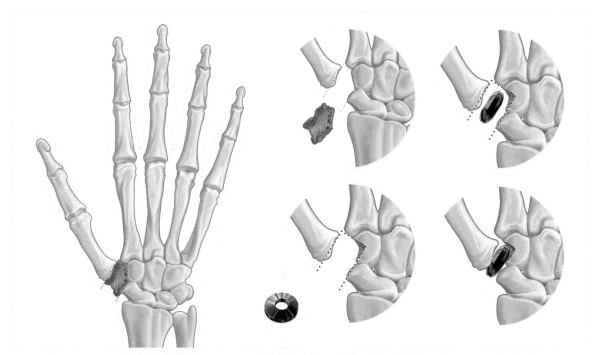

Fig. 20.4 Drawing of the principles of the procedure of Pyrodisk implant with total trapeziectomy.

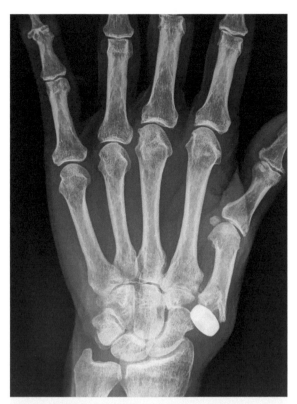

Fig. 20.5 Radiograph showing instability of the metacarpal and the Pyrodisk implant occurring with time.

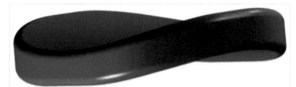

Fig. 20.6 Pyrocardan implant.

20.3 Pyrocardan

20.3.1 Characteristics of the Implant

Pyrocardan implant (Wright Medical-Tornier SAS, Bioprofile, Grenoble, France) (▶ Fig. 20.6) is an intra-articular interfacing unconstrained interposition of the TMC joint.[3] It is rectangular-shaped with two perpendicularly opposing tubular concave faces. This geometry is supposed to replicate the carpometacarpal (CMC) joint movements. The implant has a 1-mm central thickness regardless of size. There are 7 variants, between 12 and 18 mm wide. The thickness of the exterior edges is proportional to the implant size. Its placement requires minimal intra-articular bone resection that respects the capsuloligamentary muscle insertions outside the joint space area.[10] Stabilization ligamentoplasty is, therefore, not necessary.

20.3.2 Indications

This minimally invasive arthroplasty is indicated in minimally destroyed CMC joint as found in the early stages of OA, Eaton's stages 1 and 2, or even in some early stage 3 cases. In fact, most of the patients we see in our practice for a chronic and painful OA of the CMC joint are eligible for a Pyrocardan arthroplasty which is now our treatment of choice.

There is no restriction of age or activity of the patient. Young or active patients are not a contraindication.

However, this implant is not indicated in case of severe collapse or core modification (cyst) of the trapezium or in the case of a subluxation of more than one-third of the metacarpal base.

We recommend not using Pyrocardan implants in case of severe Z-deformity of the thumb column. This implant is not able to restore thumb length and realign correctly the metacarpal base.

20.3.3 Surgical Technique (▶ Fig. 20.7)

We recommend a dorsal approach to the CMC joint with a skin incision of about 30 mm.[11] The capsule is opened and released from the dorsal aspect of the metacarpal with a longitudinal medial joint opening delimiting two dorsal capsular flaps prolonged with the periosteum of the dorsal metacarpal (▶ Fig. 20.8). Using a thin oscillating saw, the dorsal and palmar beaks of the metacarpal saddle are resected, thereby altering the saddle shape of the metacarpal surface. Then with the saw, the lateral and medial horns of the trapezium are resected, noting that the medial horn is often more prominent than the lateral horn, due to the joint space obliquity and to the presence of an internal osteophyte. Cuts of the metacarpal and the trapezium surfaces must be orthogonal to the thumb column's axis. This allows metacarpal realignment in case of preoperative dislocation (less or equal to one-third). A complete joint synovectomy is then performed, respecting the continuity of the capsule. Using a burr, all irregularities of the bone cuts are removed. The metacarpal surface is remodeled into a slightly spherical convex surface (like a top of a Champagne cork), and the trapezium is remodeled to an anteroposterior cylindrical slightly convex surface. The trial implant is then positioned and can be checked under fluoroscopy. The implant size is selected so that it completely covers the trapezium. After placement of the final implant, the dorsal capsuloperiosteal flaps are repositioned and sutured to one another without excessive tension, eventually assisted by an intraosseous anchorage at the metacarpal base and reinforced with a running suture on the periosteum.

Postoperative care has been standardized, by immobilization using a thermoformed orthosis worn constantly for 2 weeks. Self-rehabilitation is then started and the

20

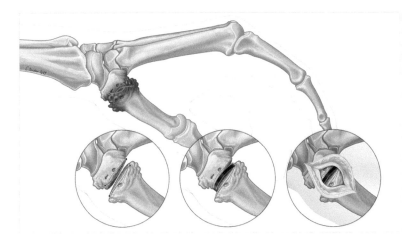

Fig. 20.7 Drawing of the principles of the procedure of Pyrocardan implant in carpometacarpal (CMC) joint.

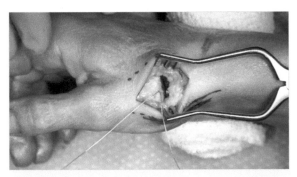

Fig. 20.8 Operative view of Pyrocardan implant in carpometacarpal (CMC) joint before closing the two longitudinal capsular flaps prolongated with the dorsal periosteal of the metacarpal. The threads come from a bone anchor.

orthosis is worn overnight and occasionally during the day until the fourth week. There is no systematic postoperative physiotherapy protocol, and no restrictions for the use of the thumb after the sixth week.

The implant can also be placed by an anterior or an arthroscopic approach but we found these two approaches more difficult to perform than the dorsal one for a perfect bone surfaces preparation and adequate positioning of the implant.

20.3.4 Results in the Literature

Final outcomes seem to be influenced by the indications and the surgical technique.

In a series comparing 25 Pyrocardan and 36 Pyrodisk implants, placed in cases of stage 1 to 3 rhizarthrosis, Odella et al[7] got better results with the Pyrodisk. However, the series was biased by the respective indications of the two implants: Pyrocardan being indicated only in cases of metacarpal dislocation while Pyrodisk reserved for well-centered joint.

Lauwers et al[12] performed 25 Pyrocardan implants by extensive anterior approach associated with FCR ligamentoplasty. They reported 18.5% failure rate at 25 months

follow-up. They explain the divergence between their results and those of our initial series[3] by the difference in operative technique and the necessity of a learning curve for the placement of this implant.

The series by Russo et al[13] that assessed 36 cases of stage 1 to 3 rhizarthrosis showed good results at an average follow-up of 31.5 months. Two cases required implant repositioning after early dislocation, although the stage of CMC OA was not reported.

Erne et al[14] compared a small Pyrocardan implant series with Lundborg's trapeziectomy-ligamentoplasty series. At an average 1.5-year follow-up, the Pyrocardan series has a significantly faster asymptomatic functional recovery time.

In a prospective case series of 40 Pyrocardan with a mean follow-up of 29 months, Logan et al[15] reported comparable clinical outcomes to our original series.[3] Moreover, grip and pinch strength were superior to LRTI procedure in a match cohort.

20.3.5 Author's Experience

The results of our preliminary series of 27 patients,[3] with an average follow-up of 16.6 months, showed 100% of patients satisfied or very satisfied. VAS measured 1.6, and Quick-DASH and Patient Rated Wrist Evaluation (PRWE) scores were 10.1 and 12.9, respectively. Comparable mobility was on the opposite side, while grip strength of 25 kg and pinch strength of 6.7 kg were 97 and 100% on the opposite side, respectively. No revision was needed and no radiological dislocation or loosening was found.

We studied at a minimum 5-year follow-up, 103 case series (unpublished study yet),[16] including the cohort of our initial series, with a minimal follow-up of 70 months. In this midterm series, there were 27% manual workers (▶ Fig. 20.9) and 39% preoperative subluxation of the first metacarpal. This study demonstrated improvement in values of pain, strength, and function between the short and the long term. Final outcomes showed significant improvement in postoperative value for pain of 0.6 on

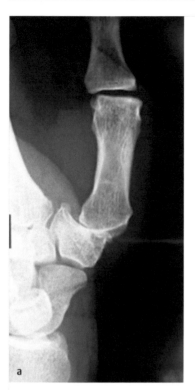

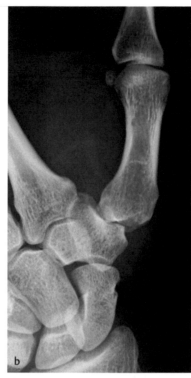

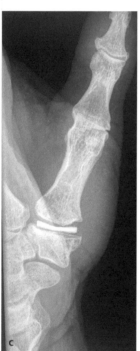

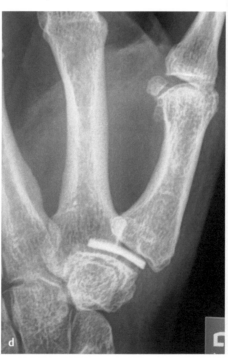

Fig. 20.9 Carpometacarpal (CMC) osteoarthritis (OA) with subluxation of the metacarpal in a 47-year-old heavy manual worker treated with Pyrocardan implant. No ligamentoplasty was performed. Return to work was 3.5 months postoperatively. After 7 years, the patient is pain free; thumb range of motion (ROM), and pinch and grip strength are comparable to the opposite side. **(a, b)** Preoperative view showing metacarpal subluxation. **(c, d)** Postoperative radiographs after 7 years.

VAS scale (7 preoperatively), PRWE of 4 (58 preoperatively), Quick-DASH of 9 (52 preoperatively), and tip-pinch strength of 7 kg (5 preoperatively). There were no significant differences in key-pinch (8 kg) strength, grip strength (27 kg postoperatively), and mobility compared to the opposite side. The average return to work time for nonheavy manual workers was 12 weeks and for heavy manual workers 13.5 weeks. Satisfaction rate was 96%.

Preoperative metacarpal subluxation was reduced postoperatively in 80% of patients. No significant bone remodeling or implant instability was found in the follow-up (▶ Fig. 20.10).

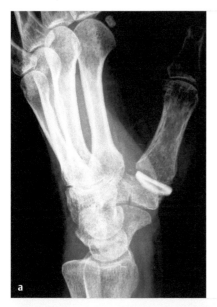
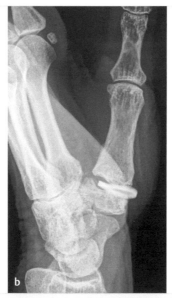
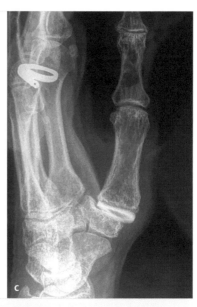

Fig. 20.10 Long-term results in a dominant hand of a 60-year-old retired woman. Pyrocardan implant is not perfectly positioned because the trapezial articulating surface is not enough prepared on its medial side. **(a)** Postoperative radiograph after 1 month. Note the subluxation of the implant and the base of the metacarpal. **(b)** Postoperative radiograph after 5 years. No worsening of the malposition. **(c)** Postoperative radiograph after 10 years. The implant is perfectly well tolerated. The patient is pain free with Kapandji scoring at 10, tip pinch of 8 kg, key pinch of 10 kg, grip pinch of 30 kg, Quick-DASH = 9.09, PRWE = 2.

Two patients had reoperation for changing the size of the implant and remodeling the shape of the articulating bone surfaces.

Two patients had to have their implant removed and converted to a trapeziectomy after about 1 year due to chronic pain. The 5-year implant survival rate was 96.2 %.

20.4 Tips and Tricks for Pyrodisk and Pyrocardan Implants

- Orientation of the articulating surfaces after bone preparation should be perpendicular to the axis of the thumb column including longitudinal axis of the scaphoid.
- Sizing of the implant should fully cover the trapezium surface.
- Avoid overstuffing joint. If so, change the thickness of the implant in case of Pyrodisk, or remove more articulating surfaces in case of Pyrocardan.
- Use peroperative fluoroscopy to check the positioning of the trial implant, the correct bone preparation especially on its medial side and the collinearity of the metacarpal, the implant and the trapezium (or the scaphoid in case of Pyrodisk after trapeziectomy).
- Do not tighten longitudinally the ligamentoplasty of the Pyrodisk implant, or the capsule closure of the Pyrocardan implant to avoid an overstuffed joint.
- Surgical technique may require a learning curve. Attendance at a cadaver laboratory may be beneficial to shorten it.[15]

20.5 Conclusion

Pyrodisk and Pyrocardan implants are effective in terms of pain relief and function improvement for the treatment of CMC joint OA. They both preserve the length of the thumb column providing better improvement in strength and quicker function recovery without pain compared to trapeziectomy. Complication rates are low. Due to pyrocarbon material these interposition arthroplasties are well tolerated and have eliminated the problems encountered with silicone implants or metallic and polyethylene prosthesis used in CMC joint.

References

[1] Bellemère P. Pyrocarbon implants for the hand and wrist. Hand Surg Rehabil. 2018; 37(3):129–154
[2] Barrera-Ochoa S, Vidal-Tarrason N, Correa-Vázquez E, Reverte-Vinaixa MM, Font-Segura J, Mir-Bullo X. Pyrocarbon interposition (PyroDisk) implant for trapeziometacarpal osteoarthritis: minimum 5-year follow-up. J Hand Surg Am. 2014; 39(11):2150–2160
[3] Bellemère P, Gaisne E, Loubersac T, Ardouin L, Collon S, Maes C. Pyrocardan implant: free pyrocarbon interposition for resurfacing trapeziometacarpal joint. Chir Main. 2011; 30:S28–S35
[4] Oh WT, Chun YM, Koh IH, Shin JK, Choi YR, Kang HJ. Tendon versus pyrocarbon interpositional arthroplasty in the treatment of trapeziometacarpal osteoarthritis. BioMed Res Int. 2019; 10. Article ID 7961507
[5] Smeraglia F, Barrera-Ochoa S, Mendez-Sanchez G, Basso MA, Balato G, Mir-Bullo X. Partial trapeziectomy and pyrocarbon interpositional arthroplasty for trapeziometacarpal osteoarthritis: minimum 8-year follow-up. J Hand Surg Eur. 2020;45:472–476
[6] Mariconda M, Russo S, Smeraglia F, Busco G. Partial trapeziectomy and pyrocarbon interpositional arthroplasty for trapeziometacarpal

joint osteoarthritis: results after minimum 2 years of follow-up. J Hand Surg Eur Vol. 2014; 39(6):604–610

[7] Odella S, Querenghi AM, Sartore R, DE Felice A, Dacatra U. Trapeziometacarpal osteoarthritis: pyrocarbon interposition implants. Joints. 2015; 2(4):154–158

[8] Vitale MA, Taylor F, Ross M, Moran SL. Trapezium prosthetic arthroplasty (silicone, Artelon, metal, and pyrocarbon). Hand Clin. 2013; 29 (1):37–55

[9] Chaise F. Les arthroplasties d'interposition trapézométacarpiennes au Pyrodisk. Résultats de 40 interventions avec 1 an de recul minimum. Chir Main. 2011; 30:S24–S27– (in French)

[10] Maes-Clavier C, Bellemère P, Gabrion A, David E, Rotari V, Havet E. Anatomical study of the ligamentous attachments and articular surfaces of the trapeziometacarpal joint: consequences on surgical management of its osteoarthrosis. Chir Main. 2014; 33(2):118–123

[11] Video of the current surgical technique of Pyrocardan interposition in TMC joint. Available at: https://youtu.be/_pOgo7qW27Y

[12] Lauwers TM, Brouwers K, Staal H, Hoekstra LT, van der Hulst RR. Early outcomes of Pyrocardan® implants for trapeziometacarpal osteoarthritis. Hand Surg Rehabil. 2016; 35(6):407–412

[13] Russo S, Bernasconi A, Busco G, Sadile F. Treatment of the trapeziometacarpal osteoarthritis by arthroplasty with a pyrocarbon implant. Int Orthop. 2016; 40(7):1465–1471

[14] Erne HC, Schmauß D, Cerny M, et al. Lundborg's resection arthroplasty vs. Pyrocarbon spacer (Pyrocardan®) for the treatment of trapeziometacarpal joint osteoarthritis: a two-centre study. Handchir Mikrochir Plast Chir. 2017; 49(3):175–180– (in German)

[15] Logan J, Peters S, Strauss R, Manzanero S, Couzens G, Ross M. Pyrocardan trapeziometacarpal joint arthroplasty: medium term outcomes. J Wrist Surg. 2020;9(6):509–517

[16] Gerace E, Royaux D, Gaisne E, Ardouin L, Bellemere P. Pyrocardan® implant arthroplasty for trapeziometacarpal osteoarthritis with a minimum of five years of follow-up. Hand Surg and Rehabil. 2020; 39(6):528–538

20

21 Total Thumb CMC Arthroplasty

Bruno Lussiez

Abstract

Trapeziometacarpal prostheses, along with trapeziectomies and interposition arthroplasties, are one of the modern surgical options for the treatment of trapeziometacarpal osteoarthritis. The short-term and medium-term results have been improved by modifications of the initial models (modularity, anatomic stems, bony fixation, surgical technique) and their indications have now been extended. The level of complications is acceptable for many of the models. Dislocations are uncommon (single and double mobility principle). The future improvements will focus on durability of polyethylene and bony fixation of the trapezial cup. Indications are actually based on the level of activity of the patient, and radiological aspect of the osteoarthritis and the trapezium.

Keywords: trapeziometacarpal osteoarthritis, surgical treatment, prosthesis, arthroplasty

21.1 Introduction

Osteoarthritis of first carpometacarpal (CMC) joint is the second most common location of degenerative arthritis of the hand.[1] It is in fact a regional condition, with consequences on the constitutive elements of the thumb: metacarpophalangeal (MCP) joint, extensor and flexor tendons, tendons of the first compartment, muscles of the first web, carpal tunnel. It may create instability of the first column with different consequences: functional (pain), biomechanical (strength), anatomical (mobility), and esthetic (Z-deformation). First treatment is conservative, and surgical procedure is only proposed in case of failure. Indications are then high level of pain, decrease of strength (key-pinch, grasp), stiffness of the first ray, and sometimes esthetic aspect (Z-deformation). Trapeziectomy and arthrodesis of the CMC joint were the first procedures to be proposed,[2,3] followed by several modifications of trapeziectomy, such as tendon interposition, chondrocostal interposition, and ligamentoplasty (abductor pollicis longus [APL], flexor carpi radialis [FCR] tendons). CMC arthrodesis causes significant decrease in mobility and high level of complications.[4]

Outcomes of the different trapeziectomy procedures are generally reliable, but with some drawbacks (irreversible osseous resection, shortening of the thumb, Z-deformation, intracarpal instability, delay of recovery, low strength). In early cases of osteoarthritis, with dysplasia of the trapezium, different types of osteotomy have been proposed, with long-term good results.

For better preservation of length of the first ray, two other types of surgical procedure have been more recently introduced: interposition implants and coupled prosthesis. Implants may be associated with partial (resurfacing) or total (interposition spacer) trapeziectomy. Most of them are now made of pyrolytic carbon, with a compatible module of elasticity and optimal wear resistance.[5] Instability of some types of these implants[6] limits their indications.

Total trapeziometacarpal joint "ball-and-socket" prosthesis was proposed in the early 1970s. The aim is to give a stable fulcrum between trapezium and first metacarpal, allowing conservation of centers of rotation of the joint for optimal muscular action, and conservation of length of first ray.

21.2 Historical Aspects

Jean-Yves de la Caffinière,[7] a French orthopaedic surgeon, designed in 1971 (▸ Fig. 21.1), and published in 1973 the first total CMC 1 prosthesis, based on the principle of "ball-and-socket." This prosthesis was made of chromium-cobalt alloy, cemented with a straight neck, straight stem, polyethylene cup, and single size. First results are disappointing, with high levels of loosening of the cup.[8] Modification of this first implant was made and results published by de la Caffinière.[9] Long-term results were good[10,11,12] or moderate,[13] limiting the use of this prosthesis in elderly low-demanding patients. In 1982 Braun analyzed the results of 29 "Braun-Cutter" implants and later Badia and Sambandam[14] reviewed 26 cases with good results, recommending this technic for low-activity-demanding old patients. Then a second generation of ball-and-socket prosthesis appeared in the 1990s, with modifications in the design and fixation. Some types were evolution of same initial implants (GUEPAR); others were modifications of other

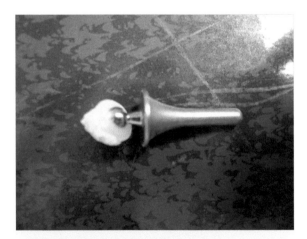

Fig. 21.1 de La Caffinière carpometacarpal (CMC) 1 prosthesis.

initial implants (Maia, modification of initial Arpe, Isis evolution of GUEPAR II). Some of them disappeared due to commercial failure or high level of complications.[15,16,17,18,19] Although a number of reports were made by the original conceptors, there were few cases and few prospective analyses, making the analysis of these different implants difficult. Then long-term follow-up of some of these prostheses[20,21,22,23,24,25,26,27] allowed accurate choice of the implants, and were followed by ultimate modifications (semiretentivity, double mobility) in the concept of the prosthesis (▶ Fig. 21.2).

Actually most of the main models are native from Europe, especially from France, explaining the important differences between the rules of hand and orthopaedic surgeons in surgical treatment of CMC 1 arthritis. Trapeziectomy (with or without ligament reconstruction and tendon interposition [LRTI]) remains the commonest surgical option for the majority of American surgeons, and only 2% of them do prosthesis,[28] whereas the number of CMC prosthesis is between 2 and 3.5 times higher than trapeziectomy in French and Belgian hand surgeon population (▶ Fig. 21.3 and ▶ Fig. 21.4).

21.3 Different Types of Total CMC Arthroplasty (TCA)

The implants used actually are essentially based on the "ball-and-socket" principle, for replacement of the "approximate center of rotation" of normal TM joint.[29,30] Most of them get the center of rotation in the trapezium; in one type (Rubis II) the center is in the base of the first metacarpal. The "ball-and-socket" principle is a simplification of normal anatomical kinematics (nonintersecting and nonorthogonal rotation-axes). Unlike the different technics of trapeziectomy, biomechanically the TCA restores the point of support between the trapezium and the first metacarpal, and anatomically respect most of bone, tendons, and ligaments of the thumb.

The goal of TCA is to restore strength, range of motion, and remove pain.

Huang et al[18] analyzed 19 types of TCA, corresponding to evolution of initial conceptions, drawings, changing of fixation, and apparition of modularity. Certain types of TCA have disappeared due to bad results or commercialization problems.

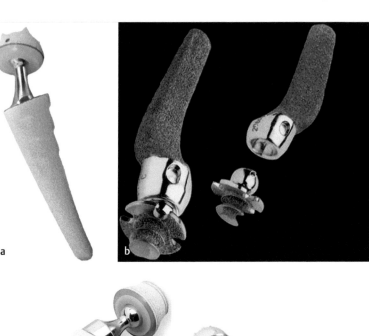
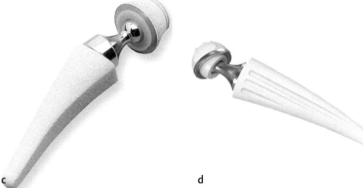

Fig. 21.2 (a–d) Different types of carpometacarpal (CMC) 1 modern arthroplasties: Maia, Rubis II, Ivory, Touch.

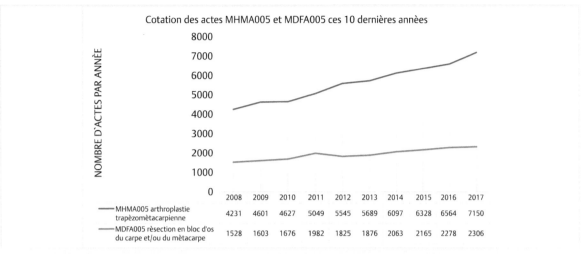

Fig. 21.3 Evolution of number of carpometacarpal (CMC) 1 prosthesis in France (2008–2017).

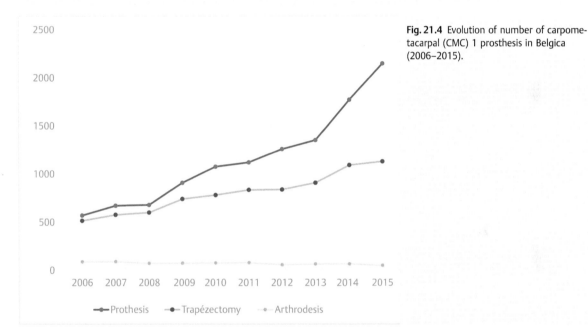

Fig. 21.4 Evolution of number of carpometacarpal (CMC) 1 prosthesis in Belgica (2006–2015).

21

Actually, most of TCA get anatomical design of the stem, with several sizes, several types of neck (length, orientation), several sizes and shapes of cup (hemispherical, cylindro-hemispherical, conical, truncated, screw), and modular construction (stem, neck, cup, insert of Polyethylene [PE]). Most of the types have a metal-polyethylene couple, some metal-on-metal couple. Some models propose semiconstrained couple, for improving stability of the prosthesis. Osteointegration after press-fit insertion is achieved by covering of cup and stem with hydroxyapatite (HA) or porous coating. Some models propose fixation with cement, in first intention or for revision.

Last modifications are applications of the principle of double-mobility, inspired by the hip prosthesis, on the TCA (Moovis, Touch), for improving stability and decreasing the shear forces between the cup and the bone trapezium.

21.3.1 The Models (▶ Table 21.1)

Metal-on-Metal

- **Elektra**[31] is modular, unconstrained, uncemented arthroplasty. Its metacarpal component is a HA-coated titanium stem (four sizes) with chrome-cobalt head and neck (four sizes). The cup (diameter 6.5 mm) is a chrome-cobalt cone-shaped press-fit screw (one size).
- **Motec (Swemac AB)**[32] is unconstrained, uncemented arthroplasty. The stem is a threaded, slightly conical component (four sizes), coated with Bonit. Trapezium is also threaded with HA-coated surface (one size).
- **Rubis I and II**[21] is an unconstrained reverse prosthesis (center of rotation in the base of the first metacarpal), coated with microporous titanium by plasma torch.

Table 21.1 Main different types of TCA

1971: Caffinière (de la) (formerly Howmedica, UK)

1982: Braun-Cutter (SBI/Avanta Orthopaedics, San Diego, CA, USA)

1985: Guepar I (Alnot), not commercialized

1986: Steffee

1987: Cooney (Mayo-Clinic prosthesis)

1989: Roseland 2 (DePuy International Ltd, Leeds, England), not commercialized

1990: MojeAcamo

1990: Ledoux/Carrat: First noncemented TCA (DIMSO/Stryker), not commercialized

1991: Arpe (Zimmer Biomet, Warsaw, IN, USA)

1994: Ivory (Stryker Corporate, Kalamazoo, MI, USA)

1996: Elektra (formerly SBI Inc., Morrisville, PA, USA)

1996: Avanta (Avanta Orthopaedics, San Diego, CA, USA)

1997: Rubis II

1999: Maia (Lepine, Lyon, France)

1999: Nahigian prosthesis

2000: Camargue (France), not commercialized

2003: Guepar II

2006: Isis (Biotech, Evolutis)

2013: Moovis (Stryker Corporate, Kalamazoo, MI, USA))

2014: Touch (Kerimedical, Geneva, Suisse)

Abbreviations: CMC, carpometacarpal; TCA, total CMC arthroplasty.

Triangular section of the stem. Range of motion: 55 degrees in all directions. Trapezial cup is a screwed circular plate.

Metal-on-Polyethylene

- **de la Caffinière**[7]: Chromium-cobalt alloy (Vitalium), cemented with a straight neck, straight stem, polyethylene cup, and single size.
- **Ledoux/Carrat**[33]: Conical cup with six wings, expanded by cylindrical polyethylene liner, producing a "plug" effect and immediate anchorage. Anatomic stem. Arc of mobility is 66 degrees.
- **Braun-Cutter**[14]: Cemented, cylindrical outer shape PE cup and titanium conical stem implants (one size). Arc of mobility is 90 degrees.
- **Roseland**[26]: Semiconstrained noncemented implant with tronco-conical cup (two sizes) and T-shape stem (three sizes), coating with HA in its proximal part. Not commercialized anymore.

- **Arpe**[20,23,27]: Uncemented titanium cup and stem. Modular, straight, and offset neck; two head length; stem (four sizes). The cup is hemispherical, HAP-coated (two sizes, 9 and 10 mm), and the liner PE may be retentive or not retentive. Arc of mobility is 120 degrees.
- **Ivory**[22,34]: Anatomical HA-covered metal stem, double-coned HA-covered cup, with PE (ultra-high molecular UHMPE) insert. The cup presents a double taper, for stable press-fit. Fixation of the neck on the stem in three rotations (−30, 0, +30 degrees). Cup and PE are separate. Arc of mobility is 91 degrees.
- **Isis**[35,36]: Evolution of the Guepar. Titanium stem, triangular, porous coated in its proximal part (five sizes); modular neck with variable length and orientation; semiretentive cup. Arc of mobility is 68 degrees. Two types of cup: cemented (two sizes), screw (one size).
- **Maia**[24,25,37]: Semiconstrained or unconstrained ball-and-socket implant, with anatomical triangular stem (four sizes), removable PE insert, hemispherical cup (two sizes), two types of neck. Arc of mobility is 110 degrees.
- **Moovis**: Double mobility principle, with short triangular stem (three sizes), and conical cup.
- **Touch**: Double mobility principle, neck with inclination of 15 degrees to counteract the horizontal stress of dorsoradial subluxation of certain types of osteoarthritis, and decrease the stress on the trapezium cup.

Ceramics

- **MojeAcamo**: Based on the principle that ceramics have the least amount of wear, and a low friction joint interface. Total ceramic implant, uncemented, coating is a glass-ceramic layer,[19] and osteointegration at the interface bone/implant is favored by roughened surface.
- Another type of TCA is based on **resurfacing prosthesis**, duplicating the double-saddle anatomy of the normal joint.
- **Camargue**: Trapezial implant with saddle shape, and PE insert with saddle shape attached to the stem. Not commercialized since 2005.
- **SR TMC** (Avanta, San Diego, CA, USA): PE metacarpal short stem and trapezium component of chrome cobalt.[38]

21.4 Surgical Technique

The "approximative" center of rotation has to be restored as far as possible during surgery. The orientation of the cup is important for prevention of eccentric wear of PE, instability of the stem, and ideal physiological range of motion of the prosthesis.[39,40]

21.4.1 Surgical Approaches for TCA

Posterolateral or Lateral (▶ Fig. 21.5)

The incision is longitudinal (3–5 cm), distal to the first tendinous compartment (abductor pollicis longus [APL] and extensor pollicis brevis tendons) (▶ Fig. 21.1). After

21

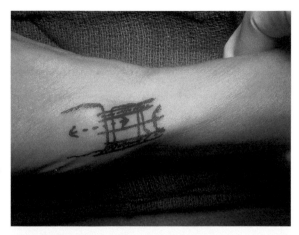

Fig. 21.5 Lateral approach.

visualization of sensitive branches of anterior and dorsal radial nerve, the approach of trapeziometacarpal joint may be of three types: longitudinal, with a proximal capsulo-ligamentar flap, or with L-shape flap. Important steps are the section of the intermetacarpal ligaments, the resection of medial osteophyte and anterior calcifications, synovectomy, and optimal exposure of the trapezium surface. Advantages of this approach are the conservation of insertions of thenar muscles and the quality of closure. Disadvantage is the technically demanding exposure of trapezium surface, especially in male-centered arthritis with strong ligaments.

Anterolateral

It is a modification of the Gedda-Moberg approach without the proximal incurved branch. After dissection of the sensitive branch of anterior radial nerve, a deinsertion of the APL tendon and the proximal insertions of lateral thenar muscles are done, then two capsulo-ligamentar flaps are elevated for optimal exposure of the joint. The main advantage of this approach is the best exposure of trapezium surface.

21.4.2 Steps for Insertion

Whatever the model of prosthesis and the surgical approach, the quality of results depends on few essential points. First of them is the maximum shortening of the learning curve, which means exercises on cadaver pieces before first case, and to be helped during the first case by a senior surgeon. Then respect the following points:

- Optimal exposure of trapezium surface.
- Section of intermetacarpal ligaments.
- Resection of medial trapezial osteophyte.
- Optimal centering and orientation of the cup.
- Intraoperative fluoroscopic control.
- Reinsertion of APL tendon to the APB muscle, or on the base of the first metacarpal, to minimize the risk of dislocation.

- Testing of stability of prosthesis in all sectors of mobility (research of "came-effect").
- Testing of tension: not too tightened to allow mobility and decrease stress on the components, and not too loose to prevent instability. Allow a piston-effect of less of half of the head.

21.4.3 Postoperative Care

Immobilization of the thumb is the rule with cast or splint for a mean period of 3 weeks, but some surgeons authorize early return of light activity of the thumb with protection by removable splint. Rehabilitation may be done after this first period, to reinforce the extrinsic and intrinsic muscle groups, but usually the patient is asked to do the exercises himself. The delay for functional recovering of the thumb is variable, around 10/12 weeks after surgery.

21.5 Results

The results of the CMC joint total arthroplasties depend on the satisfaction of the patient, the objective clinical results (pain, strength, mobility, esthetic aspect), radiological modifications, and the level of complications and revisions.

21.5.1 Results of the Prosthesis

First TCA have been inserted more than 45 years ago, and during this period, there have been good and bad results.[16,18,31,41] Bad results with unacceptable high level of failure for certain types of prosthesis, essentially metal-on-metal articulations,[15,16,17] some material (ceramic),[41,42] and these models have been abandoned because of these known poor results.[15] Actually, main types of TCA have been followed with long-term follow-up,[20,21,22,24,26] and their results are acceptable with high level of satisfaction of the patients.

21.5.2 Comparison with Trapeziectomies

Few analysis compared the two technics. In each of these comparisons the results are better for the prosthesis: strength and delay of recovery,[12,43,44,45,46,47] mobility,[47] Q-DASH, and esthetic aspect.[47]

21.5.3 Complications (▶ Table 21.2)
Related to the Prosthesis

Some complications have almost disappeared: related to the stem (anatomical stem), fracture of the trapezium (best ancillary), related to cement fixation (press-fit/HA/porous-coated fixation). The main problems are localized

21

Table 21.2 Complications related to the prosthesis

	Author	Follow-Up	Kaplan/Meier	Dislocation	Loosening	Revision
Caffiniere de la	Soondergaar 1991	9 yr	82 %			
	Boeckstyn 1989	5 yr	80 %			
	Van Cappelle 1999	16 yr	72 %			
	Johnston 2011	26 yr	74.00 %			
Ledoux/Carat	Ledoux (24 cases) 1997			1.50 %	7 %	12.70 %
Elektra	Klahn (39 cases) 2012	5 yr	60 %	0–7 %	3–47 %	44 %
	Regnard (100 cases) 2006	54 mo	83 %	7 %	15 %	
	Hansen 2013	55 mo				38 %
	Hernandez-Cortes (19 cases) 2012	2 yr			47 %	
Arpe	Ferrero (69 cases) 2014	130 mo	94 %	3–9 %	5–9 %	4.60 %
	Cootjans (120 cases) 2017	80 mo	96 %	4.80 %	0.60 %	3 %
	Apard (32 cases) 2007	5 yr	85 %		15.50 %	22 %
Maia	Bricout (156 cases) 2016	62 mo	90.80 %	4.50 %	2.60 %	11.50 %
	Toffoli (80 cases) 2017	76 mo	93.00 %	1 %	Linear-lucent line 17.6 %	4.20 %
	Andrzejewski 2019	60 mo	92.20 %	9.70 %	Linear-lucent line 5.3 %	12.40 %
Isis	Seng (30 cases) 2013	30 mo	93 %	0 %	10 %	
					Linear-lucent line 20 %	
Ivory	Vissers (26 cases) 2019	130 mo	85 %		Linear-line lucent 30.7 %	15 %
	Goubau (24 cases) 2013	5 yr	95 %			4 %
	Spaans (20 cases) 2016	37 mo		10 %		15 %
Rubis II	Dehl (104 cases) 2017	10 yr	89 %	13 %	1 %	8.70 %
Roseland	Moutet (127 cases) 2011	37 mo		0.80 %	3.20 %	
					Linear-lucent line 6.3 %	
Motec	Hansen (22 cases) 2013	24 mo				27 %
		29 mo				32 %
	Thillemann (42 cases) 2016	2 yr		18 %%	53 %	42 %
Braun-Cutter	Badia (26 cases) 2006	59 mo		3.80 %		3.80 %
MojeAcamo	Kazscap (12 cases) 2012	50 mo				42 %
	Hansen (9 cases) 2008	1 yr				88 %
SR TMC	Ten Brinke (10 cases) 2016	5 yr	80 %			20 %

21

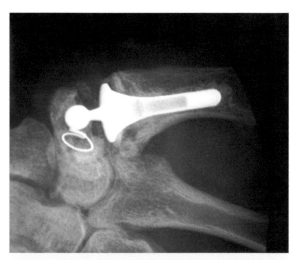

Fig. 21.6 Loosening/tilting of a cup (de La Caffinière).

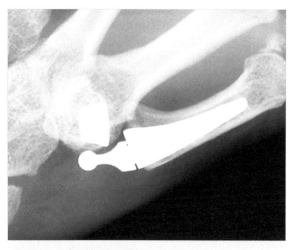

Fig. 21.7 Dislocation (Ivory).

around the cup: failure of fixation (radiolucent lines/loosening, tilting, subsidence),[52] wear of PE, and dislocation (▶ Fig. 21.6 and ▶ Fig. 21.7). The problems of fixation are various: mechanical properties of the material (elasticity), quality of bone in trapezium, quality of osteointegration, level of stress at the interface bone/cup (level of activity), design of the cup, and quality of positioning of the cup at implantation. Wear of PE is frequent after several years, depending on the quality and the thickness of material, but also by penetration of the cup by head of prosthesis.[48] Double mobility and modification of PE (cross-linked) should decrease the incidence of this problem. Dislocation may occur early, due to traumatism or technical error: orientation of the cup, cam-effect with medial osteophyte. Dislocation may appear after several years, related to wear of PE and instability.

De Quervain tenosynovitis is frequent with certain series, related to excessive tension of the implant.

Elevated serum chrome and cobalt values for patients with metal-on-metal articulation (Elektra, Motec), without being a general health risk.[41]

Related to Surgery

Other complications are uncommon: hematoma, infection, allergia, irritation of sensitive branches of radial nerve.

21.5.4 Revision

Thumb CMC joint total exchange arthroplasty may be an option after failed primary arthroplasty, with or without trapezium bone grafting. Changing of the cup (larger cup), replacement of PE, trapeziectomy with suspension plasty, and/or interposition with tendon or spacer are other options, depending on the quality of trapezium. Stem can be left in case of trapeziectomy if no impingement. CMC fusion may be an option in case of irreducible closing of the first web.

The main reason for revision was loosening of the trapezium component, up to 76%[17,41] and dislocation. *Early loosening* (1–2 yr), with migration and/or tilting of the cup, related to no fixation of the cup by absence of osteointegration or trauma, and *late loosening*, totally different, with metal-on-metal prosthesis and metal debris,[33] and metal-on-PE prosthesis with wear of PE and debris of PE at interface bone/cup.

21.6 Indications

To select the best candidate for TCA, the first general considerations to be taken into account are diabetes, smoking, intoxication, number of preoperative injections of corticosteroids or hyaluronic acid.

Then clinical indications are considered: age, level of pain and its tolerance, level of impairment in daily activities such as work, sports, and hobbies, significant decrease in strength, level of activities (low, medium, high), loss of autonomia for elderly people, decrease in mobility. In rare cases, esthetic reason (Z-deformation) is also considered.

Then radiological indications are considered depending on the classification used.[49,50,51] There are technical contraindications: height of trapezium, quality of bone (mediocre quality of trapezium bone is a statistically significant factor),[37] number of infiltrations, known as allergia.

Eaton grade III or some IV for patients with medium-to-high level of functional demand[20] and grade III and selected IV (scapho-trapezo-trapezoidal joint [STT] painless osteoarthritis) for Badia.[14] Dell stages II and III for Vissers.[22] Discrete degenerative changes in STT joint (sclerotic changes and narrowing without osteophytes) appear not to be a contraindication for using TCA. In case of more important changes in STT joint (Dell IV, Eaton IV), clinical examination of this joint determines if pain is reproduced by palpation and mobilization of this joint.

21

21.7 Conclusion

Trapeziometacarpal prosthesis is actually one of the modern options for surgical treatment of CMC 1 osteoarthritis. Since first implantations, the rate of survey of the main types of actual TM prosthesis is similar to the prosthesis of the big joints.

The indications depend on the patient, his age, his level of activity, and the impairment in his daily activities. The patient must be informed of advantages and disadvantages of this technique. Then the radiological aspect of his trapezium and the joints around are the technical judges.

To improve the results, and try to approach the "ideal prosthesis," the construction of a European Joint Registry for prosthesis and implants of CMC 1 joint is an urgent requirement.

References

[1] Batra S, Kanvinde R. Osteoarthritis of the thumb trapeziometacarpal joint. Curr Orthop. 2007; 21:135–144

[2] Gervis WH. Excision of the trapezium for osteoarthritis of the trapezio-metacarpal joint. J Bone Joint Surg Br. 1949; 31B(4):537–539, illust

[3] Muller GM. Arthrodesis of the trapezio-metacarpal joint for osteoarthritis. J Bone Joint Surg Br. 1949; 31B(4):540–542, illust

[4] Rizzo M, Moran SL, Shin AY. Long-term outcomes of trapeziometacarpal arthrodesis in the management of trapeziometacarpal arthritis. J Hand Surg Am. 2009; 34(1):20–26

[5] Bellemère P, Gaisne E, Loubersac T. Pyrocardan implant: free pyrocarbon interposition for resurfacingtrapeziometacarpal joint. Chir Main. 2011; 30:S28–S35

[6] Maru M, Jettoo P, Tourret L, Jones M, Irwin L. Thumb carpometacarpal osteoarthritis: trapeziectomy versus pyrocarbon interposition implant (Pi2) arthroplasty. J Hand Surg Eur Vol. 2012; 37(7):617–620

[7] Caffinière de la JY. Prothèse totale trapézo-métacarpienne. RevChir Ortho. 1973; 59:299–308

[8] Wachtl SW, Guggenheim PR, Sennwald GR. Cemented and noncemented replacements of the trapeziometacarpal joint. J Bone Joint Surg Br. 1998; 80(1):121–125

[9] de la Caffinière JY. Facteurs de longévité des prothèses totales trapézométacarpiennes. Chir Main. 2001; 20(1):63–67

[10] Johnston P, Getgood A, Larson D, Chojnowski AJ, Chakrabarti AJ, Chapman PG. De la Caffinière thumb trapeziometacarpal joint arthroplasty: 16–26 year follow-up. J Hand Surg Eur Vol. 2012; 37(7):621–624

[11] Chakrabarti AJ, Robinson AH, Gallagher P. De la Caffinière thumb carpometacarpal replacements. 93 cases at 6 to 16 years follow-up. J Hand Surg [Br]. 1997; 22(6):695–698

[12] Jager T, Barbary S, Dap F, Dautel G. Analyse de la douleur postopératoire et des résultats fonctionnels précoces dans le traitement de la rhizarthrose. Étude prospective comparative de 74 patientes trapézectomie-interposition vs prothèse MAIA(®). Chir Main. 2013; 32 (2):55–62

[13] van Cappelle HG, Elzenga P, van Horn JR. Long-term results and loosening analysis of de la Caffinière replacements of the trapeziometacarpal joint. J Hand Surg Am. 1999; 24(3):476–482

[14] Badia A, Sambandam SN. Total joint arthroplasty in the treatment of advanced stages of thumb carpometacarpal joint osteoarthritis. J Hand Surg Am. 2006; 31(10):1605–1614

[15] Hernández-Cortés P, Pajares-López M, Robles-Molina MJ, Gómez-Sánchez R, Toledo-Romero MA, De Torres-Urrea J. Two-year outcomes of Elektra prosthesis for trapeziometacarpal osteoarthritis: a longitudinal cohort study. J Hand Surg Eur Vol. 2012; 37(2):130–137

[16] Klahn A, Nygaard M, Gvozdenovic R, Boeckstyns ME. Elektra prosthesis for trapeziometacarpal osteoarthritis: a follow-up of 39 consecutive cases. J Hand Surg Eur Vol. 2012; 37(7):605–609

[17] Thillemann JK, Thillemann TM, Munk B, Kroner K. High revision rates with the meta-on-metal Motec® carpometacarpal joint prosthesis. J Hand Surg Am. 2016; 41E(3):322–327

[18] Huang K, Hollevoet N, Giddins G. Thumb carpometacarpal joint total arthroplasty: a systematic review. J Hand Surg Eur Vol. 2015; 40(4):338–350

[19] Kaszap B, Daecke W, Jung M. High frequency failure of the Moje thumb carpometacarpal joint arthroplasty. J Hand Surg Eur Vol. 2012; 37(7):610–616

[20] Martin-Ferrero M. Ten-year long-term results of total joint arthroplasties with ARPE® implant in the treatment of trapeziometacarpal osteoarthritis. J Hand Surg Eur Vol. 2014; 39(8):826–832

[21] Dehl M, Chelli M, Lippmann S, Benaissa S, Rotari V, Moughabghab M. Results of 115 Rubis II reverse thumb carpometacarpal joint prostheses with a mean follow-up of 10 years. J Hand Surg Eur Vol. 2017; 42(6):592–598

[22] Vissers G, Goorens CK, Vanmierlo B, et al. Ivory arthroplasty for trapeziometacarpal osteoarthritis: 10-year follow-up. J Hand Surg Eur Vol. 2019; 44(2):138–145

[23] Cootjans K, Vanhaecke J, Dezillie M, Barth J, Pottel H, Stockmans F. Joint survival analysis and clinical outcome of total joint arthroplasties with the ARPE® implant in the treatment of trapeziometacarpal osteoarthritis with a minimal follow-up of 5 years. J Hand Surg Am. 2017; 42(8):630–638

[24] Toffoli A, Teissier J. Maia®trapeziometacarpal joint arthroplasty: clinical and radiological outcomes of 80 patients with more than 6 years of follow-up. J Hand Surg Am. 2017; 42(10):838.e1–838.e8

[25] Andrzejewski A, Ledoux P. Maïa® trapeziometacarpal joint arthroplasty: Survival and clinical outcomes at 5 years' follow-up. Hand Surg Rehabil. 2019; 38(3):169–173

[26] Semere A, Vuillerme N, Corcella D, Forli A, Moutet F. Results with the Roseland(®) HAC trapeziometacarpal prosthesis after more than 10 years. Chir Main. 2015; 34(2):59–66

[27] Apard T, Saint-Cast Y. Results of a 5 years follow-up of Arpe prosthesis for the basal thumb osteoarthritis. Chir Main. 2007; 26(2):88–94

[28] Wolf JM, Delaronde S. Current trends in nonoperative and operative treatment of trapeziometacarpal osteoarthritis: a survey of US hand surgeons. J Hand Surg Am. 2012; 37(1):77–82

[29] Comtet JJ, Cheze L, Rumelhart C, Dumas R. Proposition d'un système d'axes articulaires pour l'étude des mobilités de l'articulation trapézo-métacarpienne. Chir Main. 2006; 25:22–25

[30] Hollister A, Buford WL, Myers LM, Giurintano DJ, Novick A. The axes of rotation of the thumb carpometacarpal joint. J Orthop Res. 1992; 10(3):454–460

[31] Regnard PJ. Electra trapezio metacarpal prosthesis: results of the first 100 cases. J Hand Surg [Br]. 2006; 31(6):621–628

[32] Krukhaug Y, Lie SA, Havelin LI, Furnes O, Hove LM, Hallan G. The results of 479 thumb carpometacarpal joint replacements reported in the Norwegian Arthroplasty Register. J Hand Surg Eur Vol. 2014; 39(8):819–825

[33] Ledoux P. Echec de prothèse totale trapézo-métacarpienne non cimentée. Etude multicentrique. Ann Chir Main. 1997; 16:215–221

[34] Spaans AJ, van Minnen LP, Weijns ME, Braakenburg A, van der Molen AB. Retrospective study of a series of 20 Ivory® prosthesis in the treatment of trapeziometacarpal osteoarthritis. J Wrist Surg. 2016; 5(2):131–136

[35] Obert L, Couturier C, Marzouki A, et al. Prothèse ISIS®: évaluation biomécanique et clinique multicentrique préliminaire. Chir Main. 2011; 30 suppl:136–143

[36] Seng VS, Chantelot C. La prothèse trapézométacarpienne Isis(®) dans la rhizarthrose : à propos de 30 cas à 30 mois de recul moyen. Chir Main. 2013; 32(1):8–16

[37] Bricout M, Rezzouk J. Complications and failures of the trapeziometacarpal Maia® prosthesis: a series of 156 cases. Hand Surg Rehabil. 2016; 35(3):190–198

21

[38] Ten Brinke B, Mathijssen NM, Blom I, Deijkers RLM, Ooms EM, Kraan GA. Model-based roentgen stereophotogrammetric analysis of the surface replacement trapeziometacarpal total joint arthroplasty. J Hand Surg Eur Vol. 2016; 41(9):925–929

[39] Duerinckx J, Caekebeke P. Trapezium anatomy as a radiographic reference for optimal cup orientation in total trapeziometacarpal joint arthroplasty. J Hand Surg Eur Vol. 2016; 41(9):939–943

[40] Lussiez B. Radiological analysis of two types of trapezium cup: .about 50 cases. Chir Main. 2011; 30:86–90

[41] Hansen TB, Dremstrup L, Stilling M. Patients with metal-on-metal articulation in trapeziometacarpal total joint arthroplasty may have elevated serum chrome and cobalt. J Hand Surg Eur Vol. 2013; 38(8):860–865

[42] Kollig E, Weber W, Bieler D, Franke A. Failure of an uncemented thumb carpometacarpal joint ceramic prosthesis. J Hand Surg Eur Vol. 2017; 42(6):599–604

[43] Ulrich-Vinther M, Puggaard H, Lange B. Prospective 1-year follow-up study comparing joint prosthesis with tendon interposition arthroplasty in treatment of trapeziometacarpal osteoarthritis. J Hand Surg Am. 2008; 33(8):1369–1377

[44] Cebrian-Gomez R, Lizaur-Utrilla A, Sebastia-Forcada E, Lopez-Prats FA. Outcomes of cementless joint prosthesis versus tendon interposition for trapeziometacarpal osteoarthritis: a prospective study. J Hand Surg Am. 2019; 44(2):151–158

[45] Robles-Molina MJ, López-Caba F, Gómez-Sánchez RC, Cárdenas-Grande E, Pajares-López M, Hernández-Cortés P. Trapeziectomy with ligament reconstruction and tendon interposition versus a trapeziometacarpal prosthesis for the treatment of thumb basal joint osteoarthritis. Orthopedics. 2017; 40(4):e681–e686

[46] Vandenberghe L, Degreef I, Didden K, Fiews S, De Smet L. Long term outcome of trapeziectomy with ligament reconstruction/tendon interposition versus thumb basal joint prosthesis. J Hand Surg Eur Vol. 2013; 38(8):839–843

[47] De Smet L, Vandenberghe L, Degreef I. Long-term outcome of trapeziectomy with ligament reconstruction and tendon interposition (LRTI) versus prosthesis arthroplasty for basal joint osteoarthritis of the thumb. Acta Orthop Belg. 2013; 79(2):146–149

[48] Spartacus V, Mayoly A, Gay A, Le Corroller T, Némoz-Gaillard M, Roffino S, Chabrand P. Biomechanical causes of trapeziometacarpal arthroplasty failure. Computer methods in biomechanics engineering; 2017, doi:10:1080/10255842

[49] Dell PC, Brushart TM, Smith RJ. Treatment of trapeziometacarpal arthritis: results of resection arthroplasty. J Hand Surg Am. 1978; 3(3):243–249

[50] Eaton RG, Glickel SZ. Trapeziometacarpal osteoarthritis: staging as a rationale for treatment. Hand Clin. 1987; 3(4):455–471

[51] Allieu Y. Classifiactiondseformsanatomo-radiologiques de la rhizarthrose. In: Prothèses et Implants de la trapézo-métacarpienne. Montpellier Sauramps médical; 2009:29–42

[52] Ledoux P. M1/M2 ratio for radiological follow-up of trapeziometacarpal surgery. Hand Surg Rehabil. 2017; 36(2):146–147

21

22 STT and Peritrapezium Joints Arthroplasties

Philippe Bellemère

Abstract

STT joint arthroplasty has been proposed alternatively to the simple resection arthroplasty for the treatment of STT osteoarthritis. Pyrocarbon free interposition of the STT joint has replaced silicon interposition which is not used anymore. Aim of pyrocarbon STT arthroplasty is to relieve pain and preserve wrist motion and function by maintaining height and kinematic of the scaphoid.

Severe midcarpal instability associated with STT joint destruction is a contraindication of pyrocarbon interposition. Pyrocarbon interposition of the STT joint may use two types of implants: a concave-convex-shaped disk (STPI); and a thinner one (Pyrocardan), rectangular and biconcave-shaped. Open or arthroscopic implantation of these implants are possible. STPI interposition requires distal scaphoid resection while Pyrocardan interposition spares the scaphoid but remodels the articular trapezio-trapezoid surface.

Pyrocarbon implants for STT arthroplasty give reliable outcomes. Pain relief is effective, wrist and thumb motion and strength are preserved, and intracarpal stability of the wrist does not deteriorate. Complications are rare. The most frequent is implant instability more likely encountered with STPI interposition especially after inappropriate scaphoid preparation on its medial side. Thin implant like Pyrocardan seems particularly adapted to the anatomy and the kinematic of the narrow STT joint.

In select cases of pantrapezium osteoarthritis, double arthroplasty of STT and TM joints with Pyrocardan implant may be an efficient trapezium-preserving procedure.

Keywords: pyrocarbon, STT joint, implant, arthroplasty, interposition, arthritis, Pyrocardan, STPI

22.1 Introduction

Scaphotrapeziotrapezoid (STT) osteoarthritis (OA) is the second most frequent arthritic location in the wrist and is mainly isolated and idiopathic (▶ Fig. 22.1).[1] Painful STT OA must be initially treated conservatively with medical treatment. When it fails, surgical treatment is recommended. Several surgical techniques may be proposed: triscaphoid arthrodesis, bone resection (trapeziectomy with partial trapezoidal excision or distal pole of the scaphoid) with or without suspension ligamentoplasty and tendon interposition, arthroscopic debridement or partial joint resection with or without interposition, and arthroplasty using a pyrocarbon implant interposition. Silicone implant interposition arthroplasty is not used anymore in STT joint.

Radiographic occurrence of concomitant STT OA to painful trapeziometacarpal (TM) has been found in 60 %.[2] Such peritrapezial OA may be symptomatic at the STT and TM levels and trapeziectomy with partial trapezoidal excision with or without suspension ligamentoplasty and tendon interposition is the classical surgical option after failed medical treatment. Nevertheless, in some conditions, a double implant arthroplasty of the STT and TM joints may be proposed.[3]

22.2 Pyrocarbon Implants for STT Arthroplasty

STT implant interposition arthroplasty aims to relieve pain and preserve wrist motion and function. The mechanical goals of the implant are to maintain scaphoid mobility and scaphoid length. Therefore the implant allows compressive forces to be dissipated from the implant to the scaphoid, hence limiting the likelihood of intracarpal instabilities, especially a dorsal intercalated segment instability (DISI) malalignment, exacerbated by excessive scaphoid flexion or height loss.

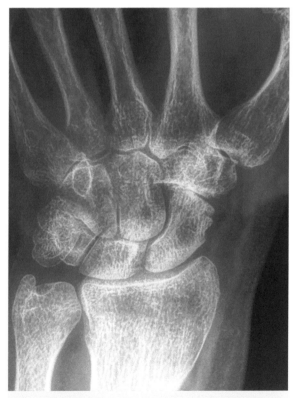

Fig. 22.1 Isolated idiopathic osteoarthritis of the scaphotrapeziotrapezoid (STT) joint.

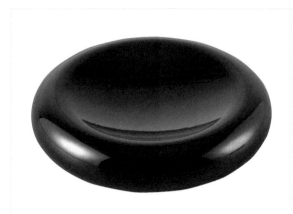

Fig. 22.2 STPI (scaphotrapezial pyrocarbon implant).

22.2.1 Indications

Failure or conservative treatment (splinting, anti-inflammatory drugs, intra-articular corticoid injections, and physiotherapy) of painful idiopathic STT OA is an indication of STT arthroplasty. Some authors limit their indication of STT pyrocarbon spacer after resection arthroplasty in case of wide scapholunate angle or in the presence of DISI deformity to give more stability and height to the scaphoid.[4] Chronic inflammatory process such as chondrocalcinosis and rheumatoid arthritis may induce preoperative distal resorption of the scaphoid and midcarpal instability with important dorsal subluxation of the capitate and DISI malrotation. Clinical signs of midcarpal instability may be present and such instable wrist is a contraindication of pyrocarbon interposition in the STT joint. STT arthrodesis may be a better option.[5]

22.2.2 STPI

The first pyrocarbon implant for the STT joint, called STPI (Scaphoid Trapezium Pyrocarbon Implant) (Wright Medical-Tornier SAS, Bioprofile, Grenoble, France) was proposed in 2000 by Péquignot et al.[6] This discoid implant has two joint surfaces, one convex for the trapeziotrapezoidal surface, and the other concave for the distal scaphoid articular surface (▶ Fig. 22.2). This implant is available in three sizes varying in diameter and thickness (from 3 to 4 mm). It is a mobile spacer requiring for its implantation the resection of the distal scaphoid (▶ Fig. 22.3).

Surgical Technique

Dorsal implantation is recommended by Péquignot. The capsular approach is between the tendons of the extensor pollicis longus on the radial side and the extensor carpi radialis brevis on the ulnar side. Capsular incision is made longitudinally and the distal portion of the scaphoid is exposed.

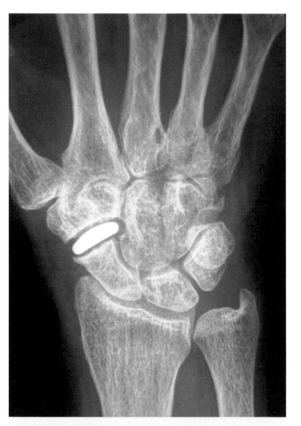

Fig. 22.3 Radiographic view of the scaphoid trapezium pyrocarbon implant (STPI) in the scaphotrapeziotrapezoid (STT) joint.

Palmar implantation is another option made with a longitudinal skin incision on the volar aspect between the flexor carpi radialis (FCR) tendon and the radial artery.[7] After reaching the plane of radiocarpal joint, a longitudinal incision is made on the STT joint distal to the radioscaphocapitate ligament.

Whatever the side of the approach chosen, about one-quarter of the scaphoid length (3 to 4 mm) is removed distally after a bone cut is made with an oscillating saw perpendicularly to the axis of the scaphoid.

The appropriate implant size is chosen using trial implants under fluoroscopic control to confirm that enough bone has been removed on the medial side and to check the absence of impingement of the implant especially on its radial side. The implant should be mobile and self-stabilizing.

After closure of the capsule, no ligamentoplasty is required.

Postoperative permanent splinting of the wrist does not exceed 2 to 3 weeks. After this time period passive and active motion exercises of the wrist and the thumb are allowed, and a removable splint is worn for protection for 3 weeks.

Arthroscopic implantation of the STPI spacer has been proposed after arthroscopic debridement and partial

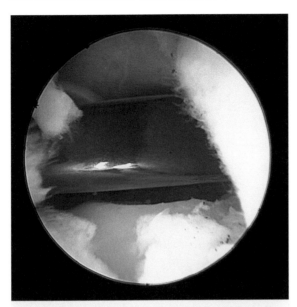

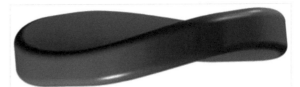

Fig. 22.5 Pyrocardan implant.

Fig. 22.4 Arthroscopic view of a pyrocarbon implant in the scaphotrapeziotrapezoid (STT) joint. The scaphoid is at the bottom, trapezoid at the top, and capitate on the right. (This image is provided courtesy of Christophe Mathoulin, Institut de la Main, clinique Bizet, Paris, France.)

22

resection of the STT joint especially in case of instability of the scaphoid seen with DISI deformity.[8,9] The arthroscopic portals are located dorsally. One STT portal (ulnar to the tendons of the first compartment) is used as the working portal with a 2.5-mm shaver and burr and occasionally a 3.5-burr, and the second arthroscopic portal (radial to the tendons of the third compartment) is used as the viewing portal using a 1.9-mm arthroscope. A volar portal can be used as if there is difficulty visualizing the dorsoulnar portion of the STT joint.[10] Joint debridement, synovectomy, and resection of 3 to 4 mm of the distal scaphoid are performed. A small transverse incision can join the two dorsal arthroscopic portals for inserting the implant (▶ Fig. 22.4). Postoperative protocol is same as the open procedure.

Results of the Literature

Several STPI interposition studies have been published[6,7,8,9,11] with small cohort and an average follow-up of 1.5 to over 6 years. Satisfactory short- and medium-term clinical results were achieved in all the studies; these studies found much improvement in pain and function.

Mobility was not significantly changed, and the grip strength was preserved or even improved. Implant instability was reported in two arthroscopy studies[8,9] and one open surgery study[7] at a rate of 20, 15.4, and 4%, respectively. These were attributed to technical errors related to insufficient medial scaphoid resection.

Pre-existing intracarpal misalignment was controlled or corrected in all series. No failure requiring conversion of this arthroplasty to another surgical solution has been reported in the literature.

Author's Experience

Good clinical results were also achieved in our experience of 24 STPI interposition. However, two cases of implant luxation required reoperation for repositioning. We do not use the STPI implant anymore because we find this implant to be thick and potentially instable. We prefer to use a thinner and more stable pyrocarbon implant such as the Pyrocardan.[12]

22.2.3 Pyrocardan Implant in STT Joint

Since March 2010, we have used the Pyrocardan implant (Wright Medical-Tornier SAS, Bioprofile, Grenoble, France) in the STT joint because its two concave surfaces make it stable under axial loads, its rectangular shape is closer to that of the STT joint, its minimal thickness reduces bone resection, and its implantation saves the scaphoid surface and its distal ligament attachments, thereby preserving its height and kinematics (▶ Fig. 22.5). The Pyrocardan implant is available in seven sizes, defined by the longest implant length, from 12 mm (XXS) to 18 mm (XXL). The implant is 1 mm thick at its center. The thickness of the exterior edges is proportional to the implant size (see ▶ Fig. 22.6).

Surgical Technique (▶ Fig. 22.7)

The approach is an anterior curved incision of about 4 cm centered on the scaphotrapezoid space, delimited by the FCR tendon, and the volar tubercles of the scaphoid and trapezium (▶ Fig. 22.8A).[13] The FCR sheath is opened to treat tenosynovitis or to remove the synovial cysts often associated with arthritis. Partial detachment of the proximal insertions of the thenar muscles from the trapezium tubercle is required to access the STT joint, which is then opened longitudinally between the distal flange of the FCR tendon and the scaphoid and trapezium tubercles. Axial traction is placed on the thumb to expose the STT joint space. The aim of joint preparation is to spare the articular surface of the scaphoid and the ligament insertions at the distal pole, while removing the double

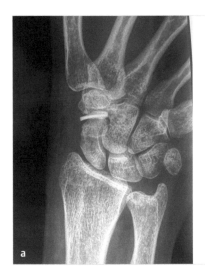
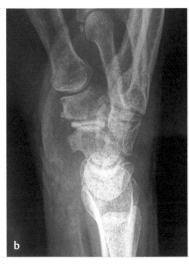

Fig. 22.6 Radiographic views of the Pyrocardan implant in the scaphotrapeziotrapezoid (STT) joint. **(a)** Anteroposterior (A-P) view. **(b)** Lateral view.

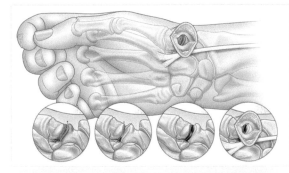

Fig. 22.7 Drawing of the principles of the procedure of Pyrocardan implant in scaphotrapeziotrapezoid (STT) joint.

concavity of the trapeziotrapezoid surface. Resection is performed using a thin oscillating saw, starting with the extremities of the lateral edge of the trapezium, followed by the medial edge, which is relative to the trapezoid (▶ Fig. 22.8b). The articular trapeziotrapezoid surface is then remodeled using a reamer to obtain a slight mediolateral and anteroposterior convexity (▶ Fig. 22.8c). The trial implant is then positioned along its long axis mediolaterally with its concavity facing the new trapeziotrapezoid surface. The size of the implant is chosen to ensure optimal trapeziotrapezoid articular coverage over the scaphoid. A majority of implants used in our practice range from size 14 to size 15. Fluoroscopic control is required to check the bone preparation, especially of the most medial part of the joint and the position of the trial implant during flexion–extension and ulnar and radial deviation movements of the wrist. Kinematics of the distal pole of the scaphoid on the implant surface is also evaluated under visual examination. The final implant is inserted and the articular capsule is closed with resorbable suture. No ligamentoplasty is required even in case the capsule is not closable.

Arthroscopic implantation of Pyrocardan implant in STT joint is also possible but has not yet been reported in the literature.

Postoperative permanent splinting of the wrist does not exceed 2 to 3 weeks. After this time period passive and active motion exercises of the wrist and the thumb are allowed, and a removable splint is worn for protection for 3 weeks.

Results in the Literature and Author's Experience

Relief of pain and function recovery were achieved with significant improvement in our 22 case series of Pyrocardan implant in STT joint reviewed at a mean follow-up of 36 months.[12] Grip and pinch strengths improved as well. Thumb and wrist motions did not change. Average time for functional recovery was 7.2 weeks and the patient satisfaction score was 9.5/10. No implant instability was found and preoperative intracarpal instability was partially or completely corrected. Carpal height was maintained and the capitolunar angle improved slightly. One revision with implant removal was performed on a patient who complained of persistent pain. This was probably the consequence of an overloaded arthroplasty.

22.3 Double Pyrocarbon Interposition for Peritrapezial OA: "Burger Arthroplasty"

In case of symptomatic pantrapezium OA (▶ Fig. 22.9), trapeziectomy with or without interposition (tendon or pyrocarbon implant) is the most frequently used treatment.

Trapezium-preserving procedure such as combined resection arthroplasty of TM and STT joints with or without tendon interposition (FCR) or soft tissue allograft has

22

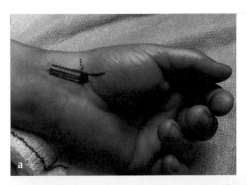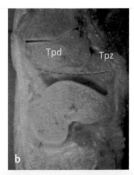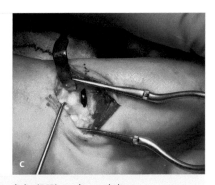

Fig. 22.8 Surgical technique. **(a)** Palmar incision allowing the access of the flexor carpi radialis (FCR) tendon and the scaphotrapeziotrapezoid (STT) joint. **(b)** Bones resection (dotted line) of the trapezium and trapezoid on a cadaveric specimen. Tpd, trapezoid; Tpz, trapezium. **(c)** Pyrocardan implant in the STT joint.

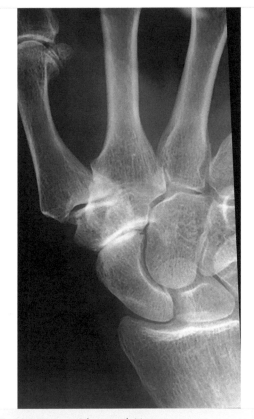

Fig. 22.9 Pantrapezial osteoarthritis.

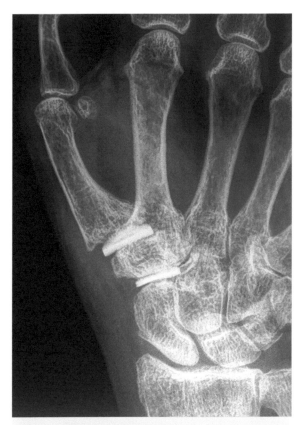

Fig. 22.10 Double pyrocarbon arthroplasty called "burger arthroplasty" with Pyrocardan implant for the treatment of pantrapezial osteoarthritis.

been proposed to avoid the loss of height of the radial column after total trapeziectomy.[14,15,16]

A double pyrocarbon arthroplasty (TM and STT) using the Pyrocardan implant interposition is also possible in a procedure that we call "burger arthroplasty" (▶ Fig. 22.10).

22.3.1 Indications

This procedure is possible only in the early stages of peritrapezium OA in which the height and the trabecular structure of the trapezium are preserved (▶ Fig. 22.9). Otherwise in more severe stages the risk after the "burger arthroplasty" could be a trapezium collapse. In case of doubt we recommend to check preoperatively the status of the trapezium with a computed tomography (CT) scan. Any intraosseous cyst, bone rarefaction, or loss of height of the trapezium should be a contraindication for a "burger arthroplasty."

22.3.2 Surgical Technique

We recommend performing the procedure with two skin incisions, allowing the approaches as described above for the STT joint and as described in Chapter 20 for the TM joint. In order to preserve the trapezium vascularization, caution must be paid to avoid extensive soft tissue dissection during the procedure. The TM joint is prepared first and the trial TM implant is left in the joint during the preparation of the STT joint. Fluoroscopic control is made with the trial implants in each joint and the size of each implant is chosen. Final implant is first placed into the STT joint and the joint is closed. Arthroplasty of the TM joint is then performed with the final implant.

For the postoperative period, patient is immobilized with a thumb splint for 2 weeks and only overnight for 2 consecutive weeks while active motion is encouraged during the day.

Double arthroplasty of peritrapezium osteoarthritis may also be performed with total prosthesis in TM joint and Pyrocardan implant in STT joint.

22.3.3 Author's Experience

The clinical and radiological situation of peritrapezium OA for a "burger arthroplasty" is not common, and we have operated about 30 patients in the last 10 years. Our results (unpublished data) at the midterm (average follow-up of 45 mo) have shown significant pain relief and significant improvement in Quick-DASH and Patient-Rated Wrist Evaluation (PRWE) scores to 28.5 and 26.1 postoperatively, respectively; a better grip and pinch strengths of 26 and 6 kg, respectively; Kapandji score at 9.5; and no MCP joint hyperextension. One patient required revision trapeziectomy following trapezium collapse.

"Burger arthroplasty" may be a satisfactory alternative to other more invasive options for the treatment of early stages of pantrapezial OA in select cases. This technique does not burn the bridges to a trapeziectomy in case of an eventual complication.

22.4 Conclusion

Pyrocarbon implants for STT arthroplasty give reliable outcomes. Pain relief is effective, wrist and thumb motion and strength are preserved, and intracarpal stability of the wrist does not deteriorate. Thin implant like Pyrocardan seems particularly adapted to the anatomy and the kinematic of the narrow STT joint. In select cases of pantrapezium OA, double arthroplasty of STT and TM joints may be an efficient trapezium-preserving procedure.

Acknowledgments

Special thanks to Dr. C. Chaves for providing data not yet published from his work ("burger arthroplasty").

References

[1] Moritomo H, Viegas SF, Nakamura K, Dasilva MF, Patterson RM. The scaphotrapezio-trapezoidal joint. Part 1: an anatomic and radiographic study. J Hand Surg Am. 2000; 25(5):899–910
[2] Katzel EB, Bielicka D, Shakir S, Fowler J, Buterbaugh GA, Imbriglia JE. Midcarpal and scaphotrapeziotrapezoid arthritis in patients with carpometacarpal arthritis. Plast Reconstr Surg. 2016; 137(6):1793–1798
[3] Bellemère P. Pyrocarbon implants for the hand and wrist. Hand Surg Rehabil. 2018; 37(3):129–154
[4] Pegoli L, Pozzi A. Arthroscopic management of scaphoid-trapezium-trapezoid joint arthritis. Hand Clin. 2017; 33(4):813–817
[5] Garcia-Elias M. Excisional arthroplasty for scaphotrapeziotrapezoidal osteoarthritis. J Hand Surg Am. 2011; 36(3):516–520
[6] Péquignot JP, D'asnieres de Veigy L, Allieu Y. Arthroplasty for scaphotrapeziotrapezoidal arthrosis using a pyrolytic carbon implant: preliminary results. Chir Main. 2005; 24(3–4):148–152
[7] Marcuzzi A, Ozben H, Russomando A. Treatment of scaphotrapezial trapezoidal osteoarthritis with resection of the distal pole of the scaphoid. Acta Orthop Traumatol Turc. 2014; 48(4):431–436
[8] Mathoulin C, Darin F. Arthroscopic treatment of scaphotrapeziotrapezoid osteoarthritis. Hand Clin. 2011; 27(3):319–322
[9] Pegoli L, Zorli IP, Pivato G, Berto G, Pajardi G. Scaphotrapeziotrapezoid joint arthritis: a pilot study of treatment with the scaphoid trapezium pyrocarbon implant. J Hand Surg [Br]. 2006; 31(5):569–573
[10] Carro LP, Golano P, Fariñas O, Cerezal L, Hidalgo C. The radial portal for scaphotrapeziotrapezoid arthroscopy. Arthroscopy. 2003; 19(5):547–553
[11] Low AK, Edmunds IA. Isolated scaphotrapeziotrapezoid osteoarthritis: preliminary results of treatment using a pyrocarbon implant. Hand Surg. 2007; 12(2):73–77
[12] Gauthier E, Truffandier MV, Gaisne E, Bellemère P. Treatment of scaphotrapeziotrapezoid osteoarthritis with the Pyrocardan® implant: results with a minimum follow-up of 2 years. Hand Surg Rehabil. 2017; 36(2):113–121
[13] Surgical technique of STT joint arthroplasty with Pyrocardan implant. Available at: https://youtu.be/-qEwvnlOZpE
[14] Barron OA, Eaton RG. Save the trapezium: double interposition arthroplasty for the treatment of stage IV disease of the basal joint. J Hand Surg Am. 1998; 23(2):196–204
[15] Cobb T, Sterbank P, Lemke J. Arthroscopic resection arthroplasty for treatment of combined carpometacarpal and scaphotrapeziotrapezoid (pantrapezial) arthritis. J Hand Surg Am. 2011; 36(3):413–419
[16] Rubino M, Cavagnaro L, Sansone V. A new surgical technique for the treatment of scaphotrapezial arthritis associated with trapeziometacarpal arthritis: the narrow pseudoarthrosis. J Hand Surg Eur Vol. 2016; 41(7):710–718

22

23 Thumb IP Joint Arthroplasty: An Alternative to Arthrodesis

Stephan F. Schindele

Abstract

The interphalangeal (IP) joint of the thumb is, after the thumb saddle (or carpometacarpal [CMC-1]) joint, the second most important joint in the axis of the first ray. The IP joint at the end of the motion axis is responsible for the precise adjustment of the thumb. Pain-free mobility at the distal end of the thumb is important for grasping small objects, especially for pinching to the index and middle fingers, while stability is necessary in fixing those objects.

Post-traumatic destruction or primary and secondary osteoarthritis of the thumb IP joint is rare, but leads to considerable pain and limitations in functional activities. Following unsuccessful conservative treatment, arthrodesis of the destroyed joint is the preferred operative procedure to manage this condition.

Although IP arthrodesis attains a pain-free outcome with a low complication rate, there is significant functional limitation, especially associated with pinching and picking up small objects. In addition, there is an even stronger functional limitation, if there is an associated degeneration of the metacarpophalangeal (MCP) or carpometacarpal (CMC) joints in the same thumb. Joint replacement, as an alternative to arthrodesis, preserves range of motion and is well documented for the distal interphalangeal (DIP) joints in the long fingers.

To date, there is very little literature focused on the replacement of the thumb IP joint, except for two recent articles describing IP arthroplasty with either a silicone implant or a surface gliding implant originally designed for the PIP joint and made of pyrocarbon and metal-polyethylene materials.

This chapter should give an overview about technical aspects in joint replacement with a surface gliding implant originally described and developed for the proximal interphalangeal (PIP) joint. We have used it in a small series for joint replacement at the IP joint of the thumb to provide mobility and stability in selected patients with painful osteoarthritis and failed conservative therapy.

Keywords: thumb interphalangeal joint, arthroplasty, surface replacement, surgical technique, arthrodesis, surface gliding implant, metal-polyethylene, silicone

23.1 Introduction

The interphalangeal (IP) joint of the thumb is, after the thumb saddle (or carpometacarpal [CMC-1]) joint, the second most important joint in the axis of the first ray. The CMC-1 joint positions the thumb in its three-dimensional space for retropulsion, opposition, and ab- or adduction, while the metacarpophalangeal (MCP-1)

joint fixes objects toward the long fingers. The IP joint at the end of the motion axis is responsible for the precise adjustment of the thumb. Pain-free mobility at the end of the thumb is important for grasping small objects, especially for pinching to the index and middle fingers, while stability is indispensable in fixing those objects. Jemec et al highlighted the existence of IP joint rotational mobility to optimize fine and precise motor skills.[1]

23.1.1 Treatment Strategies at the Thumb IP Joint

Posttraumatic destruction or primary and secondary osteoarthritis of the thumb IP joint is rare, but leads to considerable pain and limitations in functional activities. Conservative treatment (e.g., local treatment, painkillers, and steroid injections) is the first step in dealing with the associated symptoms. Following unsuccessful conservative treatment, arthrodesis of the destroyed joint is the preferred operative procedure to manage this condition.[2,3] Arthrodesis achieves a pain-free situation, but with a limitation in functional activity, particularly in the precise pinching and picking up of small objects from the table (i.e., paper clips) or between the radial-sided fingers. Turning small objects (i.e., a Swiss fondue fork) between the thumb and index finger and holding a pen while writing requires enough mobility at the distal joints of both digits (▶ Fig. 23.1).

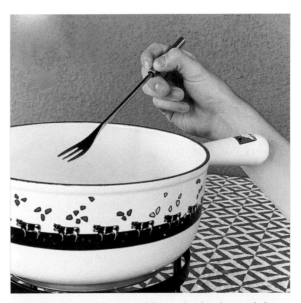

Fig. 23.1 Necessary active mobility at the thumb interphalangeal (IP) joint and distal interphalangeal (DIP) joint of the index finger for turning a Swiss fondue fork. (Copyright © Stephan Schindele.)

23.1.2 Arthroplasty

Arthroplasty with artificial replacement of the joint is well documented at the thumb level for the CMC-1 as well as for the fingers at the proximal interphalangeal (PIP) joint and MCP joint. At the distal interphalangeal (DIP) joints of the fingers, where the priority is to achieve pain-free stability, the most common treatment is arthrodesis in a straight or slightly flexed position. Joint replacement at the DIP level with a silicone spacer may be a treatment alternative, but has until now only been documented for DIP joints of the long fingers.[4,5,6,7,8] In one of the last publications focused on this topic, Sierakowski et al reported only a small number of complications for silicone joint replacements, which was comparable to the low complication rate associated with DIP arthrodesis.[9]

To date, there is very little literature focused on the replacement of the thumb IP joint, except for two recent articles describing IP arthroplasty with either a silicone implant or a surface gliding implant originally designed for the PIP joint and made of pyrocarbon and metal-polyethylene materials.[10,11]

23.2 Characteristics of Possible Implants for Thumb IP Joint Replacement

Possible implants for IP joint replacement are those that fit well into the destructed joint and have the potential to provide sufficient stability, especially for the pinch to the index finger at the ulnar side. Destructed and unstable IP joints with insufficient ulnar collateral ligaments or huge bone loss (due to inflammatory disease or of posttraumatic origin) are a contraindication for joint replacement at this level.

Based on our experience, we use the original Swanson silicone spacer (Wright Medical Group N.N.) or a metal-polyethylene nonconstrained surface replacement, which was originally developed and designed for the PIP joint (CapFlex, KLS Martin Group, Tuttlingen, Germany).[12,13,14] The latter comprises a cobalt-chrome alloy element and the corresponding surface partner is made of ultra-high molecular weight polyethylene (UHMW-PE). The back of both elements are coated with titanium to promote osteointegration (▶ Fig. 23.2).

23.3 Indications and Contraindications for Thumb IP Joint Replacement

IP joint replacement is possible for any destructed joint where mobility is needed. Especially in the case of simultaneously arthrodesis at the more proximal MCP- or CMC-1 levels, sustaining mobility at the most distal end of the thumb is important. Prerequisites for replacement

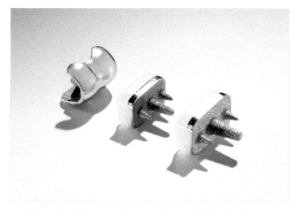

Fig. 23.2 Modular CapFlex-PIP implant for the thumb interphalangeal (IP) joint. Gliding surface metal (polished cobalt-chrome) and ultra-high molecular weight (UHMW) polyethylene. The back side of each element is coated with titanium for osteointegration. (This image is provided courtesy of KLS Martin Group, Tuttlingen, Germany.)

of the thumb IP joint are a stable joint with sufficient collateral ligaments and tendons, especially at the ulnar side, and no severe bone loss at the corresponding base or head of the first phalanx.

Contraindications include severe bone destruction with huge defects, chronic instability, or luxation of the joint, and chronic or acute infections or skin lesions at the involved thumb.

23.4 Published Outcomes and Our Own Results

Only two case reports exist in the literature to date. We recently presented one case with a Swanson silicone arthroplasty at one IP joint and a CapFlex surface replacement on the contralateral side. The postoperative follow-up time points for the silicone and metal-PE implants were 6 and 4 years, respectively.[11] The second publication presented the outcome of a pyrocarbon implant in a 15-year-old boy with posttraumatic destruction and a follow-up for 22 months.[10]

The prevalence of destructed thumb IP joints is low, and in our clinic, we can only report on a small series of patients with silicone and surface-gliding implant for IP joint replacements. Silicone has the disadvantage of being a flexible material, which contributes to a higher associated risk of implant breakage; therefore, our team no longer uses this implant type. We have observed good postoperative stability of CapFlex-PIP at the PIP level, and now use this implant for the IP joint. Although this implant is specifically made available for its application and treatment of the PIP joint, we have experience with the CapFlex-PIP as an off-label implant in the treatment of IP joints. All IP joint-treated patients are documented in a clinical registry in conjunction with our patient series receiving PIP arthroplasty.

23

Currently, we have data stemming from a small series of eight patients treated with a noncemented surface replacement at the IP joint and a minimum follow-up of 1 year. The patient mean age is 66.4-year-old and six patients are female. The dominant hand was affected in five patients, two had an affected nondominant hand, and the last patient is ambidextrous (i.e., right and left hand were affected in five and three patients, respectively). We reported one complication involving dorsal luxation of the joint within the first 6-week postoperative control period. Because the affected patient was dissatisfied with the outcome and a closed reduction procedure was not possible, open reduction with temporary K-wire fixation through the soft tissue was performed. A further 6 months after the second intervention, subluxation of the joint reoccurred and the patient underwent a conversion to arthrodesis.

The progression of the remaining seven patients could be followed up to a minimum period of 1 year. Active range of motion was 40 degrees (range, 10–60 degrees), which was slightly lower compared to the mean baseline

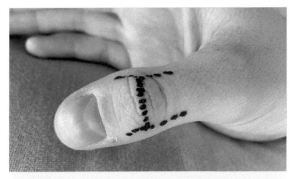

Fig. 23.3 H-shaped incision with longer proximal incisions to present the extensor pollicis longus (EPL) tendon. (Copyright © Stephan Schindele.)

value of 56 degrees. Mean postoperative pain at rest as measured on a visual analog scale decreased from 6 (baseline) to 2.5, and pinch grip to the index finger increased from a preoperative mean value of 5.5 to 6.7 kg at 1 year postsurgery. Mean baseline grip strength also increased from 18.4 to 21.8 kg at follow-up, and the mean brief Michigan Hand Outcomes Questionnaire score at baseline (where 100 indicates good overall function) increased from 43.5 to 57.1 points 1 year after surgery. All implants remained stable throughout the mean 1-year follow-up period without any radiographic signs of migration, osteolysis, or loosening.

23.5 Author's Own Experience and Preferred Technique (Tips and Tricks)

Thumb IP joint arthroplasty with the Cap-Flex implant can be performed using either a local block with tourniquet, Wide Awake Local Anesthesia No Tourniquet (WALANT) technique, regional block, or general anesthesia. It is important that the patient relaxes during the operation as stress or fear can induce tension on the thumb flexor pollicis longus tendon, which makes it difficult for the surgeon to achieve the correct overview (especially at the distal base) and tension upon insertion of the trial components.

A dorsal approach with extensor pollicis longus (EPL) tenotomy is commonly used for arthrodesis, which we also apply for our joint replacement procedures. An H- or Y-shaped skin incision is recommended and allows the surgeon to adequately prepare the distal part of the EPL tendon over a length up to 3 cm from the origin of the base distally (▶ Fig. 23.3 and ▶ Fig. 23.4).

As a next step complete synovectomy and removal of all osteophytes has to be performed to obtain a good overview of the joint (▶ Fig. 23.5). In case of stiff and very fixed

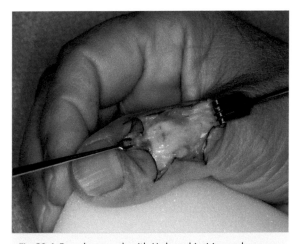

Fig. 23.4 Dorsal approach with H-shaped incision and preparation of the extensor pollicis longus (EPL) tendon over the destructed joint. (Copyright © Stephan Schindele.)

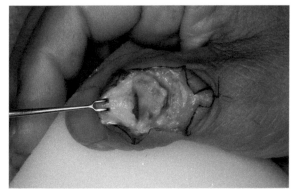

Fig. 23.5 Overview to the destructed interphalangeal (IP) joint with huge dorsal osteophytes after tenotomy of the extensor pollicis longus (EPL) tendon and synovectomy. (Copyright © Stephan Schindele.)

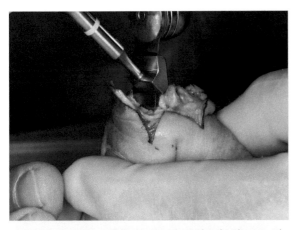

Fig. 23.6 Preparation of the bone at the P1 head with a special resection guide for the proximal interphalangeal (PIP) joint. (Copyright © Stephan Schindele.)

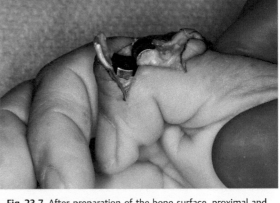

Fig. 23.7 After preparation of the bone surface, proximal and distal "trial" implants are applied to check the correct size and tension at the joint. (Copyright © Stephan Schindele.)

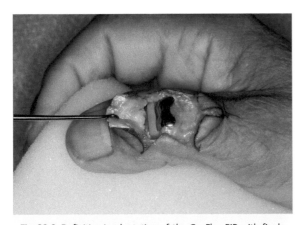

Fig. 23.8 Definitive implantation of the CapFlex-PIP with final check for correct size, fit, and tension clinically and under fluoroscopy. (Copyright © Stephan Schindele.)

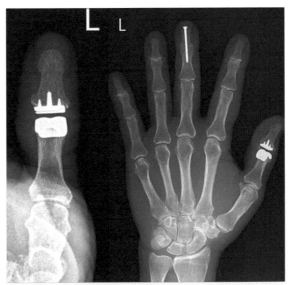

Fig. 23.9 Six-week postoperative radiographs showing correctly fitting proximal and distal components without signs of loosening or migration. (Copyright © Stephan Schindele.)

joints, the dorsal part of the radial collateral ligament can be released without handling the ulnar collateral ligament, the latter of which is responsible for maintaining correct thumb stability during pinching and grasping.

In a second step, the proximal head is prepared and modeled using existing resection guides and a modulator (impactor) in a similar manner to that described for PIP arthroplasty (▶ Fig. 23.6). The correctly sized trial implant is then inserted proximally. Thereafter, the distal base can also be prepared as described for PIP arthroplasty[12]; here it is necessary to achieve a flat platform with enough cancellous bone for good osteointegration of the implant. The height of the polyethylene component is dependent on the stability and should not choose too loose. At the end of the second step, the alignment of the correctly placed trial implant components should be checked under fluoroscopy (▶ Fig. 23.7).

For the third step, all trial implants are replaced with the actual implants and the EPL tendon is sutured

sufficiently to avoid too much tension, which can lead to hyperextension of the joint (▶ Fig. 23.8). Postoperative immobilization in a splint protects the sutured EPL tendon. In our small series, patients begin with early active mobility without load after 4 weeks and with load between the postoperative weeks 7 and 8. Final radiographic control at 6 weeks postsurgery should indicate correct angulation and well-fitted components with complete osteointegration (▶ Fig. 23.9).

An alternative implant for thumb IP joint arthroplasty is the original Swanson silicone implant, which was associated with good results for 131 DIP joints of the long fingers affected by painful osteoarthritis and posttraumatic injury.[9] Nevertheless, lateral stability at the thumb IP joint is just as important as that required for the DIP joint.

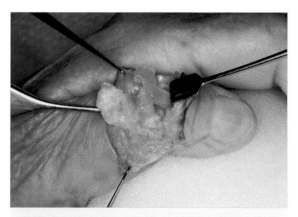

Fig. 23.10 Explantation of a broken and failed silicone implant at the thumb interphalangeal (IP) joint. (Copyright © Stephan Schindele.)

With degradation of the implant over time, we have observed cases of implant failure involving breakage and instability in our small series (▶ Fig. 23.10). The intrinsic stability of silicone implants is not as high as that of the more anatomic implants, and stability at the IP joint is of greater importance over mobility. Therefore, we now use the CapFlex-PIP implant in select cases with short spikes for noncemented use and fixation with osteointegration.

In the case of equivocal stability, especially in inflammatory arthritis, we still recommend arthrodesis as a definitive treatment solution. Based on the limited data in the literature as well as our available short-term outcome data, arthrodesis of the IP joint remains the golden standard for treating an affected and destructed thumb.

Acknowledgment

I would like to thank Dr. Melissa Wilhelmi (Zurich) and Professor Grey Giddins (Bath) for proofreading the manuscript.

References

[1] Jemec B, Verjee LS, Jain A, Sandford F. Rotation in the interphalangeal thumb joint in vivo. J Hand Surg Am. 2010; 35(3):425–429

[2] Cox C, Earp BE, Floyd WE, IV, Blazar PE. Arthrodesis of the thumb interphalangeal joint and finger distal interphalangeal joints with a headless compression screw. J Hand Surg Am. 2014; 39(1):24–28

[3] Rizzo M. Thumb arthrodesis. Tech Hand Up Extrem Surg. 2006; 10 (1):43–46

[4] Brown LG. Distal interphalangeal joint flexible implant arthroplasty. J Hand Surg Am. 1989; 14(4):653–656

[5] Schwartz DA, Peimer CA. Distal interphalangeal joint implant arthroplasty in a musician. J Hand Ther. 1998; 11(1):49–52

[6] Snow JW, Boyes JG, Jr, Greider JL, Jr. Implant arthroplasty of the distal interphalangeal joint of the finger for osteoarthritis. Plast Reconstr Surg. 1977; 60(4):558–560

[7] Wilgis EF. Distal interphalangeal joint silicone interpositional arthroplasty of the hand. Clin Orthop Relat Res. 1997(342):38–41

[8] Zimmerman NB, Suhey PV, Clark GL, Wilgis EF. Silicone interpositional arthroplasty of the distal interphalangeal joint. J Hand Surg Am. 1989; 14(5):882–887

[9] Sierakowski A, Zweifel C, Sirotakova M, Sauerland S, Elliot D. Joint replacement in 131 painful osteoarthritic and post-traumatic distal interphalangeal joints. J Hand Surg Eur Vol. 2012; 37(4):304–309

[10] McKee D, Domingo-Johnson EL. Novel use of joint replacement in a thumb interphalangeal joint. Case Rep Orthop. 2019; 2019:2603098

[11] Schindele S, Marks M, Herren DB. Thumb interphalangeal joint replacements with silicone and surface gliding implants: a case report. J Hand Surg Eur Vol. 2019; 44(6):649–651

[12] Schindele SF, Altwegg A, Hensler S. Surface replacement of proximal interphalangeal joints using CapFlex-PIP. Oper Orthop Traumatol. 2017; 29(1):86–96

[13] Schindele SF, Hensler S, Audigé L, Marks M, Herren DB. A modular surface gliding implant (CapFlex-PIP) for proximal interphalangeal joint osteoarthritis: a prospective case series. J Hand Surg Am. 2015; 40(2):334–340

[14] Schindele SF, Sprecher CM, Milz S, Hensler S. Osteointegration of a modular metal-polyethylene surface gliding finger implant: a case report. Arch Orthop Trauma Surg. 2016; 136(9):1331–1335

23

Section 4

Arthroplasty of the Wrist

24 Systematic Review of Wrist Arthroplasty

Onur Berber, Lorenzo Garagnani, and Sam Gidwani

Abstract

Total wrist arthroplasty has evolved over several decades and has made gains in outcomes and popularity. In contrast, wrist hemiarthroplasty is a more recent innovation. A systematic review of available literature has been performed to assess the clinical effectiveness of both these treatment options. A total of 38 studies were included in the qualitative analysis, representing 1,543 total wrist arthroplasty and 117 hemiarthroplasty index operations. The effects of surgery on pain, function, range of motion, and grip strength were examined. Rates of complications and implant survival were also assessed. The introduction of third- and fourth-generation implant total arthroplasty designs has led to improvements in outcomes and implant survival, although reporting of outcomes was not consistent across all studies. Only early- to mid-term outcome reporting was available for hemiarthroplasty, and results were more variable. Ongoing performance monitoring remains vital for both procedures.

Keywords: wrist arthritis, arthroplasty, hemiarthroplasty, outcome, systematic review

24.1 Introduction

24.1.1 Evolution of Total Wrist Arthroplasty

Wrist prostheses have undergone significant evolution since the earliest implant designs. The first generation of implant to receive wide commercial use was the Swanson silicone prosthesis, a flexible stemmed hinged spacer introduced in 1967.[1] Early results were promising with good pain relief and functional range of motion, but longer follow-up revealed high implant failure/fracture rates of up to 65%, and a soft tissue reactive silicone synovitis in approximately 30% of cases.[2,3,4]

Several other prostheses followed, including the Meuli wrist arthroplasty system in 1972,[5] the Volz total wrist arthroplasty (TWA) in 1973,[6,7] the Trispherical TWA in 1977,[8] the Biaxial TWA in 1989,[9] the Destot prosthesis in 1991,[10] and the Anatomic Physiologic Wrist in 1996.[11] There were three iterations of the Meuli wrist prosthesis (I–III). The first was a cemented ball-and-socket metal-on-metal articulation.[12] The ball was later changed to create a metal-on-polyethylene bearing surface and the center of rotation was altered to improve wrist alignment and stability (Meuli II).[5] Due to persisting high rates of dislocation and loosening, Meuli III was developed in 1986, with a cementless fixation and a bearing surface altered to create a metal ball on an ultra-high molecular weight polyethylene (UHMWPE) socket.[13,14]

Implants such as the Meuli II and Volz were considered the second generation of TWA, with the defining features being radial and carpal components with a ball-and-socket or hemispherical articulation.[15,16,17] The third generation of implants, such as the Meuli III, Universal, and Biaxial arthroplasties, attempted to better reproduce the center of wrist rotation so as to improve stability and reduce dislocation.[13,14,18,19] The Biaxial implant consisted of a hemispherical metal-on-polyethylene-bearing design and was developed at the Mayo clinic in the late 1970s. Results were first published by Cobb and Beckenbaugh in 1996.[9] The Universal wrist was developed by Menon; the results of the first series were published in 1998.[18] The Universal consisted of titanium radial and carpal components with a toroidal-shaped high-density polyethylene-bearing surface. The carpal component was stabilized with three screws into the carpus.

24.1.2 Current Implants

The Motec (▶ Fig. 24.1; Swemac Innovation AB), Universal 2 (▶ Fig. 24.2; Integra LifeSciences), Freedom (▶ Fig. 24.3; Integra LifeSciences), Re-Motion (Stryker), and Maestro (Biomet) are examples of fourth-generation implants. These newer implants typically require less bone resection, with removal of only the proximal carpal row. Carpal fixation distally is mostly achieved with bone screws, and proximally with a press-fit into the radius. The implants are typically porous coated to enable osseointegration.[20,21]

The Motec prosthesis (▶ Fig. 24.1), although considered a fourth-generation implant, has some design features reflecting earlier generation principles with an articulation which is a metal-on-metal ball-and-socket bearing.[16,22] A new screw fixation concept was introduced for the radial and carpal components. The screws are manufactured from a grit-blasted titanium alloy, coated with a resorbable calcium phosphate (Bonit; DOT Medical Solutions Laboratories Gmbh, Rostock, Germany) to encourage osseointegration.[22] The Motec, previously called the Gibbon, evolved from the Elos prosthesis, which was in use between 2000 and 2005. The performance of the Elos and Gibbon has been described by Krukhaug et al in their report on the Norwegian Arthroplasty Register.[23]

The Universal was initially designed with a toroidal articulation but was later changed to an ellipsoidal shape to improve stability and reduce the risk of dislocation.[24] This was one of the changes that led to the development of the contemporary Universal 2 (▶ Fig. 24.2), which features a titanium alloy carpal component with two screws and a central peg, and a cobalt-chrome alloy radial component. The Universal 2 wrist arthroplasty has been further modified to produce the Freedom wrist arthroplasty (▶ Fig. 24.3). The design changes include a shorter, more

24

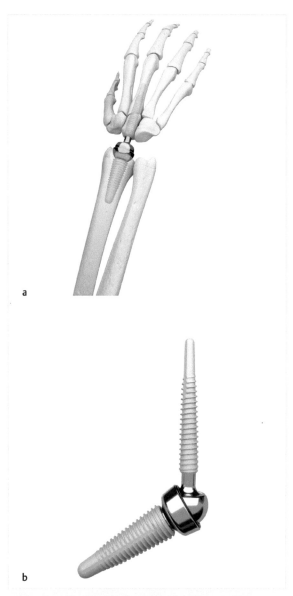

a

b

Fig. 24.1 (a, b) Motec wrist joint prosthesis. (Courtesy of Swemac.)

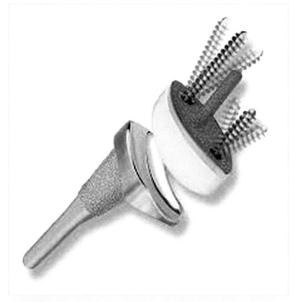

Fig. 24.2 Universal 2 total wrist implant system. (Courtesy of Integra.)

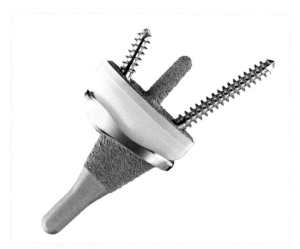

Fig. 24.3 Freedom total wrist arthroplasty. (Courtesy of Integra.)

tapered carpal stem, a lower profile radial tray with a 5-degree rotation relative to the radial stem for slight supination of the wrist at rest and a shorter less invasive radial stem. The Re-Motion arthroplasty system (see ▶ Fig. 25.1) has cobalt-chrome alloy radial and carpal components, with titanium coated to the undersurface of the carpal component. The articulation is a metal on UHMWPE. The results of the first patient series was published by Herzberg et al.[25] The Maestro wrist system incorporates an uncemented titanium alloy stem articulating with a cobalt-chrome radial body. An UHMWPE-bearing surface is fixed to the radial body. The carpal component is a monoblock of cobalt-chrome with a titanium alloy central-capitate peg.

Currently, the four commercially available wrist implants in the United States are the Universal 2, Freedom, Re-Motion, and Maestro. In Europe the Motec is also approved for use. More recently, a new wrist implant was introduced, named the Prosthelast (Argomedical).[26] It consists of a titanium radial implant fixed to an elastic intramedullary wire that rests on the subchondral bone of the radial head, aiming to preventing axial migration of the radial component. The carpal component has a polyethylene-bearing surface which attaches to a titanium plate. Only preliminary data with short-term follow-up are available, so this implant was not included in this study.

Wrist arthroplasties have been analyzed in several reviews.[27,28,29,30] Cavaliere and Chung performed a comparative review of wrist arthroplasty versus wrist arthrodesis.[27] No pain or mild pain was experienced by 90% of patients in the arthroplasty group, but the rates of major complication were higher in the arthroplasty group (25%) compared to the arthrodesis group (13%). Newer third-generation prostheses had lower major complication rates (21%) than older generation implants. The systematic review by Yeoh and Tourret had similar findings with arthroplasties having higher complication rates.[29] A more recent systematic review by Berber et al demonstrated that newer fourth-generation implants had lower complication rates (range 0.1–2.9%) than earlier designs (range 0.2–8.1%; p = 0.002).[30] Maintenance of a range of motion is seen as the clear advantage of wrist arthroplasty over arthrodesis, yet this benefit is not always shown in objective assessment. A functional range of motion, as defined by Palmer et al is 5 degrees of flexion, 30 degrees of extension, 10 degrees of radial deviation, and 15 degrees of ulnar deviation,[31] was achieved in only 3 of the 14 studies in the review by Cavaliere and Chung with similar findings reported by Berber et al.[27,30]

Wrist hemiarthroplasty is an emerging management option for wrist arthritis and wrist trauma. To date there have been several publications reporting early to midterm outcomes.[32,33,34,35,36,37,38,39] Studies have also reported on the early clinical results of hemiarthroplasty in elderly patients with acute non-reconstructable distal radial fractures, as first described by Roux.[32,36,37,38,39,40] Anneberg et al reported on the outcomes of a new hemiarthroplasty system, KinematX (Extremity Medical, LLC).[35] The remaining studies typically utilized the radial or carpal components of a current TWA system.

Since the most recent review by Berber et al,[30] there have been several new publications with greater data available on current fourth-generation wrist arthroplasty systems, as well as on wrist hemiarthroplasties.

The proposed research question forming the basis for this review is: "What is the clinical effectiveness of TWA and wrist hemiarthroplasty?"

24.2 Objectives

The objective of this review was to evaluate the clinical effectiveness of TWA, defined as the effect of TWA on the specific outcomes listed below:
- Outcome 1: Pain.
- Outcome 2: Secondary measures of function (e. g., grip strength) and quality of life.
- Outcome 3: The frequency of treatment failure/implant survival and adverse events.

We also wished to assess whether the use of fourth-generation wrist arthroplasty systems was associated with improved clinical effectiveness.

24.3 Methods

A study protocol was created prior to undertaking this review. This was modified from a previous protocol published on the National Institute for Health Research PROSPERO Database (CRD42017067377). Preferred Reporting Items for Systematic Reviews and Meta-Analyses (PRISMA) guidelines were adhered to.

24.3.1 Study Inclusion Criteria

Types of Participants

Studies were included if participants were adults over the age of 16 years and of any gender. The underlying clinical diagnosis was arthritis of the wrist. The cause of arthritis was kept broad to reflect common daily practice in most orthopaedic clinics, including both inflammatory and noninflammatory arthritis.

Types of Interventions

The two interventions were TWA and wrist hemiarthroplasty. There have been four generations of TWA, with only the latest generation of implants still commercially available. Subgroup analysis by generation was performed to assess whether the performance of the latest implants has improved.

Types of Outcome Measures

The core measures used as a basis for defining the primary and secondary outcomes in this study originated from recommendations established by the OMERACT (Outcome Measures in Rheumatoid Arthritis Clinical Trials) conference in 1992. These were first approved by the American College of Rheumatology[41] and later published under WHO and ILAR endorsement.[42] The core end points were also refined for osteoarthritis in general[43] and hand osteoarthritis[44] in particular.

Primary and Secondary Outcome Measures

Pain relief was chosen as the primary outcome in this study. Pain is commonly reported as a continuous variable on a "visual analog scale" (VAS) or on a categorical scale. Secondary outcome measures included function, grip strength, wrist motion, adverse events, and implant survival.

Inclusion and Exclusion Criteria

The studies chosen for inclusion in this review include randomized control trials, cohort studies, case–control studies, and case series. Case reports and abstracts were excluded from this review. Studies with fewer than five patients and studies failing to report on any of the primary or secondary outcomes were excluded. The minimum duration of follow-up was chosen as 1 year.

24

24.3.2 Search Methods

Several databases were searched on the 20th of May 2019, including OVID Medline (dates: 1946 to present), OVID Excerpta Medica Database (EMBASE) (dates: 1974 to present), Cochrane Central Register of Controlled Trials (Issue 6 of 12, June 2019), NICE Database, Cumulative Index to Nursing and Allied Health Literature (CINAHL) (1981 to present), and British Nursing Index (BNI) (1992 to present). Trial registers were also searched for relevant studies including ClinicalTrials.gov and the World Health Organization International Clinical Trials Registry Platform (ICTRP).

The reference lists from the papers identified in the above searches were reviewed for potential studies of interest. The "PICOS" elements (Population, Intervention, Comparator, and Outcomes) were used to construct an effective search strategy. Other search filters included studies published in the English language only; animal or cadaveric studies were excluded. No date restrictions were applied to maximize search numbers.

24.3.3 Data Collection and Analysis

Study Selection, Data Extraction, and Management

Studies were selected through two stages of screening. The first stage involved a review of the study title and abstracts to remove obviously irrelevant articles. The full text of the remaining articles was then reviewed in more detail by

the study authors. The basic dataset for extraction was adapted from recommendations in the Cochrane Handbook for Systematic Review of Interventions.[45]

Assessment of Risk of Bias and Quality of Evidence

The GRADE system was chosen to perform a quality appraisal of case series.[46] This system specifies four levels of quality (high, moderate, low, very low) based on five factors including study design (randomized controlled trials vs. observational studies), study quality (bias, loss to follow-up, sparse data), consistency of results (degree of consistency of effect between or within studies), directness of evidence (generalizability of population and outcomes to population of interest), and effect size.

24.4 Results

24.4.1 Description of Studies

Search Results

The results returned from the database searches are summarized in ► Fig. 24.4. Of the 38 articles, 31 reported the outcomes of wrist arthroplasty,[10,11,14,15,16,17,18,19,20,21,23,33, 47,48,49,50,51,52,53,54,55,56,57,58,59,60,61,62,63,64,65] two undertook a retrospective matched cohort review of arthroplasty against arthrodesis cases[66,67] and five reviewed the outcomes of wrist hemiarthroplasty.[32,33,34,35,37]

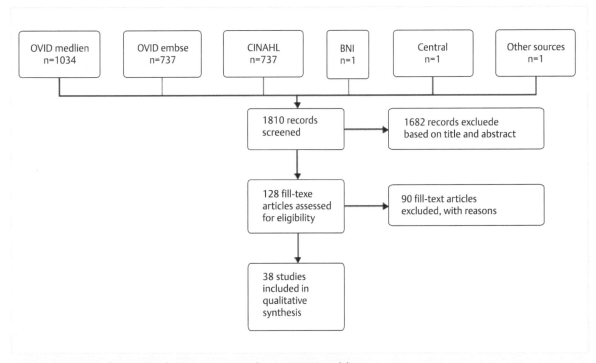

Fig. 24.4 Summary of the study selection process according to PRISMA guidelines.

Table 24.1 Patient demographics

	Wrist hemiarthroplasty	Total wrist arthroplasty
Total number of patients	117	1,414
Total index operations	117	1,543
Male:Female	1:2.0	1:2.8
Mean age	63 yr	59 yr
Underlying pathology		
• *Inflammatory arthritis*	***2.7%***	***60.8%***
◦ Rheumatoid arthritis	0.9%	60.1%
◦ Psoriatic arthritis	1.8%	0.4%
◦ Other	–	0.3%
• *Noninflammatory*	***45.5%***	***17.6%***
◦ Acute traumatic	21.4%	–
◦ Posttraumatic arthritis	18.8%	8.5%
◦ Degenerative arthritis	5.4%	8.3%
◦ Lunate AVN	–	0.6%
◦ Other	–	0.2%
• *Not classified*	***51.8%***	***21.6%***

Abbreviation: AVN, avascular necrosis.
Note: Mean age calculated through weighted average.

▶ Table 24.1 summarizes the overall patient demographics of both the TWA and hemiarthroplasty patient cohorts.

Included Studies

Total Wrist Arthroplasty

The underlying wrist pathology in the TWA studies was a mix of inflammatory and noninflammatory causes in the majority of the studies. However, in some, a TWA was performed only on patients with noninflammatory wrist arthritis.[10,16,60,62,65,67] Two studies undertook a retrospective matched cohort review of arthroplasty against arthrodesis.[66,67] Both were included as the TWA data could be extracted for analysis.

Common reasons for excluding studies from this analysis included patient follow-up of less than 1 year and a lack of outcome measurements and reporting of revision wrist arthroplasty. Four studies were excluded as more recent data have been published.[8,56,68,69] Botero et al from Strasbourg, France was the first to report on a new TWA implant (Prosthelast).[26] Patient follow-up was less than 1 year and so the paper was rejected from this review.

Wrist Hemiarthroplasty

The majority of wrist hemiarthroplasties were performed on patients with noninflammatory wrist pathology (▶ Table 24.1). In two studies, wrist hemiarthroplasty was performed on elderly patients with acute non-reconstructable distal radius fractures.[32,38] This was first reported by Roux et al; however, the paper was in French and hence is not included in this review.[39] This was also reported by Vergnenegre et al; this paper was also rejected as patient follow-up was less than 1 year.[40] There was an updated publication by Herzberg et al on earlier results and therefore only this most recent article was included.[36,37]

Wrist Arthroplasty Implants

Total Wrist Arthroplasty

▶ Table 24.2 provides a summary of the TWA studies. Fourteen different implants were used, ranging from earlier second-generation prostheses such as the Meuli and Volz to contemporary fourth-generation systems such as the Universal 2, Maestro, Re-Motion, and Motec.

Hemiarthroplasty

Wrist hemiarthroplasty was reported in five studies summarized in ▶ Table 24.3. Herzberg et al and Ichihara et al both reported on wrist hemiarthroplasty for acute non-reconstructable distal radial fractures in elderly patients.[32,37] The implants included the radial (DRH) or carpal components (CH) of pre-existing TWA systems such as the radial component of the Maestro[33,34] or Re-Motion[33,37] wrist systems; the carpal component of the Maestro[33]; and more recently the KinematX[35], the Cobra[37] (GroupeLepine), and the radial component of the Prosthelast system.[32]

Quality of Evidence

Several study authors were involved in product design[10,14,16,18,55,59,65] and Divelbiss et al received benefits for their work.[54] The GRADE quality assessment was of "moderate grade" in several studies as the risk of bias was

24

Table 24.2 Summary of the included total wrist arthroplasty studies

Study	Wrist arthroplasty implant	Underlying pathology (often the primary diagnosis was not recorded)	Generation of implant	Number of index procedures	Length of follow-up: mean and (range)
Menon[15]	Volz	RA n = 14; PA n = 1; OA n = 1	2	18	40 (24–66) mo
Figgie et al[55]	Trispherical	RA	2	35	9 (5–11) yr
Meuli and Fernandez[14]	MWP II Meuli	RA n = 33; Posttraumatic n = 12	2	49	4.5 (2–6) yr
Gellman et al[53]	Volz	RA = 12; PA n = 1; Posttraumatic n = 1	2	14	6.5 (3.5–11.5) yr
Menon[18]	Universal	RA n = 23; OA n = 8	3	37	79.4 (48–120) mo
Takwale et al[19]	Biaxial	RA	3	66	52 (12–99) mo
Divelbiss et al[54]	Universal	RA	3	22	1–2 yr
Levadoux and Legre[10]	Destot	Posttraumatic	3	28	47 (12–72) mo
Rahimtoola and Rozing[17]	RWS	RA n = 24; PA n = 1; OA n = 2	2	27	4 (2–8) yr
Radmer et al[11]	APH	Seropositive RA n = 36, seronegative RA n = 4	3	40	52 (24–73) mo
Murphy et al[66]	Universal	RA	3	27	26 +/– 16 mo
Ward et al[51]	Universal	RA	3	19	7.3 (5–10.8) yr
Reigstad et al[16]	Motec	Posttraumatic arthritis including SLAC/SNAC	4	8	7.6 (7–9) yr
Ferreres et al[20]	Universal 2 n = 19 Universal n = 2	RA n = 15; PA n = 1; and other inflammatory n = 2; Keinbock's n = 2; Noninflammatory other n = 2	4 3	21	5.5 (3–8) yr
Krukhaug et al[23]	1. Biaxial n = 90 (80/90 uncemented) 2. Elos n = 23 (3 versions preceding Gibbon v1 = 2, v2 = 6, v3 = 15) 3. Gibbon n = 76 (later called the Motec)	Inflammatory (RA, PA) n = 116; Noninflammatory (OA, posttraumatic, ligamentous, postinfective) n = 73	3 3 3	189	
Cooney et al[47]	1. Biaxial n = 16 2. Re-Motion n = 22 3. Universal 2 n = 8	RA n = 29; Posttraumatic n = 10	3 4 4	46	6.0 (3.5–15) yr
Ekroth et al[50]	1. Biaxial n = 6 2. Volz n = 1	RA	3 2	12	17.8 (11.7–28.3) yr
Herzberg et al[64]	Re-Motion	RA n = 129 (60 %); Non-RA n = 86 (40 %)	4	215	4 (2–8) yr
Morapudi et al[61]	Universal 2	RA n = 19; Posttraumatic n = 2	4	19	3.1 (1.8–3.9) yr
Bidwai et al[52]	Re-Motion	RA	4	13	33 (14–56) mo
Boeckstyns et al[56]	Re-Motion	RA n = 50; OA n = 6; Posttraumatic n = 8; Keinbock's n = 1	4	52	6.5 (5–9) yr
Nydick et al[67]	Maestro	Posttraumatic	4	7	56 +/– 10 mo

(Continued)

Table 24.2 (*Continued*) Summary of the included total wrist arthroplasty studies

Study	Wrist arthroplasty implant	Underlying pathology (often the primary diagnosis was not recorded)	Generation of implant	Number of index procedures	Length of follow-up: mean and (range)
Sagerfors et al[21]	1. Biaxial n = 52 2. Universal 2 n = 12 3. Re-Motion n = 87 4. Maestro n = 68	RA n = 185; OA n = 34	3 4 4 4	219	7 (2–13) yr
Badge et al[48]	Universal 2	RA	4	95	53 (24–120) mo
Chevrollier et al[49]	1. Universal n = 10 2. Re-Motion n = 7	RA n = 6; Other n = 1; Post-traumatic n = 8; Keinbock's n = 1, Postseptic n = 1	3 4	17	5.2 (1.1–10) yr
Gaspar et al[33]	Maestro	Inflammatory and noninflammatory	4	47	35 (12–151) mo
Gil et al[63]	Universal 2	RA n = 29, PA n = 1, JIA n = 1; Degenerative OA (including posttraumatic) n = 8	4	39	9 (4.8–14.7) yr
Reigstad et al[65]	Motec	Degenerative OA	4	56	8 (5–11) yr
Singh et al[60]	Universal 2	Posttraumatic	4	12	30 (12–50) mo
Pfanner et al[58]	Universal 2	RA	4	23	82.3 mo (2–12 yr)
Giwa et al[57]	Motec	RA n = 4, PA n = 1; Posttraumatic n = 12; Degenerative OA n = 7; Other n = 1	4	25	50 (26–66) mo
Brinkhorst et al[62]	Universal 2	Posttraumatic n = 21; Keinbock's n = 2	4	23	24 (24–50) mo
Honecker et al[59]	Re-Motion	RA n = 19; Keinbock's n = 3; Posttraumatic n = 1		23	6 yr
			Total	1543	

Abbreviations: APH, Anatomic Physiologic Wrist; JIA, juvenile idiopathic arthritis; MWP, Meuli Wrist Prosthesis; OA, osteoarthritis; PA, psoriatic arthritis; RA, rheumatoid arthritis.

low and the reported outcome effect sizes were sufficient.[21,23,46,49,56,57,58,60,62,65,66,67] The remaining studies were "very low" to "low" grade. These studies were generally retrospective observational studies, with no blinding and often with missing data.

24.4.2 Effects of Interventions

Pain

Pre- and postoperative pain scores were often not reported. Usually scores were only measured at the latest follow-up. ▶ Table 24.4 presents studies, which reported both pre- and postoperative scores. The improvement in pain scores following surgery was significant in several cases (▶ Table 24.4).[17,21,47,48,56,58,59,62,63,65]

The study by Radmer et al was a clear outlier from the general trend.[11] Total wrist replacement was performed with the APH prosthesis, an uncemented implant that demonstrated good early results at 18 months. Follow-up

at a mean of 52 (range 24–73) months, however, demonstrated catastrophic failure of all cases with a 100% revision to arthrodesis.

Patient-reported pain scores were poorly measured in the hemiarthroplasty studies. In the study by Ichihara et al using the Prosthelast implant immediately following a distal radius fracture, patients had a mean pain score of 2.8 (0–10 severe) at a mean follow-up of 32 (range 24–42) months.[32] Herzberg et al using the radial component of the Re-Motion and the Cobra implant reported a mean postoperative pain score of 1 (0–10 severe) following surgery for acute distal radial fractures.[37] Herzberg et al reported on a further cohort of four patients in whom they performed a hemiarthroplasty for persistent symptoms after a distal radial fracture at a mean of 3 (range 1–6) months post injury.[37] They reported an improvement in pain scores from a mean of 6 to 2.5. Of note, in both these studies, the hemiarthroplasty was performed in elderly but independent patients with apparently unreconstructible distal radial fractures.

24

Table 24.3 Summary of the included hemiarthroplasty studies

Study	Wrist hemiarthroplasty implant	Underlying pathology	Number of index procedures	Length of follow-up: mean and (range)
Ichihara et al[32]	Prosthelast	Acute posttraumatic	12	32 (24–42) mo
Gaspar et al[33]	Maestro DRH n = 13; Re-Motion DRH n = 39; Maestro CH n = 6	Inflammatory and noninflammatory	58	35 (12–151) mo
Huish et al[34]	Maestro CH	Posttraumatic OA n = 10; Degenerative OA n = 1	11	4 yr
Anneberg et al[35]	KinematX	RA n = 1; PA n = 2; Degenerative OA n = 5; Posttraumatic OA n = 11	20	4.1 (2.3–5.3) yr
Herzberg et al[37]	Re-Motion DRH n = 12; Cobra n = 4	Posttraumatic—acute n = 12; chronic n = 4 (average 3 mo [range 1–6 mo])	16	32 (24–44) mo
		Total	117	

Abbreviations: CH, carpal hemiarthroplasty; DRH, distal radial hemiarthroplasty; OA, osteoarthritis; PA, psoriatic arthritis; RA, rheumatoid arthritis.

Table 24.4 Summary of the pre- and postoperative pain scores in the total wrist arthroplasty studies

Study	Arthroplasty technique (n = no. of cases)	Preoperative pain score (mean unless otherwise stated)	Postoperative pain score (mean unless otherwise stated)	Pain score scale
Rahimtoola and Rozing[17]	RWS n = 27	Moderate–severe: 22; mild: 4; occasional: 1	Significant improvement (p < 0.002)	
Cooney et al[47]	1. Biaxial n = 16 2. Re-Motion n = 22 3. Universal 2 n = 8	7	2.3	0–10 severe
Boeckstyns et al[56]	Re-Motion n = 52	67 (SD 17)	27 (SD 29) (p = 0.001)	0–100 severe
Sagerfors et al[21]	1. Biaxial n = 52 2. Universal 2 n = 12 3. Re-Motion n = 87 4. Maestro n = 68		Significant improvement at rest and activity to 5 yr (p < 0.05)	0–10 severe
Badge et al[48]	Universal 2 n = 95	8.1 (range 3–10)	5.4 (range 0–10) p < 0.001	0–10 severe
Gil et al[63]	Universal 2 n = 39	8.6 ± 1.2	0.4 ± 0.8 (p < 0.001)	0–10 severe
Reigstad et al[65]	Motec n = 56	Radially Rest: 34 (SD 23); Active: 69 (SD 20)	Radially Rest: 8 (SD 14); Active: 20 (SD 22) (p < 0.05)	0–100 severe
Pfanner et al[58]	Universal 2 n = 23	9	0.82	0–10 severe
Brinkhorst et al[62]	Universal 2 n = 23	6 (SD 1)	3 (SD 3)	0–10 severe
Honecker et al[59]	Re-Motion n = 23	6.8	2.8 (p < 0.05)	0–10 severe

Note: The scale of the scoring system is given unless a Likert system was used.

Functional Outcome

▶ Table 24.5 provides a summary of the TWA studies which used the DASH or Quick-DASH, therefore allowing more direct comparison between implants. Several arthroplasty studies reported a significant improvement in outcome scores following surgery (▶ Table 24.5).[54,56,57,59,61,65] Sagerfors et al. observed this improvement with several different implants up to 5 years after surgery in outcome measures also including the Canadian occupational performance measure (COPM) and patient-reported wrist evaluation (PRWE).[21] Herzberg et al and Boeckstyns et al reported no statistically significant difference in the Quick-DASH score for wrist arthroplasty performed for inflammatory or noninflammatory arthritis.[56,64]

Table 24.5 Summary of the DASH and Quick-DASH scores for the total wrist arthroplasty studies

Study	Arthroplasty technique (n = no. of cases)	Preoperative DASH score (range)	Postoperative DASH score (range)	Notes
Divelbiss et al[54]	Universal n = 22	46	1 yr: 32.1 (p < 0.05); 2 yr: 22.4 (8 wrists)	Significant improvement at 1 yr
Ward et al[51]	Universal n = 19	62 (42–80)	Mean 7.8 yr: 40 (18–80)	
Reigstad et al[16]	Motec n = 8	–	Mean 7.6 yr: Median 10.3 (1.7–71.2)	
Cooney et al[47]	1. Biaxial n = 16 2. Re-Motion n = 22 3. Universal 2 n = 8	–	Biaxial (n = 8) = 48; Re-Motion (n = 16) = 37; Universal 2 (n = 7) = 20.	DASH scores not available for all cases No significant difference between implants (p value = 0.07)
Ekroth et al[50]	1. Biaxial n = 6 2. Volz n = 1	–	60.7	5/7 wrists revised to arthrodesis DASH for arthrodesis patients 46.2
Herzberg et al[64]	Re-Motion n = 215	–	% Improvement Rheumatoid: 20 Non-Rheum: 21	No significant difference between rheumatoid and nonrheumatoid patients
Morapudi et al[61]	Universal 2 n = 19	55.1 (22.5–87.0)	44.8 (4.3–83.3)	p = 0.004 PRWE pre = 81.4 (44.5–100); PRWE post = 35.8 (0.0–100) p < 0.001
Boeckstyns et al[56]	Re-Motion n = 52	Quick-DASH median: 58 (14–89)	Quick-DASH median: 42 (0–84)	Significant improvement: p = 0.001
Sagerfors et al[21]	1. Biaxial n = 52 2. Universal 2 n = 12 3. Re-Motion n = 87 4. Maestro n = 68		Biax: (–)12.8 [(–)21.9 – 4.2]; Universal 2: (–)13.7 [(–27.1) – (–)6.2]; Re-Motion: (–)12.3 [(–)25.5 – (–)1.4]; Maestro: (–)16.8 [(–)29.5 – (-)5.3]	Scores reported are preoperative minus postoperative at 5 yr (median and interquartile range) All change significant p < 0.05 PRWE and COPM also significant (p < 0.05)
Badge et al[48]	Universal 2 n = 95	Quick-DASH (n = 40) = 61.3 (16–91)	Quick-DASH (n = 59) = 45.8 (0–89)	Significant improvement— p < 0.001 Wrightington wrist score also significant (p < 0.001)
Chevrollier et al[49]	1. Universal n = 10 2. Re-Motion n = 7		Quick-DASH = 29 % (2.3–65.9 %)	PRWE = 26 % (range 2–55.3 %)
Reigstad et al[65]	Motec n = 56	Quick-DASH 39 (SD 18)	25 (SD 19) p < 0.05	p < 0.05
Pfanner et al[58]	Universal 2 n = 23		Quick-DASH 49	PRWHE = 41.7 (ADL domain)
Giwa et al[57]	Motec n = 25	Quick-DASH 57.6	21.05	p = 0.001
Brinkhorst et al[62]	Universal 2 n = 23	53.2 (SD 20)	12 mo (n = 12): 30.4 (SD 20)	>2 yr (n = 8) 17.5 (3–34)
Honecker et al[59]	Re-Motion n = 23	Quick-DASH 57.9	37.9	p < 0.05

Abbreviations: ADL, activities of daily living; COPM, Canadian occupational performance measure; DASH, disabilities of the arm, shoulder, and hand; PRWE, patient reported wrist evaluation; PRWHE, patient reported wrist and hand evaluation; SD, standard deviation.
Note: Scores were presented as the mean (range) unless otherwise stated.

24

Table 24.6 Summary of the DASH and Quick-DASH scores for hemiarthroplasty studies

Study	Arthroplasty technique (n = no. of cases)	Preoperative DASH score (range)	Postoperative DASH score (range)	Notes
Ichihara et al[32]	Prosthelast n = 12		Quick-Dash 37.4	
Huish et al[34]	Maestro CH n = 11	58.3	55.7	p > 0.05
Anneberg et al[35]	KinematX n = 20	50.3	24.6	
Herzberg et al[37]	Re-Motion DRH n = 12; Cobra n = 4	Quick-DASH chronic 87.5%	38.5%	Quick-DASH acute 25% (postop)

Abbreviations: CH, carpal hemiarthroplasty; DASH, disabilities of the arm, shoulder, and hand; DRH, distal radial hemiarthroplasty; SD, standard deviation.
Note: Scores are presented as the mean (range) unless otherwise stated.

The hemiarthroplasty studies typically reported DASH or Quick-DASH scores, and in nontrauma cases, pre- and postoperative scores were provided (▶ Table 24.6). Trends were difficult to identify because of the small number of studies to date. Anneberg et al demonstrated an improvement in the DASH score using the KinematX hemiarthroplasty in 20 patients with wrist arthritis at a mean follow-up of 4.1 (range 2.3–5.3) years.[35] Huish et al, however, had contrasting findings[34]: they used the carpal component of the Maestro wrist system in 11 patients with advanced wrist arthritis. They found no significant improvement in the DASH score following surgery. A high failure rate was observed in this study (45%; 5 of 11 cases).

Range of Motion and Grip Strength

There was a general trend for the long-term postoperative ranges of motion following a TWA to reach functional levels as defined by Palmar et al (5 degrees of flexion, 30 degrees of extension, 10 degrees of radial deviation, and 15 degrees of ulnar deviation).[31] ▶ Table 24.7 summarizes the postoperative ranges of motion for studies on contemporary wrist implants. A significant improvement in range was not commonly seen (▶ Table 24.7). It is worth noting that Reigstad et al define ranges of motion as "total active motion" combining flexion, extension, and radial and ulnar deviation.[16,65] Of the historical implants, only the Destot prosthesis achieved a range of motion within the functional range: 48-degree flexion, 41-degree extension, 12-degree radial, and 22-degree ulnar deviation, 90-degree pronation, and 77-degree supination.[10]

A significant improvement in grip strength was seen by several authors: Boeckstyns et al with the Re-Motion; Sagerfors et al with the Biaxial, Re-Motion, and Maestro; Badge et al with the Universal 2; Giwa et al with the Motec; and Honecker et al with the Re-Motion.[21,48,56,57,59]

A summary of ranges of motion for wrist hemiarthroplasty is given in ▶ Table 24.8. A significant improvement in range of motion was only seen with the KinematX prosthesis.[35] The achieved ranges were to functional levels. Although Huish et al observed a high failure rate with the Maestro carpal component, the postoperative ranges of motion attained with the implant were also within functional ranges.[34] A significant improvement in grip strength was also seen with the KinematX prosthesis, from a mean of 14.1 kgf preoperatively to 20.8 kgf postoperatively (p < 0.05).

Adverse Events and Survival

▶ Table 24.9 provides an overview of the range of complications seen with TWA and wrist hemiarthroplasty. The fourth-generation total wrist implants were analyzed separately from the preceding generations. The complication rates for fourth-generation implants (range 0.1–3.4%) were marginally, but not significantly, better than those for second/third-generation designs (range 0.1–6.6%). The APH implant, a third-generation prosthesis demonstrated high failure rates.[11] This implant was revised to an arthrodesis in 100% of cases.

Osteolysis was a major issue in wrist arthroplasty, typically on the carpal (5.8%) rather than radial side (1.2%). This is less of an issue with more recent fourth-generation implants (carpal osteolysis: 1.3%; radial osteolysis: 1.2%). This was seen in many studies as well as registry data from both Norwegian and Australian registers.[23,70] Aseptic loosening (3.4%) was the most common issue reported in fourth-generation implants. Aseptic loosening[11,14,19,51] and dislocation[11,15,18,21,54] were common reasons for revision in second- and third-generation implants across many studies.

The adverse event profile for the hemiarthroplasty cases should be used as a guide only because not all studies provided sufficient detail to perform an in-depth analysis. The study by Huish et al for example reported a high complication rate but little detail on individual complication types.[34] In their case series of 11 patients treated with the Maestro carpal implant, they reported a 45% failure rate at a mean of 19 (range 12–24) months. Cases were revised for ulnar-sided wrist pain. Ulnar subsidence and sclerosis of the lunate facet were seen in the failures.

Table 24.7 Summary of the range of motion for contemporary total wrist arthroplasty systems

Study	Technique (n = no. of cases)	Flexion	Extension	Radial deviation	Ulna deviation	Pronation	Supination	Total active range
Reigstad et al[16]	Motec n = 8							F/E/R/U 125 (100–48)
Ferreres[20]	Universal 2 n = 19; Universal n = 2	42 (SD 10)	26 (SD 14)	1 (SD 7)	26 (SD 9)			Flex–ext arc 68
Cooney et al[47]	1. Biaxial n = 16 2. Re-Motion n = 22 3. Universal 2 n = 8	30	38	8	20	75	70	
Herzberg et al[64]	Re-Motion n = 215	Rheum: 29 Non-Rh: 37	29 36	5 10	24 28			
Morapudi et al[61]	Universal 2 n = 19	31[a]	22[a]					Flex–ext arc 53[a]
Bidwai et al[52]	Re-Motion n = 13	23	35	7	15			Flex–ext arc 47
Boeckstyns et al[56]	Re-Motion n = 52	29 (SD 19)	31 (SD 18)	6 (SD 8)	22 (SD 14)[a]	81 (SD 11)	83 (SD 12)[a]	
Sagerfors et al[21]	1. Biaxial n = 52 2. Universal 2 n = 12 3. Re-Motion n = 87 4. Maestro n = 68	No significant improvement	Significant improvement for Biax and Maestro only.	Significant improvement for Maestro only	Significant improvement for Maestro and Re-Motion	Significant improvement for Biax	Significant improvement for Re-Motion	
Badge et al[48]	Universal 2 n = 95	31[b]	29[a]	4	14	82	76	
Chevrollier et al[49]	1. Universal n = 10 2. Re-Motion n = 7							Flex–ext arc 33
Gil et al[63]	Universal 2 n = 39	37 (SD 14)	29 (SD 13)					
Reigstad et al[65]	Motec n = 56					83 (SD 7)	83 (SD 11)	F/E/R/U 126 (SD 37)[a]
Singh et al[60]	Universal 2 n = 12	Flex–ext arc 49 (SD 16)		Radial–ulna arc 30 (SD 16)				
Pfanner et al[58]	Universal 2 n = 23	Flex–ext arc 72		Radial–ulna arc 25				
Giwa et al[57]	Motec n = 25	Flex–ext arc 112[b]		Radial–ulna arc 40		Pronation–supination arc 137		
Brinkhorst et al[62]	Universal 2 n = 23	Flex–ext arc 71 (SD 25)		Radial–ulna arc 54 (SD 18)				
Honecker et al[59]	Re-Motion n = 23	39	44[a]			75	78	

Abbreviations: F/E, flexion–extension; R/U, radial–ulna; SD, standard deviation.
Note: All measures are in degrees, and all values are rounded to nearest degree for simplicity.
[a]p < 0.05.
[b]p < 0.001.

24

Table 24.8 Summary of the range of motion for wrist hemiarthroplasty systems

Study	Technique (n = no. of cases)	Flexion	Extension	Radial deviation	Ulna deviation	Pronation	Supination
Ichihara et al[32]	Prosthelast n = 12	56.1 % of CL	79.3 % of CL			91 % of CL	87.7 % of CL
Huish et al[34]	Maestro n = 11	40	39	15	14	78	87
Anneberg et al[35]	KinematX n = 20	Flex–ext arc 96[a]		Radial–ulna arc 32.4[a]			
Herzberg et al[37]	Re-Motion n = 12; Cobra n = 4	Flex–ext arc: Acute fracture 62 Chronic 62				Pronation–supination arc: Acute fracture 149 Chronic 150	

Abbreviations: CL, contralateral side; F/E, flexion–extension; R/U, radial–ulna; SD, standard deviation.
Note: All measures are in degrees, and all values are rounded to nearest degree for simplicity.
[a]$p < 0.05$.
[b](+)$p < 0.001$.

Table 24.9 Specific complication rates (results given in %)

Complication	Second- and third-generation TWA prosthesis (total cases 663)	Fourth-generation TWA prosthesis (total cases 880)	Hemiarthroplasty (total cases 117)
Fracture	0.3	0.5	–
Nerve problems	0.6	0.3	1.7
CRPS	0.1	0.1	6.0
Wound problems	0.7	0.3	–
Superficial infection	0.3	0.5	1.7
Deep infection	0.7	0.7	0.9
Tendon problems	0.5	0.8	–
Impingement	0.3	0.8	6.0
Pain and stiffness	2.6	2.1	15.4
DRUJ symptoms	–	0.7	0.9
Metalwork breakage	0.3	0.1	–
Instability/Imbalance	1.3	0.3	3.4
Malalignment	1.1	0.3	–
Dislocation	1.6	0.4	–
Aseptic loosening	6.6	3.4	6.0
Radiological			
Radial osteolysis	1.2	1.2	–
Carpal/metacarpal osteolysis	5.8	1.3	–
General osteolysis	3.6	2.5	2.6
Implant migration	2.6	0.2	3.4
Other[a]	1.0	0.1	–
Range	0.1–6.6 %[b]	0.1–3.4 %[b]	0.9–15.4 %

Abbreviations: CRPS, chronic regional pain syndrome; DRUJ, distal radioulnar joint; TWA, total wrist arthroplasty.
[a]E.g., screw loosening, polyethylene linear wear.
[b]Mann-Whitney U-test—no significant difference ($p > 0.05$) between second/third-generation and fourth-generation TWA.

24

Other notable complications commonly observed in wrist hemiarthroplasty were pain and stiffness (15.4%), impingement (6.0%), and aseptic loosening (6.0%). Impingement in this review was taken as implant abutment against opposing carpal or radius bone(s) leading to bone erosion. This was predominantly reported by Gaspar et al in both distal radial hemiarthroplasty and carpal hemiarthroplasty cases.[33] The KinematX, designed purely as a radial hemiarthroplasty, was followed up for 4.1 years (range 2.3–5.3); it

had a lower complication profile compared to the Maestro and Re-Motion systems.[35] In the 20 patients managed with this prosthesis, two cases were revised to a TWA (one for aseptic loosening and the second for chronic regional pain syndrome) and one case to a total wrist arthrodesis for ulna-sided pain. Three patients required a manipulation under anesthesia for wrist stiffness. ▶ Table 24.10 provides a summary of the revision and arthrodesis conversion rates across the studies.

Table 24.10 Revision rates and conversion to arthrodesis rates for total wrist arthroplasty

Study	Implant (n = no. of cases)	Implant generation	Revision rate (%)	Conversion to arthrodesis (%)	Length of follow-up: mean and (range)
Menon[15]	Volz n = 18	2	33	0	40 (24–66) mo
Figgie et al[55]	Trispherical n = 35	2	5.7	5.7	9 (5–11) yr
Meuli and Fernandez[14]	MWP II Meuli n = 49	2	18	12.2	4.5 (2–6) yr
Gellman et al[53]	Volz n = 14	2	13.3	7.1	6.5 (3.5–11.5) yr
Menon[18]	Universal n = 37	3	26	5.4	79.4 (48–120) mo
Takwale et al[19]	Biaxial n = 66	3	7.6	4.5	52 (12–99) mo
Divelbiss et al[54]	Universal n = 22	3	18.2	4.5	1–2 yr
Levadoux and Legre[10]	Destot n = 28	3	14.3	14.3	47 (12–72) mo
Rahimtoola and Rozing[17]	RWS n = 27	2	3.7	3.7	4 (2–8) yr
Radmer et al[11]	*APH n = 40*	*3*	*0*	*100*	*52 (24–73) mo*
Murphy et al[66]	Universal n = 27	3	3.7	3.7	26 ± 16 mo
Ward et al[51]	Universal n = 19	3	52.6	42.1	7.3 (5–10.8) yr
Reigstad et al[16]	Motec n = 8	2	37.5	25	7.6 (7–9) yr
Ferreres[20]	Universal 2 n = 19 Universal n = 2	4	4.8	0	5.5 (3–8) yr
Krukhaug et al[23]	1. Biaxial n = 90 (80/90 uncemented) 2. Elos n = 23 3. Gibbon n = 76	3 3 3	21 (Elos = 10, Gibbon = 11, Biax = 18)	0	
Cooney et al[47]	1. Biaxial n = 16 2. Re-Motion n = 22 3. Universal 2 n = 8	3 4 4	19.6 (Biaxial = 8; Universal 2 = 1)	13.0	6.0 (3.5–15) yr
Ekroth et al[50]	1. Biaxial n = 6 2. Volz n = 1	3 2	41.7	41.7	17.8 (11.7–28.3) yr
Herzberg et al[64]	Re-Motion n = 215	3	5.1	2.3	4 (2–8) yr
Morapudi et al[61]	Universal 2 n = 19	4	0	0	3.1 (1.8–3.9) yr
Bidwai et al[52]	Re-Motion n = 13	4	7.7	0	33 (14–56) mo
Boeckstyns et al[56]	Re-Motion n = 52	4	9.6	5.8	6.5 (5–9) yr
Nydick et al[67]	Maestro n = 7	4	14.3	14.3	56 ± 10 mo

(Continued)

24

Table 24.10 (*Continued*) Revision rates and conversion to arthrodesis rates for total wrist arthroplasty

Study	Implant (n = no. of cases)		Implant generation	Revision rate (%)	Conversion to arthrodesis (%)	Length of follow-up: mean and (range)
Sagerfors et al[21]	1. Biaxial n = 52	3		8.7	0	7 (2–13) yr
	2. Universal 2 n = 12	4				
	3. Re-Motion n = 87	4				
	4. Maestro n = 68	4				
Badge et al[48]	Universal 2 n = 95	4		3.5	3.5	53 (24–120) mo
Chevrollier et al[49]	1. Universal n = 10	3		23.5	17.6	5.2 (1.1–10) yr
	2. Re-Motion n = 7	4				
Gaspar et al[33]	Maestro n = 47	4		47	Unclear	
Gil et al[63]	Universal 2 n = 39	4		7.7	0	9 (4.8–14.7) yr
Reigstad et al[65]	Motec n = 56	2		7.1	7.1	8 (5–11) yr
Singh et al[60]	Universal 2 n = 23	4		0	0	30 (12–50) mo
Pfanner et al[58]	Universal 2 n = 23	4		26	4.3	82.3 mo (2–12) yr
Giwa et al[57]	Motec n = 25	4		16.7	8	50 (26–66) mo
Brinkhorst et al[62]	Universal 2 n = 23	4		0	0	24 (24–50) mo
Honecker et al[59]	Re-Motion n = 23	4		13.0	8.7	6 yr
			Range[a]	0–52.6%	0–42.1%	

[a]Excluding Radmer et al.[11]

Survival

The revision rate for fourth-generation TWA implants ranged from 0 to 47%, and for second- and third-generation implants from 3.7 to 52.6%. The rates of conversion to arthrodesis ranged from 0 to 14.3% and 0 to 42.1%, respectively. These figures do not include the outcomes from the study by Radmer et al with the APH prosthesis which had a 100% failure rate at 52 (range 24–73) months.[11]

In the wrist hemiarthroplasty studies, Huish et al reported a 45% failure rate with the Maestro carpal component; this was managed by conversion to wrist arthrodesis in 3 (of 11) cases and conversion to a TWA in 2 (of 11) cases.[34] Gaspar et al reported their hemiarthroplasty experience with the Maestro radial component (13), Re-Motion radial component (39), and Maestro carpal component (6).[33] They reported a 29% revision rate for radial hemiarthroplasty and 67% revision rate for carpal hemiarthroplasty. The rate of conversion to arthrodesis was unclear. Anneberg et al reported a conversion to TWA in 2 of 20 cases and conversion to total wrist arthrodesis in 1 of 20 with the KinematX implant.[35]

Implant Survival

Increasingly, studies are reporting survival data. Prosthesis survival is defined as the time to implant revision for any cause. The data should be interpreted with caution as often they are obtained from small case series. Data over 10 years are now available on most of the currently available implants (▶ Table 24.11). The Universal 2 has reported survival rates of 78% at 15 years.[63] The Re-Motion on one study was noted to have 90% survival at 9 years[56]; however, more recent data by Honecker et al suggest a less impressive survival rate of 69% at 10 years.[59] The Maestro has a reported survival of 95% at 8 years,[21] while the Motec has a reported survival of 86% at 10 years, in a cohort of mostly osteoarthritic patients.[65]

Wrist hemiarthroplasty is relatively new compared to TWA. Survival data have been reported infrequently. Anneberg et al reported 80% survivorship at 5 years with the KinematX.[35] Survival data are not available in the other studies.

24.5 Discussion

A total of 1,543 TWA procedures and 117 hemiarthroplasty procedures were analyzed qualitatively in this review, representing the largest study of its kind to date.

There are now survival data of over 10 years for three of the currently available implants. Gil et al reported a 78% survival rate at 15 years with the Universal 2; Reigstad et al demonstrated an 86% survival of the Motec; and Honecker et al reported 69% with the Re-Motion both at 10 years.[59,63,65] The revision rates in these studies were 7.7% (3 of 38 cases), 7.1% (4 of 56 cases), and 13.0% (3 of 23 cases), respectively.[59,63,65]

Improvements in osseointegration technology with fourth-generation implants are reflected in a mean aseptic loosening rate requiring revision surgery of only 3.4%,

Table 24.11 Implant survival

Study	Implant	Total no. of cases	Survival	
Takwale et al[19]	Biaxial	224	83% at 8 yr	–
Krukhaug et al[23]			85% at 5 yr	–
Cooney et al[47]			50% at 6 yr	–
Sagerfors et al[21]			81% at 8 yr	78% at 12 yr
Levadoux and Legre[10]	Destot	28	85% 4 yr	
Radmer et al[11]	APH	40	100% failure 52 mo (range 24–73)	
Krukhaug et al[23]	Elos	23	57% at 5 yr	
Krukhaug et al[23]	Gibbon	76	77% at 4 yr	
Ward et al[51]	Universal	29	75% at 5 yr	60% at 7 yr
Chevrollier et al[49]			90% at 5 yr	50% at 10 yr
Morapudi et al[61]	Universal 2	230	100% at 3.9 yr	
Singh et al[60]			100% at 4 yr	
Brinkhorst et al[62]			100% at 4 yr	
Cooney et al[47]			97% at 6 yr	
Badge et al[48]			91% at 7.8 yr	
Pfanner et al[58]			64% at 12 yr	
Gil et al[63]			78% at 15 yr	
Cooney et al[47]	Re-Motion	406	97% at 6 yr	–
Herzberg et al (2012)			92% at 8 yr	–
Boeckstyns et al[56]			90% at 9 yr	94% at 8 yr
Sagerfors et al[21]			99% at 5 yr	75% 6 yr (est)
Chevrollier et al[49]			100% at 6 yr	
Honecker et al[59]			69% at 10 yr	
Sagerfors et al[21]	Maestro	68	95% at 8 yr	
Reigstad et al[16]	Motec	64	93.3% at 6 yr	
Reigstad et al[65]			86% at 10 yr	

compared to 6.6% in second/third-generation implants. Design changes to the Motec, including screw shape change and implant coating technology, have led to improved survival. The Elos, which was the early iteration of the Motec, had a survival of only 57% at 5 years according to data from the Norwegian Joint Registry.[23]

The earlier second- and third-generation systems have also been prone to instability (1.3%), malalignment (1.1%), and dislocation (1.6%). These complications together with implant loosening were the commonly reported reasons for implant revision across the studies reviewed. Dislocation has been well documented for the Volz, Universal, and Biaxial implants.[15,18,19,54] The articular bearing shape of the Universal was modified from a toroidal to an ellipsoidal shape in the Universal 2 to counteract this problem.[24] Better capsular repair techniques and soft tissue balancing have also helped improve stability.[54] Third-generation implants attempted to better reproduce the anatomic center of wrist motion to further improve stability.[13,14,18,19] Osteolysis seen on radiological assessment is a common occurrence. The osteolysis rates, comparing second/third-generation implants to fourth generation, have improved from 10.6 to 5% and reported

implant migration from 2.6 to 0.2%, respectively (▶ Table 24.9). In a previous systematic review, the complication rates for fourth-generation implants were significantly lower than preceding generations.[30] In this study, the complication rates were less in fourth-generation implants; however, this difference did not reach significance (0.1–6.6% vs. 0.1–3.4%, p > 0.05).

Ongoing disease activity in rheumatoid arthritis may be a contributing factor in implant performance; this was a particular issue in the series by Pfanner et al reporting on the Universal 2.[58] This finding is, however, not consistently seen across all studies.[21,33] National joint registry data from Norway has found no association between survival of wrist implants and underlying disease etiology for the Biax, Elos, and Gibbon prostheses.[23]

Postoperative pain scores after TWA improved significantly in several series (▶ Table 24.4).[17,21,48,56,59,63,65] A significant improvement in functional outcome was also reported with several implants including the Re-Motion,[21,56,59] Motec,[57,65] Universal 2,[21,48,61] and Maestro.[21] A significant improvement in ranges of motion was not typically reported, although preoperative motion was generally preserved following a TWA. In contrast, grip strength was reported to improve significantly with the Re-Motion wrist,[21,56,59] Motec,[57] Universal 2[48], Biaxial,[21] and the Maestro wrist arthroplasties.[21]

Clinical outcomes of wrist hemiarthroplasty have been mixed. There have been several publications reporting early to midterm outcomes only.[32,33,34,35,36,37,38,39] Huish et al reported a high failure rate with the Maestro as a carpal hemiarthroplasty in 11 patients at 4 years follow-up.[34] Despite promising early results, 5 of the 11 patients were revised for ulnar-sided wrist pain to either an arthrodesis (n = 3) or a TWA (n = 2). Ulnar subsidence and sclerosis of the lunate facet of the radius were reported. It was speculated that poor congruency between the implant and the lunate facet led to unequal loading and failure. The group discontinued the use of the implant. Gaspar et al also reflected these findings with a 10 % (5 cases) failure rate in their series of radial hemiarthroplasties (n = 52; Maestro DRH = 13, Re-Motion DRH = 39).[33] The majority of major complications (80 %, including component failure and deep infection) occurred in the Maestro DRH subgroup. Various newer implants have also been introduced including the KinematX,[35] the Cobra,[37] and the radial component of the Prosthelast system.[32] The KinematX seems to be the most promising system according to the published data. Anneberg et al demonstrated an early improvement in motion, grip strength, and function at a mean follow-up of 4.1 (range 2.3–5.3) years for patients with wrist arthritis of various causes.[35] Of the 20 cases, 2 were revised to a TWA and 1 to a total wrist arthrodesis for osteolysis, chronic regional pain syndrome, and ulnar-sided pain, respectively. Early clinical outcomes of wrist hemiarthroplasty for non-reconstructable distal radial fractures in elderly patients are emerging.[32,36,37,38,39,40] This was first described by Roux in 2011 and subsequently popularized by Herzberg.[36,37,38,39] It is currently too early to establish any trends in clinical outcomes at this stage. Overall, there are some notable complications seen with wrist hemiarthroplasty, including chronic regional pain syndrome (6 %), impingement (6 %), aseptic loosening (6 %), and pain and stiffness (15.4 %) (▶ Table 24.9). As with all new treatments, patients should be thoroughly counseled before wrist hemiarthroplasty and monitored closely after the procedure.

In general, TWA is reported to reduce pain markedly, improve grip strength, and preserve motion in patients with a symptomatic arthritic wrist. The complication rates appear to be improving, but not dramatically. Survival rates have also improved with the newer fourth-generation implants. TWA has become a more established treatment option and a valid alternative to wrist arthrodesis in appropriate patients. Early to midterm outcome data on wrist hemiarthroplasty have been mixed. There are only a small number of published studies, with relatively small numbers of cases especially compared to lower limb arthroplasty.

References

[1] Swanson AB. Flexible implant arthroplasty for arthritic disabilities of the radiocarpal joint: a silicone rubber intramedullary stemmed flexible hinge implant for the wrist joint. Orthop Clin North Am. 1973; 4 (2):383–394

[2] Swanson AB, de Groot Swanson G, Maupin BK. Flexible implant arthroplasty of the radiocarpal joint: surgical technique and long-term study. Clin Orthop Relat Res. 1984(187):94–106

[3] Comstock CP, Louis DS, Eckenrode JF. Silicone wrist implant: long-term follow-up study. J Hand Surg Am. 1988; 13(2):201–205

[4] Haloua JP, Collin JP, Schernberg F, Sandre J. Arthroplasty of the rheumatoid wrist with Swanson implant: long-term results and complications. Ann Chir Main. 1989; 8(2):124–134

[5] Meuli HC. Meuli total wrist arthroplasty. Clin Orthop Relat Res. 1984 (187):107–111

[6] Volz RG. The development of a total wrist arthroplasty. Clin Orthop Relat Res. 1976(116):209–214

[7] Volz RG. Total wrist arthroplasty: a new approach to wrist disability. Clin Orthop Relat Res. 1977(128):180–189

[8] Figgie HE, III, Ranawat CS, Inglis AE, Straub LR, Mow C. Preliminary results of total wrist arthroplasty in rheumatoid arthritis using the Trispherical total wrist arthroplasty. J Arthroplasty. 1988; 3(1):9–15

[9] Cobb TK, Beckenbaugh RD. Biaxial total-wrist arthroplasty. J Hand Surg Am. 1996; 21(6):1011–1021

[10] Levadoux M, Legré R. Total wrist arthroplasty with Destot prostheses in patients with posttraumatic arthritis. J Hand Surg Am. 2003; 28 (3):405–413

[11] Radmer S, Andresen R, Sparmann M. Total wrist arthroplasty in patients with rheumatoid arthritis. J Hand Surg Am. 2003; 28 (5):789–794

[12] Meuli HC. Arthroplasty of the wrist. Clin Orthop Relat Res. 1980 (149):118–125

[13] Meuli HC. Total wrist arthroplasty: experience with a noncemented wrist prosthesis. Clin Orthop Relat Res. 1997(342):77–83

[14] Meuli HC, Fernandez DL. Uncemented total wrist arthroplasty. J Hand Surg Am. 1995; 20(1):115–122

[15] Menon J. Total wrist replacement using the modified Volz prosthesis. J Bone Joint Surg Am. 1987; 69(7):998–1006

[16] Reigstad A, Reigstad O, Grimsgaard C, Røkkum M. New concept for total wrist replacement. J Plast Surg Hand Surg. 2011; 45(3):148–156

[17] Rahimtoola ZO, Rozing PM. Preliminary results of total wrist arthroplasty using the RWS Prosthesis. J Hand Surg [Br]. 2003; 28(1):54–60

[18] Menon J. Universal total wrist implant: experience with a carpal component fixed with three screws. J Arthroplasty. 1998; 13(5):515–523

[19] Takwale VJ, Nuttall D, Trail IA, Stanley JK. Biaxial total wrist replacement in patients with rheumatoid arthritis: clinical review, survivorship and radiological analysis. J Bone Joint Surg Br. 2002; 84(5):692–699

[20] Ferreres A, Lluch A, Del Valle M. Universal total wrist arthroplasty: midterm follow-up study. J Hand Surg Am. 2011; 36(6):967–973

[21] Sagerfors M, Gupta A, Brus O, Pettersson K. Total wrist arthroplasty: a single-center study of 219 cases with 5-year follow-up. J Hand Surg Am. 2015; 40(12):2380–2387

[22] Reigstad O. Wrist arthroplasty: bone fixation, clinical development and mid to long term results. Acta Orthop Suppl. 2014; 85(354):1–53

[23] Krukhaug Y, Lie SA, Havelin LI, Furnes O, Hove LM. Results of 189 wrist replacements: a report from the Norwegian Arthroplasty Register. Acta Orthop. 2011; 82(4):405–409

[24] Grosland NM, Rogge RD, Adams BD. Influence of articular geometry on prosthetic wrist stability. Clin Orthop Relat Res. 2004(421):134–142

[25] Herzberg G. Prospective study of a new total wrist arthroplasty: short term results. Chir Main. 2011; 30(1):20–25

[26] Botero S, Igeta Y, Facca S, Pizza C, Hidalgo Diaz JJ, Liverneaux PA. Surgical technique: about a new total and isoelastic wrist implant (Prosthelast®). Eur J Orthop Surg Traumatol. 2018; 28(8):1525–1530

[27] Cavaliere CM, Chung KC. A systematic review of total wrist arthroplasty compared with total wrist arthrodesis for rheumatoid arthritis. Plast Reconstr Surg. 2008; 122(3):813–825

[28] Boeckstyns ME. Wrist arthroplasty: a systematic review. Dan Med J. 2014; 61(5):A4834

[29] Yeoh D, Tourret L. Total wrist arthroplasty: a systematic review of the evidence from the last 5 years. J Hand Surg Eur Vol. 2015; 40(5):458–468

[30] Berber O, Garagnani L, Gidwani S. Systematic review of total wrist arthroplasty and arthrodesis in wrist arthritis. J Wrist Surg. 2018; 7 (5):424–440

[31] Palmer AK, Werner FW, Murphy D, Glisson R. Functional wrist motion: a biomechanical study. J Hand Surg Am. 1985; 10(1):39–46

[32] Ichihara S, Díaz JJ, Peterson B, Facca S, Bodin F, Liverneaux P. Distal radius isoelastic resurfacing prosthesis: a preliminary report. J Wrist Surg. 2015; 4(3):150–155

[33] Gaspar MP, Lou J, Kane PM, Jacoby SM, Osterman AL, Culp RW. Complications following partial and total wrist arthroplasty: a single-center retrospective review. J Hand Surg Am. 2016; 41(1):47–53.e4

[34] Huish EG, Jr, Lum Z, Bamberger HB, Trzeciak MA. Failure of wrist hemiarthroplasty. Hand (N Y). 2017; 12(4):369–375

[35] Anneberg M, Packer G, Crisco JJ, Wolfe S. Four-year outcomes of midcarpal hemiarthroplasty for wrist arthritis. J Hand Surg Am. 2017; 42 (11):894–903

[36] Herzberg G, Burnier M, Marc A, Izem Y. Primary wrist hemiarthroplasty for irreparable distal radius fracture in the independent elderly. J Wrist Surg. 2015; 4(3):156–163

[37] Herzberg G, Merlini L, Burnier M. Hemi-arthroplasty for distal radius fracture in the independent elderly. Orthop Traumatol Surg Res. 2017; 103(6):915–918

[38] Herzberg G, Walch A, Burnier M. Wrist hemiarthroplasty for irreparable DRF in the elderly. Eur J Orthop Surg Traumatol. 2018; 28 (8):1499–1503

[39] Roux JL. Traitement des fractures intra-articulaires du radius distal par remplacement et resurfaçage prothétique. Revue de chirurgie orthopédique et traumatologique. 2011; 97; S:S:46–S–53

[40] Vergnenègre G, Mabit C, Charissoux JL, Arnaud JP, Marcheix PS. Treatment of comminuted distal radius fractures by resurfacing prosthesis in elderly patients. Chir Main. 2014; 33(2):112–117

[41] Felson DT, Anderson JJ, Boers M, et al. The Committee on Outcome Measures in Rheumatoid Arthritis Clinical Trials. The American College of Rheumatology preliminary core set of disease activity measures for rheumatoid arthritis clinical trials. Arthritis Rheum. 1993; 36(6):729–740

[42] Boers M, Tugwell P, Felson DT, et al. World Health Organization and International League of Associations for Rheumatology core endpoints for symptom modifying antirheumatic drugs in rheumatoid arthritis clinical trials. J Rheumatol Suppl. 1994; 41:86–89

[43] Bellamy N, Kirwan J, Boers M, et al. Recommendations for a core set of outcome measures for future phase III clinical trials in knee, hip, and hand osteoarthritis: consensus development at OMERACT III. J Rheumatol. 1997; 24(4):799–802

[44] Kloppenburg M, Bøyesen P, Visser AW, et al. Report from the OMERACT Hand Osteoarthritis Working Group: set of core domains and preliminary set of instruments for use in clinical trials and observational studies. J Rheumatol. 2015; 42(11):2190–2197

[45] Higgins JPT, Green S.Cochrane handbook for systematic reviews of interventions. In: The Cochrane Collaboration; 2011: www.handbook.cochrane.org

[46] Atkins D, Best D, Briss PA, et al. GRADE Working Group. Grading quality of evidence and strength of recommendations. BMJ. 2004; 328 (7454):1490

[47] Cooney W, Manuel J, Froelich J, Rizzo M. Total wrist replacement: a retrospective comparative study. J Wrist Surg. 2012; 1(2):165–172

[48] Badge R, Kailash K, Dickson DR, et al. Medium-term outcomes of the Universal-2 total wrist arthroplasty in patients with rheumatoid arthritis. Bone Joint J. 2016; 98-B(12):1642–1647

[49] Chevrollier J, Strugarek-Lecoanet C, Dap F, Dautel G. Results of a unicentric series of 15 wrist prosthesis implantations at a 5.2 year follow-up. Acta Orthop Belg. 2016; 82(1):31–42

[50] Ekroth SR, Werner FW, Palmer AK. Case report of long-term results of Biaxial and Volz total wrist arthroplasty. J Wrist Surg. 2012; 1 (2):177–178

[51] Ward CM, Kuhl T, Adams BD. Five to ten-year outcomes of the Universal total wrist arthroplasty in patients with rheumatoid arthritis. J Bone Joint Surg Am. 2011; 93(10):914–919

[52] Bidwai AS, Cashin F, Richards A, Brown DJ. Short to medium results using the remotion total wrist replacement for rheumatoid arthritis. Hand Surg. 2013; 18(2):175–178

[53] Gellman H, Hontas R, Brumfield RH, Jr, Tozzi J, Conaty JP. Total wrist arthroplasty in rheumatoid arthritis: a long-term clinical review. Clin Orthop Relat Res. 1997(342):71–76

[54] Divelbiss BJ, Sollerman C, Adams BD. Early results of the Universal total wrist arthroplasty in rheumatoid arthritis. J Hand Surg Am. 2002; 27(2):195–204

[55] Figgie MP, Ranawat CS, Inglis AE, Sobel M, Figgie HE, III. Trispherical total wrist arthroplasty in rheumatoid arthritis. J Hand Surg Am. 1990; 15(2):217–223

[56] Boeckstyns ME, Herzberg G, Merser S. Favorable results after total wrist arthroplasty: 65 wrists in 60 patients followed for 5–9 years. Acta Orthop. 2013; 84(4):415–419

[57] Giwa L, Siddiqui A, Packer G. Motec wrist arthroplasty: 4 years of promising results. J Hand Surg Asian Pac Vol. 2018; 23(3):364–368

[58] Pfanner S, Munz G, Guidi G, Ceruso M. Universal 2 wrist arthroplasty in rheumatoid arthritis. J Wrist Surg. 2017; 6(3):206–215

[59] Honecker S, Igeta Y, Al Hefzi A, Pizza C, Facca S, Liverneaux PA. Survival rate on a 10-year follow-up of total wrist replacement implants: a 23-patient case series. J Wrist Surg. 2019; 8(1):24–29

[60] Singh HP, Bhattacharjee D, Dias JJ, Trail I. Dynamic assessment of the wrist after total wrist arthroplasty. J Hand Surg Eur Vol. 2017; 42 (6):573–579

[61] Morapudi SP, Marlow WJ, Withers D, Ralte P, Gabr A, Waseem M. Total wrist arthroplasty using the Universal 2 prosthesis. J Orthop Surg (Hong Kong). 2012; 20(3):365–368

[62] Brinkhorst ME, Selles RW, Dias JJ, et al. Results of the Universal 2 prosthesis in noninflammatory osteoarthritic wrists. J Wrist Surg. 2018; 7(2):121–126

[63] Gil JA, Kamal RN, Cone E, Weiss AC. High survivorship and few complications with cementless total wrist arthroplasty at a mean follow-up of 9 years. Clin Orthop Relat Res. 2017; 475(12):3082–3087

[64] Herzberg G, Boeckstyns M, Sorensen AI, et al. "Remotion" total wrist arthroplasty: preliminary results of a prospective international multicenter study of 215 cases. J Wrist Surg. 2012; 1(1):17–22

[65] Reigstad O, Holm-Glad T, Bolstad B, Grimsgaard C, Thorkildsen R, Røkkum M. Five- to 10-year prospective follow-up of wrist arthroplasty in 56 nonrheumatoid patients. J Hand Surg Am. 2017; 42 (10):788–796

[66] Murphy DM, Khoury JG, Imbriglia JE, Adams BD. Comparison of arthroplasty and arthrodesis for the rheumatoid wrist. J Hand Surg Am. 2003; 28(4):570–576

[67] Nydick JA, Watt JF, Garcia MJ, Williams BD, Hess AV. Clinical outcomes of arthrodesis and arthroplasty for the treatment of posttraumatic wrist arthritis. J Hand Surg Am. 2013; 38(5):899–903

[68] Courtman NH, Sochart DH, Trail IA, Stanley JK. Biaxial wrist replacement: initial results in the rheumatoid patient. J Hand Surg [Br]. 1999; 24(1):32–34

[69] Reigstad O, Lütken T, Grimsgaard C, Bolstad B, Thorkildsen R, Røkkum M. Promising one- to six-year results with the Motec wrist arthroplasty in patients with post-traumatic osteoarthritis. J Bone Joint Surg Br. 2012; 94(11):1540–1545

[70] Registry NJR. Demographics and outcomes of elbow and wrist replacement: supplementary report 2016. 2016

24

25 Surface Replacement Wrist Arthroplasty

Michel E. H. Boeckstyns and Guillaume Herzberg

Abstract

Surface replacement of the wrist is a motion preserving solution for the salvage of a severely destroyed wrist, i.e., a pan-arthritic wrist. Until the early years of the 21st century, the main indication for prosthetic replacement was inflammatory arthritis. Since then, other conditions have increasingly been of interest, including idiopathic degenerative osteoarthritis, posttraumatic arthritis, Kienböck's disease, and others. There is no clear evidence about which indications lead to the best results and the fewest complications. With the latest generation of wrist arthroplasties the distal carpal row is preserved, onto which the carpal resurfacing component can be fixed. Fixation in the metacarpals is restricted to the index metacarpal. Proximally the radial bone resection is minimal. The implants are mostly metal-on-polyethylene and attempt to mimic the natural anatomy and biomechanics of the wrist and are largely unconstrained. Wrist arthroplasty is a good solution in elderly patients who are not too physically active, or in patients with poor function of the contralateral extremity or other joints of the ipsilateral extremity; in these cases, it may be difficult to compensate for a fused wrist. Generally, clinically and statistically significant improvement in pain scores and patient reported outcome measures are obtained. Most series show no statistically significant improvement of wrist mobility or a statistically significant improvement that is barely clinically relevant. The reported 10-year implant survival ranges from 40–92%. The authors' experience has led them to revise failed total wrist arthoplasties to total wrist arthrodesis rather than to revision arthroplasties.

Keywords: wrist, arthroplasty, replacement, arthritis, implant survival, results

25.1 Introduction

In the past century, two-component implants for total wrist replacement were characterized by extensive resection of carpal bones, bulky implants, and distal fixation in the metacarpals. Failure rates were high and occurred mainly by distal loosening. Implant durability was deceiving and revision surgery was a challenge as a consequence of the resected bone stock. The indications were mainly inflammatory arthritis. On this background, Jay Menon[1] introduced the third generation of total wrist arthroplasty (TWA). He designed a surface replacement prosthesis preserving the distal carpal row, onto which the carpal resurfacing component could be fixed. Proximally, the radial bone resection was minimal. The initial results were favorable, although a high rate of postoperative dislocations necessitated a revision of the implant design. Subsequently,

a number of resurfacing prostheses based on the same principles have been developed.

25.2 Implants

The most commonly reported resurfacing wrist implants are the Universal 2 (Integra),[2] the Re-motion (Stryker),[3] and the Maestro (Biomet).[4] They are characterized by moderate bone resection and avoid fixation in the metacarpal bones, with the exception of an optional, short length of screw fixation in the index finger metacarpal (▶ Fig. 25.1). They attempt to mimic the natural anatomy and biomechanics of the wrist and are largely unconstrained. The prostheses are metal-on-polyethylene, with the radial (proximal) part being concave (metallic in the Re-motion and the Universal, polyethylene in the Maestro) and the distal part being convex. As such, they function similarly to a wrist after proximal row carpectomy. The components are impacted in the bones, mostly without the use of cement. The carpal part is supplemented with screws in the hamate and in the scaphoid/trapezoid/index metacarpal. In recent years, an updated version of the Universal 2 has been launched: the Freedom (Integra).[5] The metal-on-metal Motec (Swemac)[6] could also be considered as a resurfacing implant but differs from the other contemporary designs in being fixated distally in the middle metacarpal and is the subject of Chapter 26.

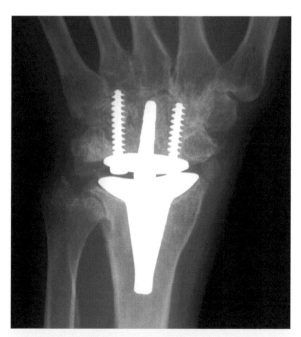

Fig. 25.1 Re-motion total wrist arthroplasty in a 45-year-old woman with rheumatoid arthritis.

The Prosthelast (Agromedical) was originally designed as a hemiarthroplasty and has now been extended to a TWA. The fixation of its carpal component is based on sagittal screw fixation in the capitate.[7]

25.3 Indications and Contraindications

Surface replacement of the wrist is a motion-preserving solution for the salvage of a severely destroyed wrist, i.e., a pan-arthritic wrist. For patients with scapholunate advanced collapse (SLAC) II or III wrists, with preserved cartilage in the midcarpal or radiolunate joints, other interventions should be considered, such as a proximal row carpectomy or a four-corner arthrodesis.[8] In cases of an irreparable joint surface of the distal radius in elderly low-demand patients with an intra-articular distal radius fracture, radiocarpal arthrodesis or distal radius hemiarthroplasty can be used.

Until the early years of the 21st century the main indication for prosthetic replacement was inflammatory arthritis. Since then, other conditions have increasingly been of interest.[9] Today, the debate over indications is polarized between the rheumatoid wrist, generally in low-demand patients but with poorer bone stock, and idiopathic or posttraumatic osteoarthritis (OA)—those patients generally having better bone stock but also being more physically active. There is no clear evidence about which indications lead to the best results and the fewest complications: it seems that carefully selected patients with rheumatoid arthritis (RA) or OA do equally well.[9]

Generally, surgeons should be very cautious about offering TWA to young patients ≤ 50-year-old) (especially for OA), patients that do heavy or moderately heavy work, patients with poor bone quality, rheumatoid patients with severe wrist instability, and patients with poor compliance. In these cases, total wrist arthrodesis is a better option. Conversely, TWA is a good solution in elderly patients who are not too physically active, or in patients with poor function of the contralateral extremity or other joints of the ipsilateral extremity: in these cases, it may be difficult to compensate for a fused wrist.

When advising patients of the options, they should always be given exhaustive and transparent information on what they can expect in terms of complications, function, and durability of TWA as well as of the other available surgical solutions; the choice of operation must be based on shared decision-making.

It seems that the use of TWA has been declining in the past decade for several reasons[10]: primarily, the number of severely destroyed rheumatoid wrists has declined due to the success of new disease-modifying drugs; the initial enthusiasm created by the promising early and medium-term results has been moderated by some longer term reports; and hemiarthroplasty has taken over some of the indications.

25.4 Results in the Literature (Short Version)

25.4.1 Complications

Early Postoperative Complications

The rate of deep postoperative infections is reported to be very low with current implant techniques including the use of perioperative antibiotics. Instability with dislocation was common with the first version of the Universal implant but this problem has been solved with the modified versions, the Universal 2 and the Freedom, and has not been a major problem with the Re-motion or the Maestro.[11] In the systematic review of the literature from 2009 to 2013,[12] the other early complications reported in the literature are: 3 to 17 % wound problems; 5 to 14 % superficial infection; 4 % synovitis; 3 to 5 % tendon laceration/rupture; 3 to 9 % nerve problems. These complications are similar to those encountered after partial and total wrist arthrodesis. Gaspar et al[13] reported a rate of complications as high as 57 % after TWA with the Maestro.

Osteolysis and Implant Loosening

Focal periprosthetic radiolucency after resurfacing arthroplasty of the wrist, with or without frank loosening of the components, has been reported repeatedly.[6,14,15,16,17,18,19,20,21,22,23] Radiolucency is the radiographical sign of periprosthetic osteolysis. In most cases, it is confined to the extremity of the implant components near the joint space and is less than 2 mm in width. In some instances it enlarges initially but stabilizes after a few years without implant loosening (▶ Fig. 25.2). In other cases it results in subsidence, mostly of the carpal components.[15] The mechanism causing osteolysis is multifactorial, including micromotion, particulate debris-induced bone resorption, stress shielding, and increased intra-articular pressure. While it is not clear how to treat asymptomatic-limited periprosthetic osteolysis, osteolysis associated with pain typically requires revision of the implant components or conversion to a wrist arthrodesis.

25.4.2 Functional Results

Generally, clinically and statistically significant improvement in pain scores and patient-reported outcome measures (PROMs) such as the Disability of the Arm, Shoulder and Hand (DASH) questionnaire, the Patient-Rated Wrist Evaluation (PRWE) questionnaire, and the Lyon wrist score can be expected after TWA.[11,12,22,24,25] These scores are comparable to the scores obtained after total wrist arthrodesis, although exact comparison is difficult due to the lack of controlled studies. Most series show no statistically significant improvement in postoperative ranges of motion or a statistically significant improvement that is barely clinically relevant.[3,4,14,18,22,23,26,27,28] Reigstad et al

25

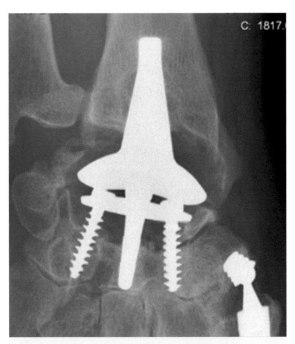

Fig. 25.2 Severe osteolysis 6 years after resurfacing arthroplasty in a patient with rheumatoid arthritis (RA).

reported significantly improved ranges of motion with the Motec prosthesis from 97 to 136 degrees (extension + flexion + ulnar + radial).[6] Changes in grip strength are difficult to evaluate in the published literature but a modest improvement is reported in some series.[12,22,25]

25.4.3 Implant Durability

Implant durability is best assessed with a cumulative survival analysis according to the Kaplan-Meier method with "revision of implant components" as the criterion for implant failure. Alternatively, the revision rate may be used. Reports are equivocal (▶ Table 25.1).

25.5 Authors' Own Experience and Preferred Technique (Tips and Tricks)

25.5.1 Personal Experience

We have been using the Re-motion implant since 2003 at the Gentofte University Hospital, Denmark, after a few years of using the Universal 1 and 2, and at the Lyon University Hospital, France since 2004. One hundred and

Table 25.1 Diagnosis, revision rate, and cumulative survival of the most commonly used resurfacing implants

Publication	Implant	Diagnosis (percentage of inflammatory arthritis)	Cumulative survival (%)[a]			Revision rate (%)	Follow-up period, mean and range (y)
			At 5 y	At 8 y	At ≥ 10 y		
Menon[1]	Universal 1	74	–	–	–	3	6.7 (4–10)
Ward et al[23]	Universal 1	100	75	62	40	42	7.3 (5–11)
Ferreres et al[17]	Universal 1 and 2	68	100	100	–	0	5.5 (3–9)
Herzberg et al[9]	Re-motion	67	92	–	–	5	4 (2–8)
Morapudi et al[29]	Universal 2	90	–	–	–	0	3.1 (2–4)
Nydick et al[4]	Maestro	22	–	–	–	4	2.3 (0–5)
Nicoloff[28]	Re-motion	59	–	–	–	1	5 (4–7)
Sagerfors et al[22]	Universal 2	100	92	92	92	8	8 (2–?)
	Re-motion	78	99	94	94	3	7 (2–?)
	Maestro	81	95	95	–	4	5 (2–?)
Chevrollier et al[16]	Universal 1	50	90	–	50	30	6.5 (2–10)
Badge et al[14]	Universal 2	100	–	91	–	7	4.4 (2–10)
Gaspar et al[13]	Maestro	62	63	55	–	47	3 (1–5)
Weiss et al[30]	Universal 2	79	100	92	92	8	9 (5–15)
Reigstad et al[31]	Motec	0	88	86	86	14	8 (5–10)
Pfanner et al[21]	Universal 2	100	82	74	64	26	6.9 (2–12)
Kennedy et al[20]	Universal 2	71	–	–	–	15	7 (4–11)
Honecker et al[19]	Re-motion	83	91	69	69	18	6 (1–10)

[a]According to the Kaplan-Meier method.

twelve primary Re-motion prostheses have been implanted—45% in patients with inflammatory arthritis. The mean follow-up time is now 6 (range 1–15) years. We have 12 drop-outs and 17 revisions (revision rate: 15%). The cumulative implant survival is 82% at 6 years and 70% at 10 and 15 years. Eighty-one percent are pleased or very pleased with the result but 19% are disappointed. These figures are worse than we reported previously,[3,9] and we are nowhere near approaching the results obtained with total knee or hip arthroplasty but are comparable to ankle or elbow resurfacing. Recently, the frequency of TWA has declined at our department, partly due to the improved medical treatment of rheumatoid joint destruction and partly due to a more stringent patient selection. We tend to operate on older patients and patients with less physical demands (like rheumatoid patients) than we used to do, hoping to diminish the need

of revision surgery. For primary cases, especially in younger patients, we now may consider interposition arthroplasty with the Amandys pyrocarbon implant (Tornier [Bioprofile]).

25.5.2 Revision Surgery

Failed TWA may be revised to a new TWA (▶ Fig. 25.3) or to a wrist arthrodesis.

Our experience has led us to revise failed TWAs to total wrist arthrodesis rather than to revision arthroplasties. Of the thirteen revision arthroplasties we performed, six needed subsequent major surgery (four total wrist arthrodeses, one re-revision arthroplasty, and one grafting of a large osteolytic lesion), while the six failed TWAs that were primarily revised to an arthrodesis healed without further need of surgery. The preferred technique

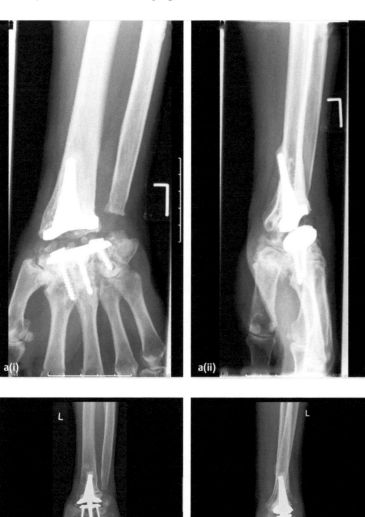

Fig. 25.3 Revision arthroplasty. **(a)** Failed Universal 1 prosthesis, 6 years after implantation for SLAC grade 4. **(b)** Seven years after revision to a Re-motion with a cemented technique and cancellous bone grafting.

25

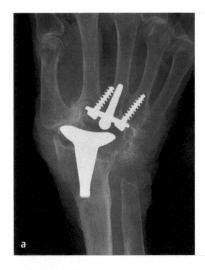
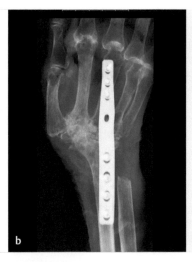

Fig. 25.4 Revision to arthrodesis. **(a)** Failed Re-motion prosthesis, 8 years after implantation in a rheumatoid wrist. Very poor carpal bone stock. **(b)** Revision to arthrodesis with bone allograft and plate-and-screw fixation.

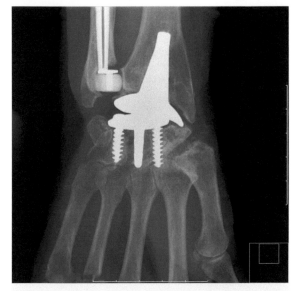

Fig. 25.5 Painful impingement between the radial component of the Re-motion prosthesis and the remaining scaphoid. This problem should be avoided by careful perioperative visual and radiographical examination. Supplementary resection of the scaphoid solved the issue.

always be relied upon uncritically. Each operative step must be checked with the image intensifier.

3. Proper tensioning of a TWA is dependent on the amount of resected bone and the size of the prosthetic components. If the reconstructed joint is too loose, it may dislocate. If it is too tight, motion is restricted. Achieving the right tension is based on a subjective assessment gained with experience.

4. Capsular repair is also important for the stability and mobility of the joint. If the capsule is inadequate, it may be reinforced by part of the extensor retinaculum.

5. Before capsular closure, it is important to check for impaction of the remaining distal scaphoid against the radial component during radial deviation. This may lead to painful impingement (▶ Fig. 25.5). Resection of more of the scaphoid may be necessary.

6. The current prosthetic designs allow for sparing of the distal radioulnar joint (DRUJ). If there is painful arthritis in the DRUJ and restricted forearm rotation, we usually advise a simple resection of the ulnar head (Darrach procedure) rather than an ulnar head replacement. There is no evidence that a more demanding procedure on top of a complicated index procedure offers any advantage.

is bone grafting and plate and screw fixation (▶ Fig. 25.4). A femoral head allograft is necessary in the case of a large bone defect.

25.5.3 Tips and Tricks

The following surgical steps are particularly important to obtain good results with wrist resurfacing:

1. Fusion of the carpal bones is mandatory. It is obtained by meticulous curettage and bone grafting of the intracarpal joints.

2. Wrist replacement with today's implants is facilitated by bone-cutting guides. However, these should not

References

[1] Menon J. Universal total wrist implant: experience with a carpal component fixed with three screws. J Arthroplast. 1998; 13(5):515–523

[2] Adams BD. Total wrist arthroplasty. Tech Hand Up Extrem Surg. 2004; 8(3):130–137

[3] Boeckstyns ME, Herzberg G, Merser S. Favorable results after total wrist arthroplasty: 65 wrists in 60 patients followed for 5–9 years. Acta Orthop. 2013; 84(4):415–419

[4] Nydick JA, Greenberg SM, Stone JD, Williams B, Polikandriotis JA, Hess AV. Clinical outcomes of total wrist arthroplasty. J Hand Surg Am. 2012; 37(8):1580–1584

[5] Adams BD. Total wrist arthroplasty for posttraumatic arthritis with radius deformity. J Wrist Surg. 2015; 4(3):164–168

25

[6] Reigstad O, Holm-Glad T, Bolstad B, Grimsgaard C, Thorkildsen R, Røkkum M. Five- to 10-year prospective follow-up of wrist arthroplasty in 56 nonrheumatoid patients. J Hand Surg Am. 2017; 42 (10):788–796

[7] Salazar Botero S, Igeta Y, Facca S, Pizza C, Hidalgo Diaz JJ, Liverneaux PA. Surgical technique: about a new total and isoelastic wrist implant (Prosthelast®). Eur J Orthop Surg Traumatol. 2018; 28(8):1525–1530

[8] Williams JB, Weiner H, Tyser AR. Long-term outcome and secondary operations after proximal row carpectomy or four-corner arthrodesis. J Wrist Surg. 2018; 7(1):51–56

[9] Herzberg G, Boeckstyns M, Sorensen AI, et al. "Remotion" total wrist arthroplasty: preliminary results of a prospective international multicenter study of 215 cases. J Wrist Surg. 2012; 1(1):17–22

[10] Melamed E, Marascalchi B, Hinds RM, Rizzo M, Capo JT. Trends in the utilization of total wrist arthroplasty versus wrist fusion for treatment of advanced wrist arthritis. J Wrist Surg. 2016; 5(3):211–216

[11] Boeckstyns ME. Wrist arthroplasty: a systematic review. Dan Med J. 2014; 61(5):A4834

[12] Yeoh D, Tourret L. Total wrist arthroplasty: a systematic review of the evidence from the last 5 years. J Hand Surg Eur Vol. 2014

[13] Gaspar MP, Lou J, Kane PM, Jacoby SM, Osterman AL, Culp RW. Complications following partial and total wrist arthroplasty: a single-center retrospective review. J Hand Surg Am. 2016; 41(1):47–53.e4

[14] Badge R, Kailash K, Dickson DR, et al. Medium-term outcomes of the Universal-2 total wrist arthroplasty in patients with rheumatoid arthritis. Bone Joint J. 2016; 98-B(12):1642–1647

[15] Boeckstyns MEH, Herzberg G. Periprosthetic osteolysis after total wrist arthroplasty. J Wrist Surg. 2014; 3(2):101–106

[16] Chevrollier J, Strugarek-Lecoanet C, Dap F, Dautel G. Results of a unicentric series of 15 wrist prosthesis implantations at a 5.2 year follow-up. Acta Orthop Belg. 2016; 82(1):31–42

[17] Ferreres A, Lluch A, Del Valle M. Universal total wrist arthroplasty: midterm follow-up study. J Hand Surg Am. 2011; 36(6):967–973

[18] Gil JA, Kamal RN, Cone E, Weiss AC. High survivorship and few complications with cementless total wrist arthroplasty at a mean follow-up of 9 years. Clin Orthop Relat Res. 2017; 475(12):3082–3087

[19] Honecker S, Igeta Y, Al Hefzi A, Pizza C, Facca S, Liverneaux PA. Survival rate on a 10-year follow-up of total wrist replacement implants: a 23-patient case series. J Wrist Surg. 2019; 8(1):24–29

[20] Kennedy JW, Ross A, Wright J, Martin DJ, Bransby-Zachary M, MacDonald DJ. Universal 2 total wrist arthroplasty: high satisfaction but high complication rates. J Hand Surg Eur Vol. 2018; 43(4):375–379

[21] Pfanner S, Munz G, Guidi G, Ceruso M. Universal 2 wrist arthroplasty in rheumatoid arthritis. J Wrist Surg. 2017; 6(3):206–215

[22] Sagerfors M, Gupta A, Brus O, Rizzo M, Pettersson K. Patient related functional outcome after total wrist arthroplasty: a single center study of 206 cases. Hand Surg. 2015; 20(1):81–87

[23] Ward CM, Kuhl T, Adams BD. Five to ten-year outcomes of the Universal total wrist arthroplasty in patients with rheumatoid arthritis. J Bone Joint Surg Am. 2011; 93(10):914–919

[24] Herzberg G, Burnier M, Nakamura T. A new wrist clinical evaluation score. J Wrist Surg. 2018; 7(2):109–114

[25] Berber O, Garagnani L, Gidwani S. Systematic review of total wrist arthroplasty and arthrodesis in wrist arthritis. J Wrist Surg. 2018; 7(5):424–440

[26] Brinkhorst ME, Selles RW, Dias JJ, et al. Results of the Universal 2 prosthesis in noninflammatory osteoarthritic wrists. J Wrist Surg. 2018; 7(2):121–126

[27] Cooney W, Manuel J, Froelich J, Rizzo M. Total wrist replacement: a retrospective comparative study. J Wrist Surg. 2012; 1(2):165–172

[28] Nicoloff M. Total wrist arthroplasty: indications and state of the art. Z Orthop Unfall. 2015; 153(1):38–45

[29] Morapudi SP, Marlow WJ, Withers D, Ralte P, Gabr A, Waseem M. Total wrist arthroplasty using the Universal 2 prosthesis. J Orthop Surg (Hong Kong). 2012; 20(3):365–368

[30] Weiss KE, Rodner CM. Osteoarthritis of the wrist. J Hand Surg Am. 2007; 32(5):725–746

[31] Reigstad O, Holm-Glad T, Thorkildsen R, Grimsgaard C, Røkkum M. Successful conversion of wrist prosthesis to arthrodesis in 11 patients. J Hand Surg Eur Vol. 2017; 42(1):84–89

25

26 Ball-and-Socket Wrist Arthroplasty

Ole Reigstad

Abstract

Wrist arthroplasty surgery has never achieved results similar to hip or knee arthroplasties. A variety of different arthroplasties have been introduced, used, and withdrawn after failing to give longer term pain free function. Mechanically and tribologically, a ball-and-socket provides the least resistance and the highest potential motion and has been very successful in multiplanar joints like the hip and shoulder. A total wrist arthroplasty was developed in our department during the 90s, starting out with small titanium implants for fixation in the distal radius and the capitate and an 18-mm metal-on-metal articulation. Wear studies, cadaver surgery, and finally a prospective trial in 8 patients led to changes in the implant, instruments and surgical technique and the final development was overtaken by an orthopedic company (Swemac), introducing the Motec wrist system in 2006. Rough surfaced and coated titan-alloy implants for fixation in the radius and 3 metacarpal, ball-and-socket metal-on-metal (MOM) or metal on poly-ether-ether-ketone (Mo-PEEK) comprised the implant. The experience in 130 patients reveals good, durable active wrist motion (around 130°), increased grip-strength, significantly reduced pain, Quick-DASH and PRWHE; but 20% of the patients can expect revision surgery within 10 years, 10% to arthrodesis, and 10% to a new arthroplasty. A modern uncemented ball-and-socket wrist arthroplasty can provide good, durable wrist function in the majority of patients.

Keywords: wrist, arthroplasty, uncemented, ball-and-socket, revision, Motec, arthrosis

26.1 History of Ball-and-Socket Wrist Arthroplasty

The ball-and-socket articulation appears to be the optimal mechanical choice for stable motion and minimum friction for force distribution between moving bone ends as seen in hip arthroplasties such that hip arthroplasty has been described as the operation of the twentieth century.[1]

Wrist motion occurs in three planes (flexion-extension, radial-ulnar deviation, pronation-supination). This large relatively unconstrained motion is similar to hip and shoulder motion. The articulation in most of the historical and contemporary prostheses has ranged from completely constrained (Swanson silicone arthroplasty[2]), via hinged to ovoid or rectangular semifit articulations.[3]

26.1.1 Meuli Wrist Arthroplasty

Hans Christoph Meuli from Berne, Switzerland developed and introduced three versions bearing his name starting in 1973.[4] The first version was intended for cemented fixation. It had a ball-and-socket articulation, with the ball (made out of polyester at first, then changed to ultra-high molecular weight polyethylene [UHMWPE]) on the proximal side. The proximal and distal components had two prongs, each made of Protasul 10 (a titanium alloy). Initial problems in his series of 41 patients included polyester synovitis, dislocations, technical errors, stem breakage, infection, and ulnar deviation. Modifications based upon these problems led to the final version in 1984 which was an uncemented implant. The components were made of corundum rough-blasted Protasul-100 (Ti6Al7Nb), including the ball, which was separately coated with titanium nitride for wear resistance. The UHMW polyethylene was inserted in the cup in the distal component (inverse articulation) (▶ Fig. 26.1a, b).

Meuli's own results published with the Meuli III (38 wrists) were satisfactory, with adequate pain reduction, a mean total flexion-extension range of motion (ROM) of 90 degrees and unchanged grip strength. Eight implants needed revision due to loosening during the average follow-up of 5.5 (range 3–9.5) years.[5] In a more recent report from Strunk and Bracker,[6] 15 Meuli III implanted in patients with rheumatoid arthritis (RA) fared well subjectively after 9 years, but only one was radiologically firmly attached to bone.[6] Although the final Meuli III design had some interesting features (including choice of bearing metal and ball-and-socket articulation), the two-prong fixation, the reverse articular concept, and the use of titanium in the articulation with a thin UHMWPE liner led to the failure of the whole concept and the withdrawal of the implant.

26.2 Development of a New Ball-and-Socket Arthroplasty

During the 1990s development of a new arthroplasty was undertaken in our department. The underlying idea was to merge the concepts from successful hip arthroplasties and some of the features from the Meuli arthroplasty to develop an arthroplasty for all patients with wrist degeneration.

26.2.1 Fixation

Rough-blasted titanium alloy (Ti6Al4V) was chosen as the bearing metal due to its excellent uncemented fixation properties as compared to cobalt-chrome-molybdenum (Co-Cr-Mo) or stainless steel.[7,8] The implant was screw-shaped to increase the surface for fixation and ease the insertion. The fixation was limited to the distal radius (sparing the distal radioulnar joint [DRUJ]) and the capitate

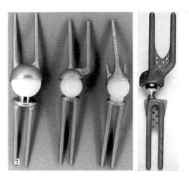
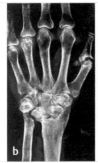
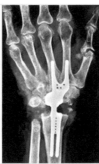

Fig. 26.1 (a) Initial Meuli I and II with a large polyester or UHMWPE head, articulation. In the Meuli II the articulation was ulnaward in the distal component. Meuli III to the right, articulation ulnaward in both components, with UHMWPE in the socket, titanium-nitride coated ball. **(b)** Preoperative RA wrist and Meuli III in situ.

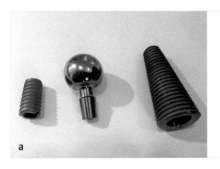
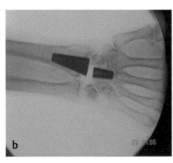

Fig. 26.2 (a) Prototypes developed and implanted in cadavers. The titanium-alloy ball coated with presumed wear-resistant titan-niobium coat was rejected after wear test failure. **(b)** Prototype implants in situ in a cadaver wrist.

in the carpus. Different surface modifications to enhance bone ingrowth were tested in rabbits; eventually we selected a resorbable 15-μm thick calcium-phosphate coating (Bonit, DOT Medical Solutions Laboratories Gmbh).[9,10]

26.2.2 Articulation

Following wear tests we rejected the use of a titanium-alloy ball coated with titan-niobium; instead we chose a highly polished 18-mm ball-and-socket metal-on-metal (MoM) articulation made of Co-Cr-Mo. It has been shown to have a very low wear rate and excellent performance in hip arthroplasties[11] and has relatively low bulk help to keep the implant small. The ball-and-socket provided almost unrestricted mobility and excellent stability. The system was modular enabling tension adjustment with different neck lengths and the potential for revision of the articulation retaining the bone-anchored implant stems (▶ Fig. 26.2).

26.3 Introduction of a New Arthroplasty

A prospective clinical trial was initiated in 2001 after receiving permission from the Regional Ethical Committee. Initially eight patients with noninflammatory wrist degeneration were selected and offered prototype wrist arthroplasty surgery as an alternative to wrist arthrodesis. The trial revealed weaknesses in the surgical method, instrumentation, and the implants.

The threads were too deep, necessitating extensive reaming to screw the implants home, sharp instruments

and sharp implant edges risked perforations in the bone, and for the distal component it was necessary to span the middle finger carpometacarpal (CMC) joint to reach the cortical part of the middle finger metacarpal in order to achieve stable fixation.[12] In 2005 the concept was overtaken by Swemac Orthopaedics AB, who did a thorough modification and included longer, thinner, and smooth-edged implants and new instruments. The principles of screwing threaded, uncemented stems into the radius and capitate/middle finger metacarpal linked with a low-friction ball-and-socket articulation were maintained.

26.3.1 The Implant

The Motec (Swemac Orthopaedics AB) wrist implant comprises a thicker, threaded proximal stem available in four different lengths (32–50 mm, in 6-mm increments), a longer and thinner, threaded distal stem available in six different lengths (40–75 mm, 5-mm increment) and two different diameters linked with a modular ball-and-socket articulation with highly polished Co-Cr-Mo MoM or Co-Cr-Mo on poly-ether-ether-ketone (PEEK). The MoPEEK is available in 15 mm and MoM in 15 and 18 mm ball diameters. There are four neck lengths on the balls for tension adjustment (▶ Fig. 26.3).

26.3.2 Patient Selection

The prerequisite for a functional wrist arthroplasty is active muscular control around the wrist. Neuromuscular imbalance or fixed malalignment of the wrist are absolute contraindications in our opinion because an unconstrained wrist implant cannot provide joint stability in

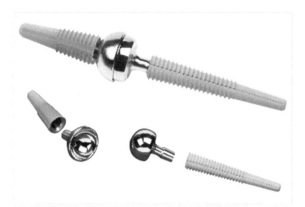

Fig. 26.3 The Motec wrist arthroplasty. Thicker, shorter, proximal component and thinner, longer, distal component. Modular metal-on-metal (MOM) articulation. (Courtesy of Swemac Orthopaedics AB.)

Table 26.1 Indications for wrist arthroplasty

	N	%
SNAC/SLAC wrist	66	51
Kienbock disease	20	15
Distal radius fracture	14	11
Primary osteoarthritis	14	11
Inflammatory arthritis	9	7
Other	7	5
Total	130	100

Abbreviations: SLAC, scapholunate advanced collapse; SNAC, scaphoid nonunion advanced collapse.

such cases. Relative contraindications include prior wrist infection or an unreliable patient. Since 2006 all patients scheduled for wrist arthrodesis in our department have been offered wrist arthroplasty; around 90% have chosen arthroplasty. So far 130 Motec have been implanted—93% in patients with noninflammatory arthritis. The mean age at surgery was 53 (range 18–79) years. The indications are shown in ▶ Table 26.1.

The patients were included in a prospective follow-up study. We recorded active ranges of motion (AROM), grip and key-pinch strength measured with JAMAR dynamometer (JA 88 Preston, Corp.), a visual analog score (VAS) for pain, the Quick-DASH (Disability of the Arm, Shoulder and Hand [DASH]) and PRWHE as subjective scores, and radiographs were evaluated preoperatively and at yearly follow-up.

26.3.3 Surgical Method and Follow-Up

The surgical method is described in detail by Reigstad and Rokkum.[13] In brief, a proximal row carpectomy (PRC) is performed, creating space for the articulation. The main surgical challenge is the position of the distal component. It is important to open the middle finger CMC joint extending the capitate to create the "one bone" between the capitate and third metacarpal necessary for optimal distal implant stability. We usually use an awl as a lever in the proximal capitate pole to confirm the ability to extend the capitate. The awl is then passed through the middle finger CMC joint, after which the blunt guidewire is introduced. We still use the fluoroscope extensively during this part of the surgery to secure the position of the guidewire. When reaming distally, use of the reamer as a lever in the capitate can result in extensive reaming dorsally and proximally (the capitate head) and reduced fit. A Homan retractor under the capitate will lift it up and reduce the lever effect. Choose the shorter implant, or ream 1 to 2 mm pass the marker to ensure burial of the

component inside the capitate. Proximally, we prefer to bury the radial component well in the distal radius (choosing one size smaller than the reamer measures on the rim of the radius). We ream until cortical engagement is confirmed on the lateral fluoroscopic view. We choose the articulation that gives the maximum ROM; if it is too tight with a medium neck we advance the screws further (they can be unscrewed and reintroduced after further reaming). A short neck is never used due to impingement between chrome-cobalt cup and the softer distal titanium-alloy screw which can give excessive metal wear.

The patients are followed-up carefully: at 2 weeks the plaster cast is changed, and stitches removed. At 6 weeks they are seen by the surgeon and by our hand therapists and allowed free weight bearing/ROM exercises. Further follow-up is scheduled at 6 and 12 months and yearly thereafter.

26.3.4 Results

On review at a mean of 8 (range 2–13) years we have found an increase in AROM from a mean of 95 degrees (range 0–190 degrees) to a mean of 130 degrees (range 13–209 degrees), a 25% increase in grip strength, a reduction in pain scores from a mean of 66 (range 10–100) to a mean of 30 (range 0–100) and improved subjective scores: the Quick-DASH improve from a mean of 43 (range 3–82) to a mean of 25 (range 0–75) and the PRWHE from a mean of 60 (range 10–96) to a mean of 28 (range 0–88) (▶ Fig. 26.4a–c).

We have seen excellent joint stability; only one dislocation was observed which was reduced, closed, and has remained stable for 6 years postreduction. Twenty percent were revised within 10-year follow-up—10% to an arthrodesis. A further 20% had additional operations including bone removal and DRUJ or tendon procedures during the follow-up period.[13,14] Similar results were described by Giwa et al[15] in 25 implants (23 patients), at follow-up at a mean of 4 years postoperatively. They had

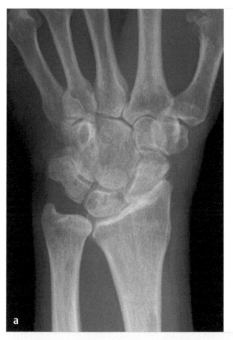
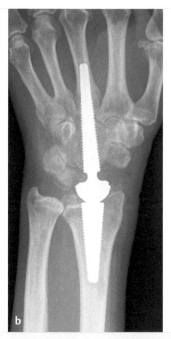
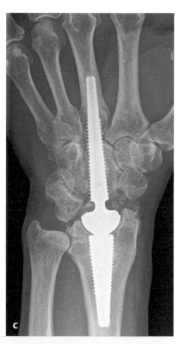

Fig. 26.4 **(a)** Posteroanterior (PA) radiographs: Preoperative scapholunate advanced collapse (SLAC) wrist in a 58-year-old carpenter. **(b)** Initial postoperative radiograph of Motec implant in situ (at the time the triquetrum was not removed as part of the primary bone resection). **(c)** Radiograph at 12 years follow-up.

a lower rate of revisions and additional operations compared to our series.

Challenges in Wrist Arthroplasties

The clinical results and performance after modern wrist arthroplasties are still inferior to hip and knee arthroplasties, and the implants are still at a developmental stage. Osteolysis and loosening are the main concerns, responsible for the deteriorating outcomes in the longer term. The primary fixation of the Motec has been excellent and early bone in-growth has been observed. We believe that the loosenings we have seen after 2 to 10 years are mainly due to wear products from the articulation, similar to loosening after years of pain-free use of well-fixed arthroplasties in the hip and knee, although this is not proven. Wear particle osteolysis has been described in other metal UHMWPE wrist arthroplasties.[16]

Metal-on-Metal/Metal-on-PEEK Wear Particles

A minimum of two chrome and cobalt blood measurements were done in all patients during the follow-up period, and the metal levels were low (f-chrome = 0.6 [range 0–1.6] µg/L and f-cobalt = 0.8 [range 0–3.2] µg/L)[14]. Nonetheless in three cases we saw evidence of painful local MOM reactions leading to revision. In less serious cases the wear from the articulation appeared to lead to asymptomatic osteolysis near the articulation. MOM implants have been discredited after failed hip resurfacing. With the alternative bearing metal-on-PEEK (MoPEEK), we have seen one case of PEEK rim wear attributed to impingement between the collar and the cup (▶ Fig. 26.5a, b).

The company has removed PEEK over the rim of the cup which, according to the company, should prevent this complication. We have less than 3 years of experience with the MoPEEK articulation.

Alternative Bearings

To increase the survival of wrist implants we believe that the developers of wrist arthroplasties should explore alternative bearings especially MoUHMWPE (in the case of the Motec), highly cross-linked polyethylene (XLPE), or ceramics to reduce wear particles and increase the longevity of the arthroplasties.

26.3.5 Revisions

In cases of loosening or articular problems we have offered revision surgery for failed Motec, Re-Motion, and Amandys wrist arthroplasties, replacing the loose implant using a longer-stemmed implant to achieve fixation (▶ Fig. 26.6). The re-revision rate, i.e., rate of second revisions is about 25% after 7-years follow-up mainly due to infections. The five infections/inflammations we found

26

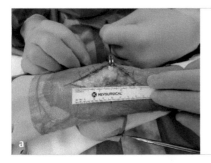
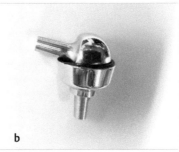

Fig. 26.5 **(a)** A dorsal pseudotumor removed 3 years after surgery, articulation changed to metal-on- poly-ether-ether-ketone (MoPEEK). **(b)** Rim wear (6 o'clock) of the PEEK articulation.

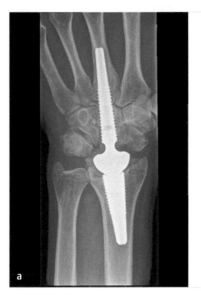
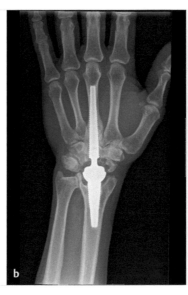

Fig. 26.6 **(a)** Loose distal Motec component after 2 years. **(b)** Eleven years follow-up with the revised longer distal component.

were diagnosed at re-revision to arthrodesis at a mean of 14 (range 4–24) months following the first revision. Caution is recommended when considering a revision.

Revision of failed Motec wrist arthroplasties to wrist arthrodesis has in our experience led to high fusion rates and clinical results similar to primary wrist arthrodesis.[17]

26.4 Conclusion

The Motec ball-and-socket wrist arthroplasty has given good clinical function and acceptable reoperation and revision rates. There is room for improvements in bone fixation and in developing the articulation.

References

[1] Learmonth ID, Young C, Rorabeck C. The operation of the century: total hip replacement. Lancet. 2007; 370(9597):1508–1519

[2] Swanson AB. Silicone arthroplasty of the wrist in rheumatoid arthritis. J Hand Surg Am. 1993; 18(1):166

[3] Sagerfors M, Gupta A, Brus O, Pettersson K. Total wrist arthroplasty: a single-center study of 219 cases with 5-year follow-up. J Hand Surg Am. 2015; 40(12):2380–2387

[4] Meuli HC. Arthroplasty of the wrist. Ann Chir. 1973; 27(5):527–530

[5] Meuli HC. Total wrist arthroplasty: experience with a noncemented wrist prosthesis. Clin Orthop Relat Res. 1997(342):77–83

[6] Strunk S, Bracker W. Wrist joint arthroplasty: results after 41 prostheses. Handchir Mikrochir Plast Chir. 2009; 41(3):141–147

[7] Williams D. The golden anniversary of titanium biomaterials. Med Device Technol. 2001; 12(7):8–11

[8] Reigstad O, Siewers P, Røkkum M, Espehaug B. Excellent long-term survival of an uncemented press-fit stem and screw cup in young patients: follow-up of 75 hips for 15–18 years. Acta Orthop. 2008; 79 (2):194–202

[9] Reigstad O, Johansson C, Stenport V, Wennerberg A, Reigstad A, Røkkum M. Different patterns of bone fixation with hydroxyapatite and resorbable CaP coatings in the rabbit tibia at 6, 12, and 52 weeks. J Biomed Mater Res B Appl Biomater. 2011; 99(1):14–20

[10] Reigstad O, Franke-Stenport V, Johansson CB, Wennerberg A, Røkkum M, Reigstad A. Improved bone ingrowth and fixation with a thin calcium phosphate coating intended for complete resorption. J Biomed Mater Res B Appl Biomater. 2007; 83(1):9–15

[11] McKellop H, Park SH, Chiesa R, et al. In vivo wear of three types of metal on metal hip prostheses during two decades of use. Clin Orthop Relat Res. 1996(329) Suppl:S128–S140

26

[12] Reigstad A, Reigstad O, Grimsgaard C, Røkkum M. New concept for total wrist replacement. J Plast Surg Hand Surg. 2011; 45(3):148–156

[13] Reigstad O, Røkkum M. Wrist arthroplasty using prosthesis as an alternative to arthrodesis: design, outcomes and future. J Hand Surg Eur Vol. 2018; 43(7):689–699

[14] Reigstad O, Holm-Glad T, Bolstad B, Grimsgaard C, Thorkildsen R, Røkkum M. Five- to 10-year prospective follow-up of wrist arthroplasty in 56 nonrheumatoid patients. J Hand Surg Am. 2017; 42 (10):788–796

[15] Giwa L, Siddiqui A, Packer G. Motec wrist arthroplasty: 4 years of promising results. J Hand Surg Asian Pac Vol. 2018; 23(3):364–368

[16] Boeckstyns ME, Toxvaerd A, Bansal M, Vadstrup LS. Wear particles and osteolysis in patients with total wrist arthroplasty. J Hand Surg Am. 2014; 39(12):2396–2404

[17] Reigstad O, Holm-Glad T, Thorkildsen R, Grimsgaard C, Røkkum M. Successful conversion of wrist prosthesis to arthrodesis in 11 patients. J Hand Surg Eur Vol. 2017; 42(1):84–89

26

27 Wrist Hemiarthroplasty for Acute Irreparable Distal Radius Fracture in the Independent Elderly

Guillaume Herzberg and Marion Burnier

Abstract

Treatment of the so-called "irreparable" distal radius fractures in the independent elderly with wrist hemiarthroplasty (WHA) is becoming a well-accepted salvage procedure when ORIF is considered too challenging. The purpose of this paper is to present our results in a single academic upper extremity unit at a minimum of 2 years' follow-up. A total of 12 female patients with a mean age of 77 years (13 wrists) fulfilled the criteria. All patients had some comorbidities, but they were all independent at home. At an average of 39 months' follow-up, the mean VAS pain was 1/10, whereas the mean PRWE was 21%, and the mean active wrist extension was 36°. There was no dislocation, loosening, infection, or removal of the implants in these 13 cases. We observed 3 cases of CRPS which resolved within 18 months. One patient was reoperated 20 months after the index operation because of finger stiffness due to tendon adhesions along with a tendency to ulnar deviation of the wrist. There is currently no good option to treat what we defined as irreparable DRF in elderly independent patients. Our data suggest that treatment of acute irreparable DRF in the independent elderly patient with a bone preserving primary WHA may be a viable option. Longer-term follow-up is needed to confirm these preliminary data.

Keywords: elderly, distal radius fracture, hemiarthroplasty, acute distal radius fracture, irreparable distal radius fracture

27.1 Introduction

Independent elderly patients presenting with acute distal radius fractures (DRF) represent a specific subgroup that has been identified previously.[1] The so-called "irreparable DRF" (IDRF) as previously defined[2] are within this subgroup.

There is a widespread use of volar plating for acute IDRF in elderly patients.[3,4] However, this is associated with a high incidence of complications and there is doubt about the clinical benefit of volar plating in the most severe acute DRF in elderly patients.[5,6]

Treating acute complex fractures of the shoulder and elbow in the elderly with primary joint hemiarthroplasty is a well-established and validated concept.[7] Several authors have recently proposed extending this concept to the wrist.[2,8,9,10]

The purpose of this chapter is to outline the benefits of treating acute IDRF in the independent elderly with immediate wrist hemiarthroplasty (WHA).

27.2 Current Therapeutic Options for Acute IDRF in the Independent Elderly

Until recently, there was no reliable option for treating IDRF in elderly patients.[2] Compared with a dependent elderly with minimal functional needs for whom a plaster cast without any trial reduction is typically the best option, an independent elderly person warrants a more ambitious treatment. Despite frequent comorbidities, they may still drive a car and participate in relatively sophisticated activities of daily living (ADL). Each possible treatment option has risks and benefits.

Closed reduction and plaster casting may give a good outcome despite very abnormal distal radial bone alignment, but some patients will have significant functional impairment as well as deformity.[6,11] Percutaneous manipulation and K-wiring works infrequently in maintaining satisfactory bone alignment due to the very limited purchase into osteoporotic fracture fragments.[3] External fixation in elderly patients is particularly cumbersome.[4] Moreover, the ligamentotaxis provided by external fixation alone allows for good reduction in the coronal plane but typically not in the sagittal plane due to the relative weakness of the dorsal ligamentous capsule compared with the volar capsule.[12]

Distraction plating has been recently proposed for IDRF in elderly patients. However in a recent paper,[13] it was reported that the postoperative immobilization period was long. The mean delay to plate removal was 30 months. Moreover, we find this carries a potential for appreciable skin complications in the elderly.

Volar plating is currently the gold standard for acute displaced DRF in the elderly whatever their severity. However, in the study by Orbay and Fernandez,[3] only 33% of fractures were classified as AO type "C" fractures. This may have skewed their results. A level I study by Arora and Gabl[5] showed that ORIF with volar plating in this group of patients did not provide any improvement in terms of function and ranges of motion when compared with closed reduction and cast immobilization. We agree that successful volar plating is very difficult to achieve in elderly IDRF cases and there is a high risk of secondary displacement as well.

Immediate distal radius replacement with a hemiarthroplasty is a new option based on a concept which is widely used for irreparable shoulder and elbow intra-articular fractures. There are already a few papers related to this topic that report favorable results.[2,8,14]

27.3 Current Evidence

In the series of Roux[8] there were six cases of acute DRF in the elderly treated with primary WHA. The results of this subgroup were not reported separately. Using the same implant, Vergnenègre et al[14] reported the outcome of WHA for acute IDRF with satisfactory functional results and no implant removal at a mean follow-up of 27 months. However, this implant is large. In the event of implant removal, the loss of bone stock would be very difficult to reconstruct. This is not the case with the bone-preserving WHA used in our series. Metal-on-cartilage contact between the implant and the convexity of the articular cartilage of the proximal carpal row is not the best contact for an arthroplasty. However, metal-on-cartilage contact is well accepted for shoulder and elbow hemiarthroplasties after acute trauma.

27.4 Authors' Experience

We have performed 24 hemiarthroplasties in 22 independent elderly women treated for acute IDRF at a single institution between April 2011 and December 2018. The senior author (GH) operated on 21 wrists; the other three wrists were operated under supervision. All patients had some comorbidities but all were independent at home. Their mean age was 77 (range 66–88) years. The mean delay from injury to surgery was 4 (range 1–7) days.

We used the radial part of the SBI-Stryker ReMotion total wrist arthroplasty in 12 wrists and a specifically designed WHA (Cobra, Groupe Lepine) in 12 wrists. Cement was used with one of the 12 ReMotion and one of the Cobra implants. Ulnar head resection was performed in 18 wrists (75%), 92% of the ReMotion, and 60% of the Cobra when the sigmoid notch was not reconstructable. We have had to revise two wrists within 2 weeks after the index operation. One radially deviated ReMotion due to implantation of a stem that was too short was replaced with a Cobra, and one small Cobra implant was replaced with a large ReMotion implant.

The surgical technique has been reported previously[2]; it is in essence the same for either implant.

We have reviewed a total of 13 patients with a minimum follow-up of 24 (mean 39; range 24–57) months. Subjectively, we assessed pain with a visual analog scale (VAS) from 0 to 10, the QuickDash, the patient-related wrist evaluation (PRWE), and a VAS evaluation of function. Objectively, we assessed forearm and wrist ranges of motion and measured grip strength. The Lyon wrist score[15] was calculated. It included a VAS for pain, a VAS of functional limitations in forearm rotation (range 0–10), and wrist flexion extension and objective measurements. The Lyon wrist score allowed a diamond-shape representation of clinical results.

The follow-up radiological criteria included periprosthetic osteolysis as defined and measured by the treating surgeon, as well as evaluation of the translation of the carpus. Coronal and sagittal inclinations of the implant were also evaluated relative to the long axis of the radius.

No dislocation, loosening, or infection was reported. Apart from the immediate replacement of two implants for mechanical reasons, we have not had to remove any implants. Three patients were diagnosed with complex regional pain syndrome type I (CRPS I). All resolved within 18 months. One patient had a further operation 20 months after the index operation because of finger stiffness due to tendon adhesions at the wrist level along with a tendency to ulnar deviation of the wrist. We performed an extensor tenolysis and transfer of the extensor carpi radialis longus (ECRL) tendon to the extensor carpi radialis brevis (ECRB) tendon. At final follow-up her clinical status was improved and she had nearly full restoration of finger flexion.

The mean VAS for pain was 1/10 (range 0–3). The mean QuickDASH score was 24% and the mean PRWE score was 21% (▶ Table 27.1). Among the 11 cases with combined WHA and ulnar head resection, no patient reported symptomatic radioulnar impingement.

Radiologically, there was no measurable subsidence of the implants, periprosthetic osteolysis, or appreciable carpal erosions. Radiographic bone healing around the implants was satisfactory in all but one case. One wrist showed a dorsal bony defect on the lateral radiograph after 1 year. This defect was present on the early postoperative radiographs suggesting insufficient dorsal bone coverage of the implant during the operation. We did not see any translation of the carpus relative to the implant in the coronal or sagittal planes (▶ Fig. 27.1, ▶ Fig. 27.2, ▶ Fig. 27.3, ▶ Fig. 27.4).

Table 27.1 Postoperative clinical data

	Postoperative data (13 patients with minimum Follow-up 2 years)	
	Average	Range
QuickDASH	24	0–50
PRWE	21	0–63
VAS Pain/10 pts	1	0–3
Pronation	72	50–85
Supination	77	70–85
Wrist Extension	36	15–50
Wrist Flexion	27	10–45
Grip Strength (Jamar) % of opposite side	72	36–100
Lyon Wrist Score (Standard)	76	63–91

27

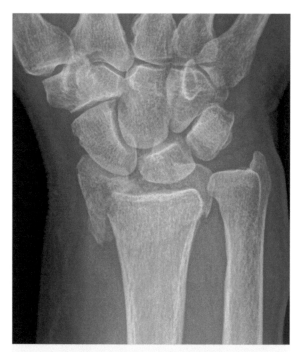

Fig. 27.1 Posteroanterior (PA) radiograph of an irreparable intra-articular distal radius fracture in an independent 70-year-old female.

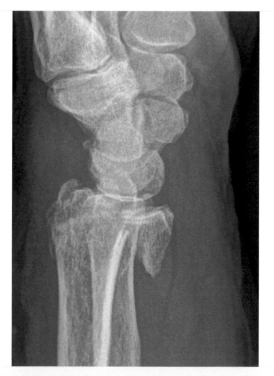

Fig. 27.2 Lateral radiograph of the same patient.

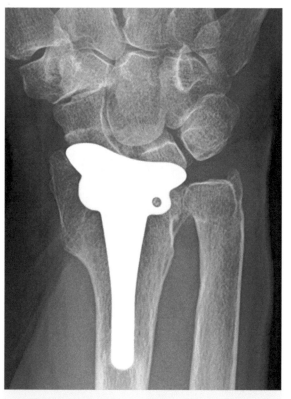

Fig. 27.3 Posteroanterior (PA) radiograph of the same patient at 3-years follow-up.

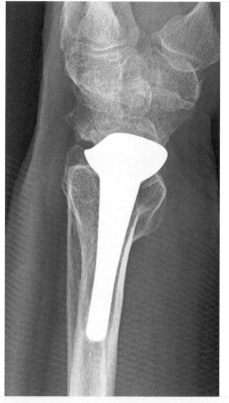

Fig. 27.4 Lateral radiograph of the same patient at 3 years.

27

27.5 Conclusion

Our current data suggest that a WHA is a reasonable and appropriate treatment for "IDRF"[2] in an independent elderly patient. Longer-term follow-up studies are needed to confirm these preliminary data.

References

[1] Herzberg G, Izem Y, Al Saati M, Plotard F. "PAF" analysis of acute distal radius fractures in adults: preliminary results. Chir Main. 2010; 29 (4):231–235

[2] Herzberg G, Burnier M, Marc A, Izem Y. Primary wrist hemiarthroplasty for irreparable distal radius fracture in the independent elderly. J Wrist Surg. 2015; 4(3):156–163

[3] Orbay JL, Fernandez DL. Volar fixed-angle plate fixation for unstable distal radius fractures in the elderly patient. J Hand Surg Am. 2004; 29(1):96–102

[4] Brogan DM, Ruch DS. DRF in the elderly. J Hand Surg Am. 2015; 40 (6):1217

[5] Arora R, Gabl M. A prospective randomized trial comparing nonoperative treatment with volar locking plate fixation for displaced and unstable DRF in patients 65 years and older. J Bone Joint Surg Am. 2011; 93A(20):2146–2153

[6] Day CS, Daly MC. Management of geriatric distal radius fractures. J Hand Surg Am. 2012; 37(12):2619–2622

[7] Park YK, Kim SH, Oh JH. Intermediate-term outcome of hemiarthroplasty for comminuted proximal humerus fractures. J Shoulder Elbow Surg. 2017; 26(1):85–91

[8] Roux JL. Treatment of intra-articular fractures of the distal radius by wrist prosthesis. Orthop Traumatol Surg Res. 2011; 97S:S46–S53

[9] Vergnenègre G, Hardy J, Mabit C, Charissoux JL, Marcheix PS. Hemiarthroplasty for complex distal radius fractures in elderly patients. J Wrist Surg. 2015; 4(3):169–173

[10] Ichihara S, Facca S, Liverneaux P. Unicompartmental isoelastic resurfacing prosthesis for malignant tumor of the distal radius: a case report with a 3 year follow-up. Orthop Traumatol Surg Res. 2015; 101(8):963: ou 663

[11] Brogan DM, Ruch DS, Kakar, P. Management of severely comminuted DRF. J Hand Surg Am. 2015; 40A(9):1905

[12] Bartosh RA. Intraarticular fractures of the distal radius: a cadaveric study to determine if ligamentotaxis restores palmar tilt. J Hand Surg Am. 1990; 15A(1):18–21

[13] Richard MJ, Ruch DS. Distraction plating for the treatment of highly comminuted DRF in elderly patients. J Hand Surg Am. 2012; 37A (5):948–956

[14] Vergnenègre G, Mabit C, Arnaud JP, Charissoux JL. Treatment of comminuted DRF by resurfacing prosthesis in elderly patients. Chir Main. 2014; 33(2):112

[15] Herzberg G, Burnier M, Nakamura T. A new wrist clinical evaluation score. J Wrist Surg. 2018; 7(2):109–114

27

28 Pyrocarbon Implants in the Wrist: Amandys and RCPI

Philippe Bellemère and Augusto Marcuzzi

Abstract

Pyrocarbon implants for the treatment of extensive wrist osteoarthritis have been recently proposed alternatively to more invasive and/or wrist motion-limiting procedures. They may also be used to salvage failed previous wrist surgery. Two type of wrist pyrocarbon implants are available: (1) The Amandys implant is a free radiocarpal interposition creating two new joint surfaces, radiocarpal, and midcarpal; (2) the RCPI implant is a stemmed hemiarthroplasty for the head of the capitate used with a proximal row carpectomy (PRC). As the arthroplasty created with these implants is nonconstrained, their indications require preoperative well-aligned wrist on radiographs.

Surgical technique for their implantation is usually performed dorsally. In any case it requires precise surgery to preserve capsule continuity and ligament attachments during the bone removal. Proper sizing of the implant must avoid overstuffing the joint and any bone impingement must be excluded.

The experience of the authors with mid-term follow-up on large series provide encouraging results which seem to not deteriorate with the follow-up. Wrist motion and function are preserved, and pain relief is achieved. Reoperation rates are low for both implants. The most frequent complication is the instability of the implant for the Amandys and the instability of the wrist for the RCPI.

Indications of each implant are not yet well defined and seem to overlap. The Amandys implant appears more suited to treat severe joint destruction while the RCPI implant particularly extends the indications of PRC in the presence of capitate head destruction.

Keywords: pyrocarbon, wrist, implant, arthroplasty, interposition, arthritis, rheumatoid, posttraumatic, Amandys, RCPI

28.1 Introduction

The properties of pyrocarbon (an elastic modulus similar to cortical bone, low roughness, a low coefficient of friction, resistance to wear, and biotolerance) make this material suitable for arthroplasty with smooth gliding interface between implant and cartilage or subchondral bone.[1]

The pyrocarbon implants contain a central core of graphite (mixed with a little tungsten powder that gives radiopacity) resurfaced with a radiolucent pyrocarbon layer.

Pyrocarbon arthroplasty for extensive joint destruction of the wrist use two implants:

- The Amandys implant which is a free spacer to create a new type of radiocarpal interposition arthroplasty.
- The RCPI implant which is a stemmed hemiarthroplasty for the head of the capitate designed to be used with a proximal row carpectomy (PRC).

In this chapter, the surgical technique and midterm results of these two implants are reported.

28.2 Amandys Implant

Philippe Bellemère

The aim of the Amandys arthroplasty is to create a radiocarpal or a midcarpal interposition arthroplasty.[2] The implant is a mobile spacer able to glide and rotate over the radius and midcarpal surfaces to dissipate and thus reduce peak loads. This arthroplasty requires minimal osseous resection at the joint margin and thus preserves the bone stock, helping to maintain the carpal height and optimize the function of the principal extrinsic carpal ligaments.

28.2.1 Characteristics of the Implant

The Amandys implant (Wright Medical-Tornier SAS, Bioprofile, Grenoble, France) is an ellipsoid spacer with a quadrielliptic surface creating two asymmetric convex joint surfaces. The two curves of the distal (carpal) surface are less pronounced than those of the proximal (radial) one (▶ Fig. 28.1). The implant has three main axes: an anterior-posterior one corresponding to its width; a transverse one corresponding to its length; and a proximal-distal one corresponding to its thickness. The implant exists in eight sizes varying in length (24–26 mm) and in four thicknesses: small (S—9 mm); medium (M—10.7 mm); large (L—12.4 mm); and extra-large (XL—14.1 mm).

The Amandys implant is used in the treatment of radiocarpal arthritis. It replaces the lunate, two-third of the proximal scaphoid, and the proximal portion of the capitate. The triquetrum is not resected in order to preserve the attachments of the dorsoradial and dorsal intercarpal extrinsic ligaments (▶ Fig. 28.2). The implant has no bone or ligament fixation so it remains free and mobile between the radius

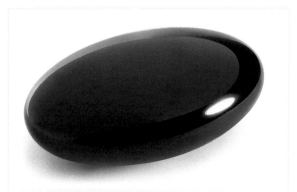

Fig. 28.1 The Amandys implant.

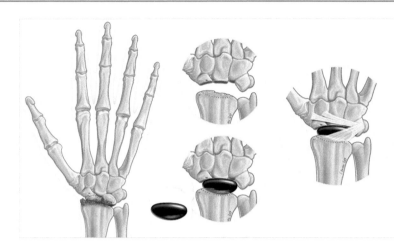

Fig. 28.2 Drawing of the Amandys arthroplasty.

and the distal carpal row. Its stability is "ensured" by its congruence with the distal radial articular surface and shaped cavity in the midcarpal bone surfaces and by the posterior and anterior capsuloligamentary structures.

28.2.2 Indications and Contraindications

Correct radiocarpal alignment, efficient capsules and ligaments, and functional wrist flexor and extensor tendons are required for an Amandys interposition implant. Major bone loss or instability as in rheumatoid or post-traumatic wrist is an absolute contraindication. The Amandys arthroplasty can be used as an alternative to a total wrist arthroplasty or total wrist arthrodesis including for radiocarpal or midcarpal osteoarthritis (OA), rheumatoid and post-traumatic arthritis, and Kienböck disease.[3] It can also be used to salvage failed previous wrist surgery, e.g., partial wrist fusion, a silicone implant, proximal row carpectomy, or even a total wrist prosthesis.[4,5]

In less severe degenerative arthritis, the Amandys arthroplasty can also be used as an alternative to partial wrist fusion, especially in the elderly.

28.2.3 Surgical Technique

Special attention must be paid to manage the periarticular soft tissue releases during the bone resections, especially the palmar capsule.[6]

Approach

A dorsal longitudinal approach centered over the middle of the wrist is usually preferred; however, if the wrist is well aligned and stable without the need for major osteoarticular reconstruction, then a radial approach with a radial styloidectomy is possible. The dorsal approach facilitates several aspects: defining the extent of bone resection; performance of bone resection and synovectomy with minimal trauma; distal radial or carpal bone grafting if necessary; preparing the joint surfaces; and

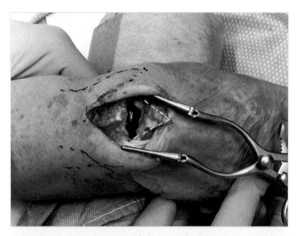

Fig. 28.3 L-shaped incision of the capsule delimiting a capsular flap outlined with dotline.

assessing the condition of the articular capsule, particularly the palmar capsule.

The dorsal approach is made with an L-shaped capsulotomy incised longitudinally over the radial side of the wrist creating a capsular flap that is reflected ulnarly (▶ Fig. 28.3).

Bone Resections

First, the proximal two-third of the scaphoid are removed with an oscillating saw just above the ligament insertions of the dorsal radiocarpal ligament and the radio-scapho-capitate ligament, which must be preserved. The saw cut is made parallel to the frontal and transversal slopes of the radial fossa, i.e., tilted volarly by c. 11 degrees and ulnarly by 22 degrees.

The lunate is then freed from all ligamentous attachments and removed. A corkscrew is used as a joystick to aid this resection. The head of the capitate is removed with a saw. The cut should be at level with that of the ulnar side of the scaphoid saw cut. The ulnar side of the saw cut is made at level with the proximal tip of the hamate.

28

Prominent osteophytes are removed, including possibly a partial radial styloidectomy.

The distal radial articular surface is then smoothed to obtain a concave ovoid surface along both axes matching the Amandys implant. This includes excision of the crest between the scaphoid and lunate fossae of the distal radius. If there is marked laxity or a tear of the palmar capsule, suture plication or reinforcement may be necessary. Any large bone cavities in the radius or the carpus can be curetted and grafted with packed cancellous graft.

Choosing the Size of the Implant

The implant must allow a range as wide as possible of passive mobility of the wrist confirmed intraoperatively with fluoroscopy. Cam effects in extreme positions of flexion, extension, and radial or ulnar deviation cause some implant rotation. They must be eliminated because they will cause implant instability postoperatively. Overstressing the implant, which can induce instability or chronic pain, should be avoided. In doubt, we recommend choosing a smaller implant size. An implant that is too thick will increase the ulnocarpal height which will result in an overconstrained wrist.

Postoperative Care

Immobilize the wrist in a neutral position with a removable plastic splint for 2 to 3 weeks and then gradually increase mobilization with no restrictions beyond 6 weeks postoperatively.

28.2.4 Associated Procedures

An Amandys arthroplasty can be combined with surgery on other joints around the wrist such as the distal radioulnar joint (DRUJ) (▶ Fig. 28.4). Partial fusion on the triquetro-hamate or scapho-trapezio-trapezoid (STT) joint or combined arthroplasties of the STT or thumb carpometacarpal (CMC) joints can also be performed.

28.2.5 Results

In the Literature

Only a few series have been published, with a maximum follow-up of 42 months.[2,8] The surgery appears to give good pain relief and wrist function measured by visual analog scale (VAS), range of motion (ROM), and grip strength. Mobility and grip strength are typically barely changed but patient satisfaction is rated as good.

Early implant instability is the most common complication. In 10% of all published cases, the implant needed repositioning. Two failures in a series of 11 (3%) were reported, both of which were converted to a total wrist arthrodesis. One was due to errors related to an inappropriate indication and inexperience, and the other for chronic pain.[7]

Cugola et al[9] compared the results of a case series of 26 total wrist prostheses with a mean follow-up of 6.5 years, to a case series of 10 Amandys implants with a mean follow-up of 3.5 years. The Amandys results gave better pain relief, mobility, and grip strength; none requiring revision. Two total wrist prostheses were revised.

Personal (PB) Experience

In our institution, the 10-year experience with the Amandys implant is based on more than 200 arthroplasties. The main indication (32%) has been degenerative such as severe scapholunate advance collapse (SLAC) or scaphoid nonunion advance collapse (SNAC) wrists, 14% were for rheumatoid arthritis, and 26% had previous wrist surgery. Two cases were converted to total wrist

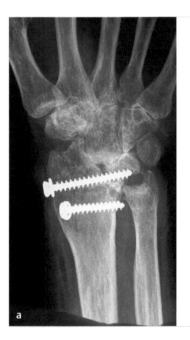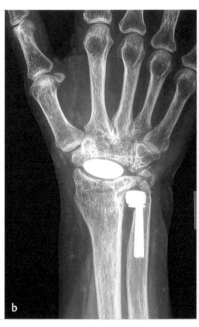

Fig. 28.4 Amandys arthroplasty with a partial distal radioulnar joint arthroplasty (Eclypse implant) in a rheumatoid wrist. **(a)** Preoperative anteroposterior (AP) radiograph. **(b)** AP radiograph after 68 months of follow-up.

arthrodesis due to implant instability with persistent pain. The revision rate for early implant instability and secondary repositioning was 6%. This rate decreased with our experience, which is indicative of a learning curve.

A series of 51 patients (55 implants) with a mean age of 58 (range 25–84) years was evaluated with a minimum of 5-year (mean 84 mo) follow-up. The results (unpublished) showed improved grip strengths at a mean of 20 kgf (68% of the opposite side) increased from 12 kgf preoperatively. The ROMs were 75 degrees of flexion-extension (66 degrees preoperatively) and 33 degrees radioulnar deviation (30 degrees preoperatively). The patient-related wrist evaluation (PRWE) improved from 63 to 27/100, the Quick-DASH improved from 63 to 34/100, and the mean visual analogue score (VAS) for pain improved from 6.5 to 2.3/10. Patients were satisfied or very satisfied in 86% of cases. A comparison of results at 2 years and at 5 years postoperatively found a significant improvement in grip strength, PRWE, and Quick-DASH scores between these two periods. The radiological results have shown no significant progressive subsidence or misalignment of the implants (▶ Fig. 28.5).

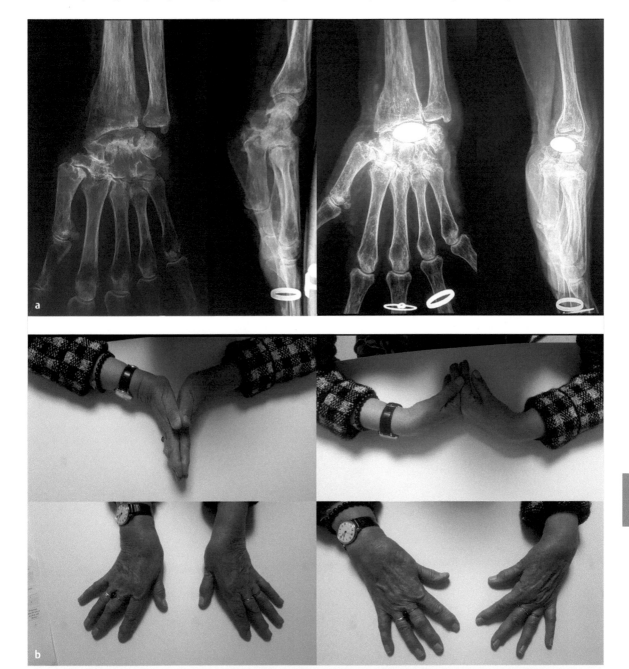

Fig. 28.5 Amandys implant for degenerative wrist on the left side. **(a)** Preoperative anteroposterior (AP) radiograph after 8 years. **(b)** Clinical results after 8 years of follow-up.

28

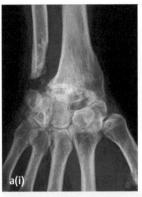
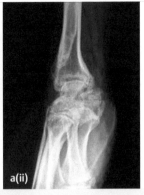
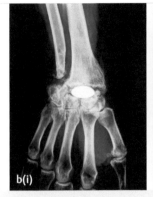
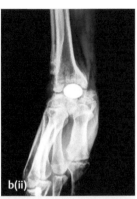

Fig. 28.6 Failure of proximal row carpectomy **(a)** treated with an Amandys implant. Postoperative radiograph after 69 months **(b)**.

A series of 28 rheumatoid wrist treated with an Amandys implant achieved similar results (unpublished data) at a mean follow-up of 45 months.

These encouraging results have prompted us to extend the indications for using the Amandys to less severe wrist damage as an alternative to a four-corner fusion procedure in grade-3 of SLAC, SCAC (scaphoid chondrocalcinosis advanced collapse), and SNAC wrists especially for patients over 60 years of age. A comparative series (unpublished) of 20 patients with a mean age of 65 years and a mean follow-up of 7 years showed a quicker functional recovery, better improvement of the ROMs, and less complication with the Amandys implant than a four-corner fusion.

28.2.6 Pitfalls, Tips, and Tricks

Proper selection of the patients is very important, in particular correct radiocarpal alignment, no major bone loss, and no carpal instability. The surgical technique must be precise particularly preserving the periarticular soft tissues especially the palmar capsule. Cam effects on the implant must be detected perioperatively primarily by checking passive joint movement.

As the implant is a mobile spacer it must not be over-constrained. The specific size should be chosen with care.

For a failed previous PRC, resection of the capitate should be extended more distally and a narrower (24-mm) implant is preferable (▶ Fig. 28.6). A radial styloidectomy may also be necessary.

For a failed previous four-corner arthrodesis, we use the standard technique if the triquetrum can be preserved (▶ Fig. 28.7). If not, the technique should be the same as for a failed previous PRC.

In the event of early instability of the implant (rotation or luxation), reoperation for implant repositioning after repeat reaming of bone surfaces and plicating the palmar capsule or changing the size of the implant has always been possible in our experience. Reoperation does not seem to adversely affect the final outcome.

28.2.7 Summary

The Amandys arthroplasty is my (PB) treatment of choice when treating severe wrist destruction. A good outcome is achieved relatively quickly and does not seem to deteriorate over the medium term. Rather the outcomes tend to improve over several years. In case of failure, this procedure does not preclude revision surgery by total wrist arthroplasty or arthrodesis.

28

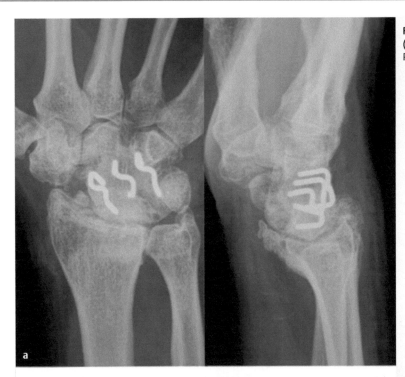

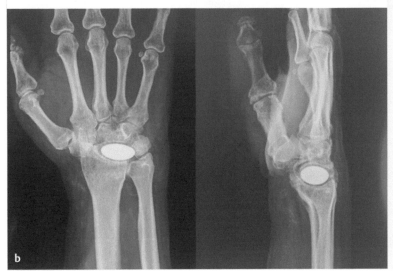

Fig. 28.7 Failure of four-bone arthrodesis **(a)** treated with an Amandys implant. Postoperative radiograph after 4.5 years **(b)**.

28

28.3 RCPI Implant

Augusto Marcuzzi

Proximal row carpectomy (PCR) is an accepted treatment for degenerative diseases of the wrist such as SNAC, SLAC, and SCAC and in the advanced stages of Kienböck's disease. When there is degeneration of the head of the capitate, a PCR is contraindicated.[10,11] In these cases the replacement of the head of the capitate with the resurfacing capitate pyrocarbon implant (RCPI) combined with PRC may be a good alternative.[11,12]

28.3.1 Characteristics of Implant

The RCPI prosthesis (Wright Medical-Tornier SAS, Bioprofile, Grenoble, France) is a single block, with a 15-degree tilt between the stem and head (▶ Fig. 28.8). It is a cementless prosthesis. The commercially available head diameter sizes are 14 mm (medium) and 16 mm (large).

28.3.2 Indications and Contraindications

The RCPI implant is indicated for SLAC, SNAC, and SCAC grades 3 and 4, and grade IV Kienböck's disease, failure of prior PRC and chronic perilunate dislocations or fracture dislocations (▶ Fig. 28.9). The contraindications are complex regional pain syndrome (CRPS); infection; poor quality of the cortical bone; inflammatory arthritis; and un-cooperative patients.

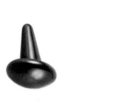

Fig. 28.8 Resurfacing capitate pyrocarbon implant (RCPI).

28.3.3 Surgical Technique

Approach

A longitudinal, dorsal wrist incision is made centered over the fourth extensor compartment. The radiocarpal joint is exposed through a dorsal capsulotomy with a proximally based capsular flap.[13] The terminal branch of posterior interosseous nerve is divided. A PRC is performed and, in some cases, a radial styloid osteotomy (▶ Fig. 28.10).

Bone Preparation

With the wrist flexed fully, the osteotomy of the head of the capitate is performed at 75 degrees to its long axis using an oscillating saw. The osteotomy line of the proximal capitate is aimed to be parallel to the lunate fossa of the distal radius. A 1.5 K-wire is inserted under fluoroscopy control in the capitate along the axis of the middle finger metacarpal as a guidewire. The cannulated RCPI reamer is drilled over the K-wire. Subchondral bone is reamed until the reamer end-stop sits flush with cut face of the capitate (▶ Fig. 28.11). Complete capitate

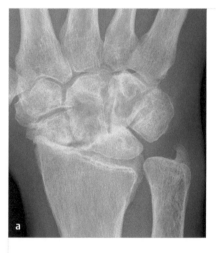
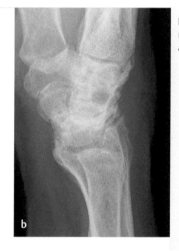
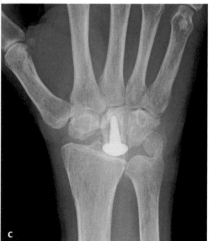
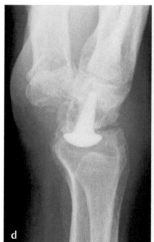

Fig. 28.9 (a–d) Pre- and postoperative radiographs of a scaphoid nonunion advance collapse (SNAC) right wrist III stage.

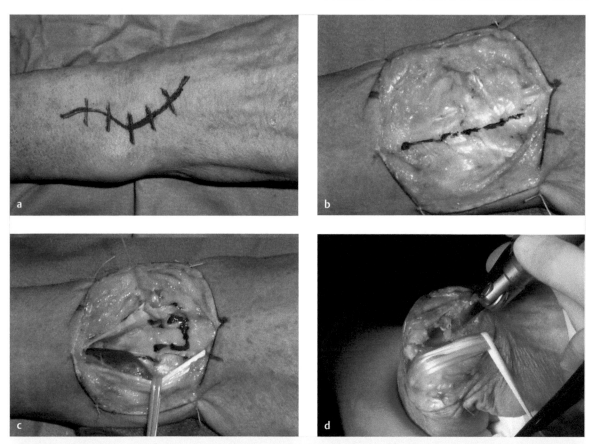

Fig. 28.10 Surgical technique for resurfacing capitate pyrocarbon implant (RCPI): Approach and proximal row carpectomy. **(a)** A dorsal skin incision on the wrist is performed. **(b)** The retinaculum of the fourth compartment of extensor tendons is opened. **(c)** A dorsal radiocarpal capsulotomy is performed. **(d)** After proximal row carpectomy, a minimal resection of the proximal capitate is performed to expose the cancellous bone.

preparation is performed to create a hole in the medullary cavity of the capitate with 14- or 16-mm broaches, taking care to avoid fracturing the capitate.

Implant Positioning

The correct sizing and positioning of the trial implant and assessment of congruency between the RCPI and lunate articular surface of the radius are evaluated using fluoroscopy. In addition to views in neutral, images are taken in maximal radial deviation to exclude radiocarpal impingement. After inserting the definitive implant the dorsal capsule and extensor retinaculum are repaired and the skin incision is closed.

Postoperative Care

The wrist is immobilized in a plaster cast in 20-degree extension and 15-degree ulnar deviation for 4 days. On the fifth day, the patients are allowed to start active wrist motion and the splint is worn during the night for 3

weeks. Four weeks after surgery, electrical stimulation (Compex) of extensor and flexor muscles of the wrist and fingers, 21 sessions daily of 30 minutes each, is started to improve ROMs and grip strength. After 45 days the patients resume normal activity.

28.3.4 Results in the Literature

There are few published papers. In 2011, Fernandes et al treated a patient with symptomatic grade IV Kienböck's with a PRC and RCPI.[14] At 12 months, the patient reported a significant improvement in pain and ROMs. In 2011, Goubier et al reported on seven patients (six men and one woman) with midcarpal and radiolunate arthritis treated with a PRC and RCPI. The mean follow-up was 30 (range 6–72) months. The mean postoperative pain measured with a VAS was 4 (range 2–5), the mean grip strength was 16 (range 5–20) kgf, and the mean ROM 25 degrees (range 20–40 degrees) for flexion, and 30 degrees (range 20–45 degrees) for extension. No carpal dislocation or radius bone erosion was noted

28

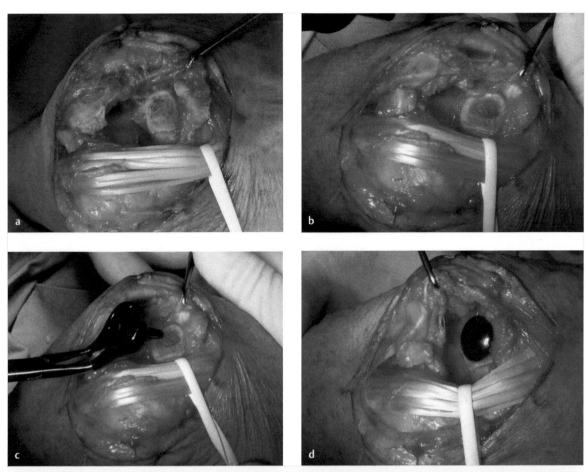

Fig. 28.11 Surgical technique for resurfacing capitate pyrocarbon implant (RCPI): Implant insertion. **(a)** The resection should be made at an angle of 15 degree matching the inclination of the distal radius. **(b)** A hole is created to receive the stem of RCPI. **(c,d)** The prosthesis is implanted giving particular attention to correct orientation of the implant: the acute angle must be dorsal.

radiologically. Six patients were satisfied with good pain relief, despite the reduced wrist motion and grip.[15] In 2012 Szalay et al reported on five patients with advanced carpal collapse treated with a PRC and RCPI. They reported that the functional capacity and wrist motion improved but they noted radiological evidence of stem loosening in two patients.[16]

In 2018 Kopel[12] reported on 33 patients (35 wrists in 20 men and 13 women) with SLAC, SNAC, and SCAC wrists treated with PRC and RCPI. The mean follow-up was 30 months. The mean postoperative pain score on a VAS was 2.8, the mean grip strength 24 kgf, and the mean ROMs 39-degree flexion, 42-degree extension, and 31-degree radioulnar deviation (only mean results were reported without the ranges). The mean postoperative DASH score was 20; 50% of the patients reported being very satisfied and 22% satisfied. Seven patients were treated with partial arthrodesis and two patients with total fusion after failure of the PRC and RCPI procedures.[12]

28.3.5 Author's Own (AM) Experience and Preferred Technique

From March 2004 to November 2018 we have treated 91 wrists (58 right and 33 left) in 91 patients (76 men and 15 women) with a mean age of 54 (range 22–81) years. The indications were: SNAC wrist (40 wrists); SLAC wrist (20); SCAC wrist (15); Kienböck's disease (7); failed PRC (3); chronic trans-scapho-perilunate dislocations (3); adaptative proximal scaphoid implant (APSI) prosthesis subluxation (2); and gout (1).

We reviewed 74 patients, at a mean follow-up of 63 (range 14–134) months. The mean postoperative pain assessed by VAS reduced from 8.4 to 1.4; complete pain relief (VAS 0) was achieved in 31 patients. The mean grip strength improved from 12 to 22 kgf. The mean ROMs improved from 52 to 78 degrees for flexion-extension and from 16 to 24 degrees for radial-ulnar deviation. The mean DASH score improved from 57 to 8.

28

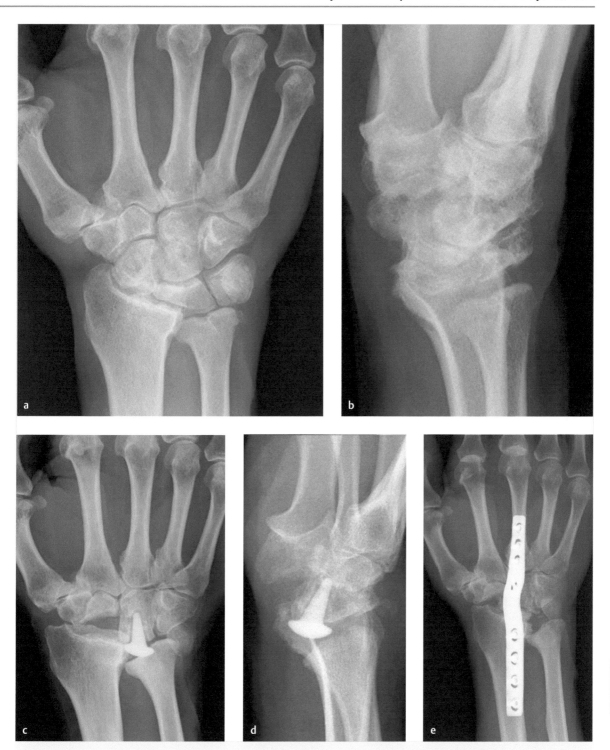

Fig. 28.12 Scapholunate advance collapse (SLAC) wrist IV stage with prior open reduction for perilunate subluxation 20 years earlier. **(a,b)** Preoperative radiographs. **(c,d)** Postoperative radiographs showing ulnar wrist instability at 24 months. **(e)** Postoperative radiographs showing conversion to a total wrist fusion.

28

The radiological examinations showed the implants were stable in the capitate and in 50 patients the implant was found to be well situated in the lunate fossa of the radius. In 19 patients a small ulnar translation of the implant was noted (less than two-third of the width of the implant centered on the lunate fossa of the radius), but without symptoms obviously related to this subluxation probably due to the support given by the triangular fibrocartilage complex (TFCC). Two patients with stage III SLAC wrist had ulnocarpal impingement within 12 months; one was converted to a total wrist arthrodesis (▶ Fig. 28.12). Only one patient has subsidence of the implant like the more common failure rate in proximal interphalangeal (PIP) joint arthroplasty. The patient treated for gout had recurrence of stiffness with gouty deposits around the implant within 2 years. One patient developed an infection 7 years postoperatively; she has been treated with removal of the implant and implantation of an antibiotic-impregnated cement spacer. Seventy-one patients reported they were satisfied; only three reported they were dissatisfied.

I favor this technique as it gives good pain relief, with preservation of wrist mobility and some improvement of grip strength with high rates of reported satisfaction. I prefer a mini-rectangular dorsal capsular approach centered on the floor of the fourth extensor compartment that preserves the dorsal intercarpal ligament and provides adequate visualization for the surgical maneuvers.[17,18] I believe it also allows early mobilization, i. e., at the fourth day to theoretically obtain a better ROM.[13] There may be a role for this implant even when there is some wear of the lunate fossa of the distal radius.[12,13,14]

28.4 Conclusion

The Amandys implant and the RCPI provide different concepts for treating wrist OA but maintaining some wrist motion. The midterm results are encouraging, acknowledging that the indications of each implant are not yet well defined and appear to overlap. The Amandys implant appears more suited to treat severe joint destruction while the RCPI implant particularly extends the indications of PRC in the presence of capitate head destruction.

Acknowledgments

Special thanks to Dr. Y. Tanwir and Dr. V. Lestienne for providing some data from their work (Amandys implant) that has not yet been published.

References

[1] Bellemère P. Pyrocarbon implants for the hand and wrist. Hand Surg Rehabil. 2018; 37(3):129–154

[2] Bellemère P, Maes-Clavier C, Loubersac T, Gaisne E, Kerjean Y. Amandys(®) implant: novel pyrocarbon arthroplasty for the wrist. Chir Main. 2012; 31(4):176–187

[3] Bellemère P, Al Hakim W, Le Corre A, Ross M. Pyrocarbon arthroplasty for Kienböck's disease. In: Bain G, Lichtman D, eds. Kienböck disease. Springer International; 2016:271–284

[4] Bellemère P, Maes-Clavier C, Loubersac T, Gaisne E, Kerjean Y, Collon S. Pyrocarbon interposition wrist arthroplasty in the treatment of failed wrist procedures. J Wrist Surg. 2012; 1(1):31–38

[5] Daruwalla ZJ, Davies KL, Shafighian A, Gillham NR. Early results of a prospective study on the pyrolytic carbon (pyrocarbon) Amandys® for osteoarthritis of the wrist. Ann R Coll Surg Engl. 2012; 94(7):496–501

[6] Video of the surgical technique of Amandys arthroplasty. Available at https://youtu.be/HhZM-JlvJXs

[7] Pierrart J, Bourgade P, Mamane W, Rousselon T, Masmejean EH. Novel approach for posttraumatic panarthritis of the wrist using a pyrocarbon interposition arthroplasty (Amandys(®)): preliminary series of 11 patients. Chir Main. 2012; 31(4):188–194

[8] Tanwin Y, Maes-Clavier C, Lestienne V, et al. Medium-term outcomes for Amandys Implant: a 5-year minimum follow-up of 63 cases. J Wrist Surg. 2021 [published online ahead of print] DOI: 10.1055/s-0041-1726406

[9] Cugola L, Testoni R, Carita E, Dib G. Total wrist arthroplasty versus Amandys. J Hand Surg Eur Vol. 2015; 40E suppl 1:S64

[10] Bedeshi P, Folloni A, Landi A. Artrosi del polso. Riv Chir Mano. 1991; 28:39–65

[11] Marcuzzi A. Utilisation of RCPI prosthesis in post-traumatic chronic disease of wrist: technique of implantation and results. In: Allieu Y (ed.), Arthroplasties radiocarpiennes: 4èmeRencontres de l'IMM, Montpellier, Paris: Sauramps Medical; 2012:101–111

[12] Kopel L. Evaluation de implant RCPI en complément de la résection de la première rangée du carpe pour l'arthrose du carpe stade III et IV. Hand Surg Rehabil. 2018; 37:390–391

[13] Marcuzzi A, Leigheb M, Russomando A, Landi A. Personal technique for wrist dorsal approach. Acta Biomed. 2014; 85(2) Suppl 2:37–45

[14] Fernandes CH, Santos JBG, Nakachima LR, Hirakawa C, Faloppa F, Albertoni WM. Resurfacing capitate pyrocarbon implant (RCPI): an alternative treatment for aseptic necrosis of the stage IV of Litchmann' classification. A case report. J Orthop. 2010; 7:10–13

[15] Goubier JN, Vogels J, Teboul F. Capitate pyrocarbon prosthesis in radiocarpal osteoarthritis. Tech Hand Up Extrem Surg. 2011; 15(1):28–31

[16] Szalay G, Stigler B, Kraus R, Böhringer G, Schnettler R. Proximal row carpectomy and replacement of the proximal pole of the capitate by means of a pyrocarbon cap (RCPI) in advanced carpal collapse. Handchir Mikrochir Plast Chir. 2012; 44(1):17–22

[17] Marcuzzi A, Ozben H, Russomando A. The use of the pyrocarbon resurfacing implant in chronic wrist disorders. Hand Surg. 2014; 39E:611–618

[18] Marcuzzi A, Colantonio F, Petrella G, Ozben H, Russomando A. Stage IV Kienböck's disease: proximal row carpectomy and application of RCPI implant. Hand Surg Rehabil. 2017; 36(2):102–108

28

29 Partial Wrist Joint Arthroplasties: APSI, Capitolunate Joint, Pisotriquetral Joint, and Little Finger Carpometacarpal Joint

Marc Leroy

Abstract

Isolated partial arthrosis of the wrist has always been a challenge. The advent of pyrocarbon in recent years has made it possible to offer therapeutic alternatives to potentially burdensome procedures.

In this chapter, we will detail our management of partial wrist arthroplasties in the most well-known cases of isolated osteoarthritis of the wrist: the use of the adaptative proximal scaphoid implant (APSI) in the scaphoid nonunion advanced collapse of the wrist, the use of pyrocarbon interposition implant (Pi2) and the resurfacing capitate pyrocarbon implant (RCPI) in isolated capitolunate arthrosis, as well as the use of Pyrocardan implant in pisotriquetral arthrosis and post-traumatic carpo-metacarpal joint of the little finger.

These arthroplasties show interesting functional results and in most cases delay the onset of osteoarthritis. In addition, these techniques are lesser intervention and burn fewer bridges than conventional treatment methods (fusion, proximal row carpectomy).

In order to avoid complications (implant dislocation), the procedures must be rigorous, accompanied by dynamic fluoroscopic control and good management of the surrounding soft tissues.

Keywords: Pyrocarbon, arthroplasties, partial wrist arthrosis

Partial wrist arthritis has always been difficult to treat. In recent years, the arrival of pyrocarbon has made it possible to offer alternative options. Because of its mechanical properties and biological tolerance, pyrocarbon is a very suitable material for interposition arthroplasties.[1]

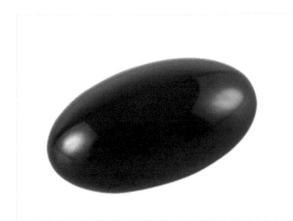

Fig. 29.1 Adaptive proximal scaphoid implant (APSI).

29.1 APSI: Adaptative Proximal Scaphoid Implant

29.1.1 Introduction

The Adaptive Proximal Scaphoid Implant (APSI) pyrocarbon implant, first developed by Péquignot and Allieu in 2000,[2] has been reported to be a very useful solution for treating wrists affected by proximal scaphoid nonunion and scaphoid nonunion advanced collapse (SNAC) wrist.[2] This ovoid-shaped implant (▶ Fig. 29.1) is intended to replace the scaphoid's proximal pole to maintain carpal height. The implant helps to restore even force distribution at the proximal carpal row and aims to reduce progression of degenerative (osteoarthritic) changes.[1] When conservative treatment is no longer beneficial, the principle is to use a spacer to preserve mobility and maintain the radial column of the carpus limiting carpal collapse (▶ Fig. 29.2a). This is an intervention that does not burn bridges other than excluding scaphoid bone union, i.e., other salvage procedures can still be undertaken if it fails.

29.1.2 Implant and Surgical Technique

The commonest approaches are radial or dorsal. A palmar approach has been used but much less commonly. We prefer the radial approach (▶ Fig. 29.2b) which easily allows for a concomitant radial styloidectomy.

Via the radial approach we protect the branches of the radial nerve and dissect down to the radiocarpal joint between the first and the second extensor compartments. If a radial styloidectomy is performed, no more than 6 mm should be removed measuring from the tip to the styloid in order to respect the anterior radiocarpal ligaments and to avoid compromising the stability of the implant (▶ Fig. 29.2c). The extent of the resection of the proximal pole of the scaphoid will depend on the initial damage: for a SNAC wrist, resection will be limited to pseudarthrosis (▶ Fig. 29.2d); for a scapholunate advanced collapse (SLAC) wrist, we recommend excising as little as possible to allow the implant to be centered and to maintain the ligament insertions of the scaphoid. The proximal end of the remaining distal scaphoid is burred to match the shape of the implant (▶ Fig. 29.2e); this aims to enhance implant stability. It is important to remove any posterior bone fragments that could generate a cam effect and cause anterior subluxation or dislocation of the implant. The implant size is based on the radiographic testing of the wrist (▶ Fig. 29.3). The aim is for the implant to be stable through the full range of wrist movement and to avoid breaching the first arc of Gilula.

29

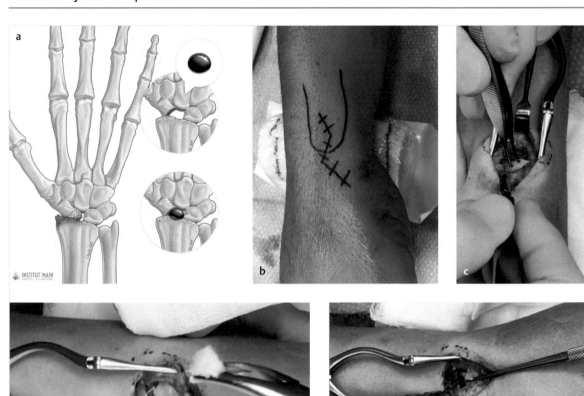

Fig. 29.2 (a) Drawings showing the use of an adaptive proximal scaphoid implant (APSI) to replace the proximal pole of the scaphoid to treat radio-scaphoid arthritis. (b) The radial approach for implantation of an APSI. (c) The styloidectomy should be no more than 6 mm from the tip of the styloid. (d) Resection of the proximal pole of the scaphoid. (e) Modeling of the proximal scaphoid to match the shape of the implant.

If, in doubt, we recommend undersizing the implant. To avoid impingement, it is necessary to ensure that the proximal scaphoid bone surface lies parallel to the slope of the distal radius in the sagittal plane. We also recommend removing a little of the capitate head of the capitate with a motorized cutter to avoid impingement with the implant. After testing with a trial, the definitive implant is inserted (▶ Fig. 29.4). The joint capsule is closed securely and if necessary the capsule can be sutured to bone (▶ Fig. 29.5). The wrist is supported in a splint/plaster for 2 weeks in a neutral position and then in a removable splint with protected mobilization for the next 4 weeks. From 6 weeks postoperatively onward the patient is encouraged to move without restriction.

29.1.3 Indication and Contraindication

For scaphoid nonunions we recommend the APSI when the proximal pole of the scaphoid is no longer suitable for reconstruction, e.g., due to fragmentation or radioscaphoid arthritis, typically SNAC stages 1 and 2. For SLAC wrists the indication for an APSI is isolated radioscaphoid osteoarthritis without associated carpal collapse. We are very cautious and generally advise against the APSI implant when there is any carpal collapse, especially any dorsal subluxation of the capitate. Small and medium bone cysts are not contraindications for the APSI, as they can be filled during the operation with bone from the scaphoid proximal pole, the radial styloid process, or a bone substitute.

29.1.4 Results in Literature

Several studies have demonstrated its effectiveness in the short and medium terms, providing good pain relief without loss of wrist mobility or strength.[2,3,4,5,6,7,8,9] The main complication is dislocation. A retrospective analysis of these implants at 10 years has shown 12% early dislocation primarily due to technical errors; and 9% reoperation for implant removal and midcarpal arthrodesis between 3 and 9 years postoperatively.[10] There is a lack of long-term follow-up using this technique[11] but the biocompatibility of pyrocarbon is well established[12] and

29

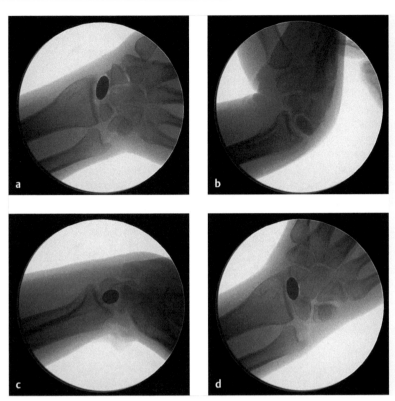

Fig. 29.3 (a–d) Dynamic testing of the wrist: the implant must be stable in all directions of wrist.

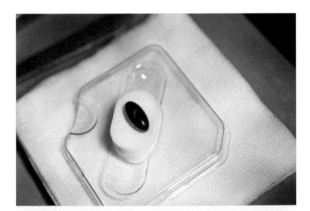

Fig. 29.4 Adaptive proximal scaphoid implant (APSI) before final implantation.

one study has suggested that it reduces the progression of osteoarthritis elsewhere in the wrist.[11]

29.1.5 Comparison with Other Techniques

Use of the APSI is a lesser intervention and burns fewer bridges than conventional treatment methods (fusion, proximal row carpectomy) and allows for various bailout options including other conventional treatments.

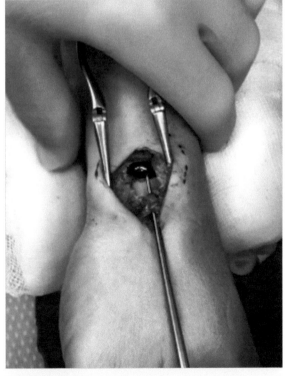

Fig. 29.5 Capsular closure.

29

Resection of the Proximal Pole of the Scaphoid and Interposition Materials

Excision of the proximal pole of the scaphoid alone with or without interposition with a "soft" material such as silicone, fascia, or tendon does not prevent progression of osteoarthritis and long-term carpal collapse.[13,14,15]

Use of the APSI appears to give better wrist mobility[11] and function than a scaphoid excision and four-corner fusion.[1,8,11] Otherwise the pain relief, patient satisfaction, and strength are similar at comparable follow-up.[16,17,18,19] The APSI appears to allow a quicker return of function but has a higher complication rate.[16,17,18,19]

Proximal Row Carpectomy (PRC)

The APSI has been reported to give better pain relief, restoration of strength, and patient satisfaction but there is no published comparative study with PRC.[1,2,3,4,5,6,7,8,9] In addition, it is a less destructive technique, but the APSI has a higher complication rate.[3,4,5,6,7] A PRC appears to be less suited to heavy manual workers and to be less durable in younger patients.[18,19]

Carpal Denervation

The APSI provides better mobility than total carpal denervation (TCD), with better pain relief and wrist function but no difference in strength and patient satisfaction.[20,21,22] Again, the rate of complications with the APSI is higher.

Rib Cartilage Autograft at the Scaphoid Proximal Pole

Insertion of a rib cartilage autograft to replace the proximal pole of the scaphoid is an attractive treatment option for early stage of radioscaphoid osteoarthritis. This technique takes longer, has risks of donor site morbidity (general anesthesia, pneumothorax), and it seems to give less good results than those of the APSI.[23,24] Even at 8 years follow-up, authors found dorsal intercalated segment instability (DISI) in 76 % of cases.[24]

In summary, we recommend using the APSI in SNAC stages 1 and 2: it is not a very invasive procedure, with a relatively short recovery time. The long-term results seem to remain reasonably good and appear to delay the progression of osteoarthritis. In addition, the procedure does not preclude further salvage procedures. We recommend a concomitant radial styloidectomy in most cases, use of a small implant where there is doubt, and performance of a detailed intraoperative evaluation of mobility and stability under fluoroscopic control.

29.2 Capitolunate Joint Arthroplasty

29.2.1 Introduction

When the capitolunate joint space is destroyed by primary osteoarthritis (OA), osteonecrosis of the capitate head or Fenton's syndrome (scaphocapitate fracture), an unconstrained capitolunate interposition arthroplasty with a pyrocarbon implant, e. g., Pi2 (*pyrocarbon interposition implant*) or RCPI (*resurfacing capitate pyrocarbon implant*) is an option to avoid a partial wrist arthrodesis.

29.2.2 Pi2 and RCPI Implants

The Pi2 ellipsoidal implant is 9 mm thick and comes in two sizes (▶ Fig. 29.6). It was originally intended for treatment of thumb carpometacarpal (CMC) joint arthritis. The RCPI is a one-piece hemiprosthesis for capitate head resurfacing (▶ Fig. 29.7). The truncated spherical head is tilted by 15 degrees and mounted on an intramedullary stem; it is press-fitted into the capitate.

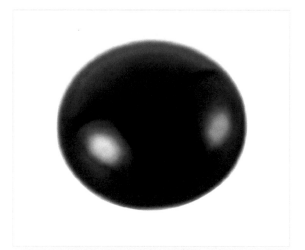

Fig. 29.6 Pyrocarbon interposition implant (Pi2).

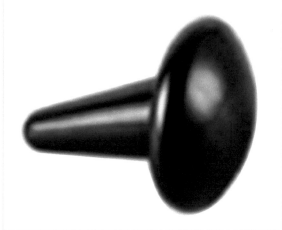

Fig. 29.7 Resurfacing capitate pyrocarbon implant (RCPI).

29.2.3 Surgical Technique and Indication

The implants are inserted by a posterior approach with transverse arthrotomy that aims to preserve the continuity of the dorsal intercarpal ligaments. The capitate head is resected by a few millimeters (no more than 5 mm to avoid damaging the extrinsic ligamentous system), and a trial implant is inserted. Similar to the APSI, care should be taken to maintain "normal" carpal alignment clinically and radiologically, particularly the medial carpal space. Typically, a smaller implant is used than for thumb CMC joint OA. The wrist is closed securely to help maintain implant stability especially for implants without a stem. The wrist is supported in a splint/plaster for 2 weeks in neutral and then a removable splint with protected mobilization for the next 4 weeks. From 6 weeks postoperatively the patient is encouraged to move without restriction.

29.2.4 Results in Literature and in Our Experience

The use of a pyrocarbon implant (RCPI) was first reported by Dereudre et al in 2010.[25] They reported good clinical results at 22-month follow-up, but dorsal translation of the distal carpal row relative to the proximal carpal row was noted radiologically. A later study reported encouraging results in a 15-year-old patient followed-up for more than 4 years; he had regained a good range of motion and grip strength and had resumed sport.[26] Our published experience is based on three cases,[27] with a mean follow-up of 4.8 (range 1–8.2) years (▶ Table 29.1).

There were improvements in functional scores and pain but not in mobility. So far, we have performed this technique in patients (unpublished) with follow-up of 10 years in one case (▶ Fig. 29.8). Resurfacing of the capitate head using a RCPI implant has been reported following trauma, i.e., Fenton's syndrome[25,28] (▶ Table 29.2). Although the functional results are good, there is little improvement in mobility.

Overall, the indications are more limited, but we believe there is a role in specific cases.

29.3 Pisotriquetral Joint Arthroplasty

29.3.1 Introduction

In cases of pisotriquetral (PT) arthrosis, a PT interface arthroplasty with a Pyrocardan implant is an alternative to PT fusion or the more conventional pisiform excision[29] (▶ Fig. 29.7). The pisiform is articulated by a small, slightly concave forward joint surface with a larger, oval, slightly convex surface of the volar and distal side of the triquetrum. It is a condylar, synovial type joint with a thin, loose capsule. It has a large proximal and a smaller distal recess. We consider that the shape of the PT joint makes it suitable for such an arthroplasty.

29.3.2 Implant Pyrocardan

This Pyrocardan implant is a biconcave implant with a rectangular cross-section (▶ Fig. 29.9, ▶ Fig. 29.10). It is available in seven sizes, from XXS to XXL. The sizes relate to the area of the surface of the implant. Whatever its

Table 29.1 Comparative clinical result of Pi2 in capitolunate arthroplasty

	Patient 1, age 29: spontaneous osteonecrosis		Patient 2, age 23: posttraumatic osteonecrosis		Patient 3, age 63: osteoarthritis	
	preop	postop	preop	postop	preop	postop
Follow-up (mo)		98		50		24
VAS	6	1	5	1	9	2
Flexion	40	35	70	50	60	50
Extension	30	55	30	45	40	60
RD	20	10	35	30	0	10
UD	20	30	10	20	25	30
Grip	8	12	26	43	12	22
DASH	68.18	25	45.45	25	72.73	2.27
PRWE	62	20	57.5	29	92	19

Abbreviations: DASH, disabilities of the arm, shoulder, and hand; Pi2, pyrocarbon interposition implant; PRWE, patient-related wrist evaluation; RD, radial deviation; UD, ulnar deviation.
Note: Age in years; follow-up in months; VAS = visual analog scale 0–10; flexion and extension in degrees; grip strength in kilograms force (kgf).

29

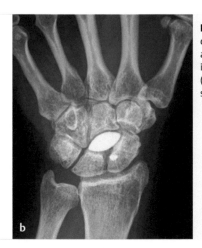

Fig. 29.8 (a, b) Idiopathic necrosis of the capitate head, treated by interposition arthroplasty with a pyrocarbon interposition implant (Pi2) after 10 years follow-up (note the radiodense bone anchor in the scaphoid).

Table 29.2 Clinical results of RCPI for treatment of chronic Fenton's syndrome

	Patient 1 Age 24	Patient 2 Age 42
Follow-up (mo)	64	48
Grip strength (kgf)	36 (90%)	38 (90%)
Flexion	40	40
Extension	45	50
RD	15	15
UD	35	35
MWS	90	95
DASH	10	12

Abbreviations: DASH, disabilities of the arm, shoulder, and hand; MWS, Mayo wrist score; RCPI, resurfacing capitate pyrocarbon implant; RD, radial deviation; UD, ulnar deviation.
Note: Age in years; follow-up in months; flexion and extension in degrees; grip in kilograms force (kgf).

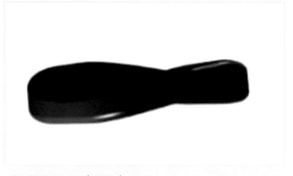

Fig. 29.9 Pyrocardan implant.

size, the thickness at the center of the implant is 1 mm, while the thickness of the outer edges of the implant is proportional to its size ranging from 12 to 18 mm.

29.3.3 Surgical Technique and Management

Via a curvilinear or zigzag incision of approximately 3.5 cm over ulnar to the pisotriquetral joint. The flexor carpi ulnaris (FCU) tendon is identified and a longitudinal arthrotomy is performed on the ulnar edge of the pisotriquetral joint (▶ Fig. 29.11a, b). After synovectomy and surgical removal of any loose bodies, the pisiform is raised and tilted radially. A fine spatula is used to assess the state of the joint capsule, particularly its strength proximally,

distally, and radially. If the capsule is deficient it is reinforced as much as possible. If it is not possible to secure the capsule, we consider it is best to change the operation, typically to pisiform excision. After resection of any osteophytes the arthritic joint surfaces are shaped with an oscillating saw or a rotary burr so that the articular surfaces of the triquetrum and the pisiform are, respectively, convex proximodistally and lateromedially, i.e., matching the implant surfaces. Trial implants are used to determine the most suitable size (▶ Fig. 29.11c), and then assessed with static and dynamic fluoroscopic images. The implants are placed without any press-fit to avoid bone impingement and the ulnar joint capsule is closed securely (▶ Fig. 29.11d). The wrist is immobilized in neutral in a thermoplastic splint worn continuously for 2 weeks. Then mobilization is encouraged with intermittent use of a removable splint. Light manual activities were allowed progressively from 4 weeks postoperatively; full unrestricted activities are allowed after 6 weeks (▶ Fig. 29.11a).

29.3.4 Results in Our Experience

Our experience is based on 14 cases with no failures. The results of our first eight cases were published at a mean

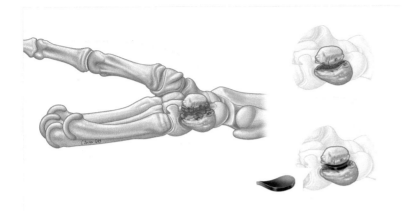

Fig. 29.10 Drawings for treatment of piso-triquetral arthroplasty with a Pyrocardan implant.

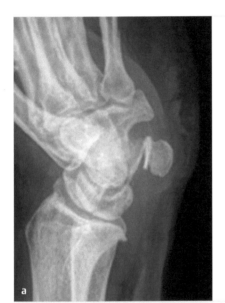

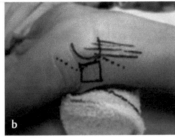

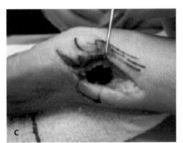

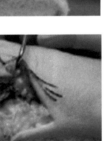

Fig. 29.11 (a) Lateral radiograph of a Pyrocardan implant in the pisotriquetral joint. **(b–d)** Operative approach and implantation of the Pyrocardan implant into the pisotriquetral joint.

follow-up of 2.8 (range 1.2–4.4) years[29] (▶ Table 29.3 and ▶ Table 29.4). The pain scores reduced from 8 to 2 out of 10 on a visual analog scale (VAS). Grip strength increased by 22% and joint mobility improved, especially in radio-ulnar deviation (+47%). The mean postoperative scores for the Mayo wrist score (MWS), QuickDASH, and patient-related wrist evaluation (PRWE) were 89, 18, and 20, respectively. All patients reported being satisfied or very satisfied. One early dislocation was seen at the first postoperative radiological examination (▶ Fig. 29.12); this implant was repositioned, and the proximal capsule strengthened, which is typically the weakest part of the PT joint capsule. So far, no other series have been reported with this implant. Compared to the excision of the pisiform, we believe that pyrocarbon interposed arthroplasty is less damaging as some pisiform is left and it provides predictable and reliable results.

29.4 Little Finger Carpometacarpal Joint Arthroplasty

29.4.1 Introduction

The carpometacarpal (CMC) joint of the little finger can develop symptomatic arthritis after fractures or dislocations. Many surgical techniques have been proposed, including arthrodesis, excision arthroplasties, and implant arthroplasties.[30,31,32,33,34,35]

29.4.2 Current Surgical Techniques

Arthrodesis of the little finger metacarpal to the hamate may treat the pain, but with loss of joint mobility. Excision arthroplasty of the little finger CMC joint with or without a soft tissue interposition may give impingement

29

Table 29.3 Clinical results of use of a Pyrocardan implant to treat pisotriquetral arthritis

Patients	Pain (VAS)	Mobility (% of ROM of affected side/CL)	Strength grip in kg (%/CL)	Satisfaction	Scores (preop value) MWS QDASH PRWE
1	Absent (0)	F/E = 85°–60° (100 %) RI/UI = 20°–50° (116 %)	28 (140 %)	Very satisfied	100 9.1 4
2	Absent (0)	F/E = 80°–70° (90 %) RI/UI = 0°–60° (100 %)	18 (100 %)	Very satisfied	100 9.1 2
3	Intermittent (5)	F/E = 70°–60° (96 %) RI/UI = 10°–50° (120 %)	28 (140 %)	Satisfied	75 47.7 (65.9) 58.5 (75.5)
4	Intermittent (2)	F/E = 50°–65° (85 %) RI/UI = 35°–50° (100 %)	30 (86 %)	Very satisfied	65 40.9 43
5	Absent (0)	F/E = X RI/UI = X	X	Very satisfied	X4.5 8 (79.5)
6	Absent (0)	F/E = 70°–70° (100 %) RI/UI ¼ 35° - 50° (121 %)	20 (133 %)	Very satisfied	100 18.2 (75) 8.5 (83.5)
7	Absent (0)	F/E = 75°–50° (100 %) RI/UI = 20°–50° (100 %)	45 (112.5 %)	Very satisfied	100 13.6 4
8	Intermittent (5)	F/E = 50°–55° (95 %) RI/UI = 10°–20° (75 %)	10 (55.5 %)	Very satisfied	70 20.5 (63.6) 56.5 (73)
Results	Mean VAS = 2 62.5 % painless	F/E = 70°–63° (99 %) RI/UI = 21°–51° (111 %)	27 ± 9 (113 %)	87.5 % Very satisfied 12.5 % Satisfied	MWS = 89 ± 15 QDASH = 18 ± 17 PRWE = 20 ± 21

Abbreviations: CL, contralateral; E, extension; F, flexion; MWS, Mayo wrist score; PRWE, patient-rated wrist evaluation; QDASH, quick disability of arm, shoulder, and hand; RI, radial inclination; ROM, range of motion; UI, ulnar inclination; VAS, visual analog scale. Note: X means no data.

pain. The alternative of excision arthroplasty of the little finger CMC joint and arthrodesis of the fifth metacarpal shaft to the ring finger metacarpal may restrict metacarpal motion and could in theory cause excessive loading of the ring finger CMC joint.[30] In addition, an arthrodesis carries the risks of nonunion or delayed union and typically requires postoperative immobilization.[31] Silicone implants have also been used but carry the risks of all implants and are not hard bearing.[34,35,36]

29.4.3 Our Approach and Management

We have performed CMC arthroplasties of the ring and little finger CMC joints with Pyrocardan implants (▶ Fig. 29.13a). The operation is performed via a dorsal approach (▶ Fig. 29.13b) between the finger extensor tendons and the extensor carpi ulnaris (ECU) tendon. After a longitudinal arthrotomy we remove any osteophytes and shape the arthritic joint surface(s) with an oscillating saw (▶ Fig. 29.13c) and a burr to create a mildly biconvex surface. The trial implant is positioned and assessed with static and dynamic fluoroscopy to determine the most suitable size (▶ Fig. 29.13d, ▶ Fig. 29.14). The final implant is inserted and the joint capsule is sutured (▶ Fig. 29.13e). The wrist is immobilized for 2 weeks in a plaster cast in neutral. Protective mobilization is performed with intermittent splint usage for the next 4 weeks. Full unrestricted activities are allowed after 6 weeks. Our unpublished experience of our first 12 cases is encouraging, with good pain relief, improvement in strength, and return to work. As yet we have not had to revise any of these cases.

Table 29.4 Preoperative and postoperative results of use of a Pyrocardan implant to treat pisotriquetral arthritis

Patients	Preoperative (%/CL)	Postoperative FU = 2.8 y (%/CL)	Gain from pre- to postoperatively (% gain)
F	65° (89)	70° (96)	
E	63° (102)	63° (101)	
ROM F–E	128° (95)	133° (99)	+5° (4) $p = 0.8$
RI	12° (71)	21° (126)	
UI	30° (62)	51° (106)	
ROM RI–UI	42° (64)	72° (111)	+30° (47) $p = 0.3$
Strength grip (kgf)	22 kg (91)	27 kg (113)	+5 kg (22) $p = 0.2$
Pain VAS	8	2	−6 (75) $p < 0.5$
QDASH	68	18	−50 (74) $p < 0.5$
PRWE	78	20	−58 (74) $p < 0.5$
MWS	57	89	32 (56) $p < 0.5$

Abbreviations: CL, contralateral; E, extension; F, flexion; FU, follow-up; Grip, hand clamping force; MWS, Mayo wrist score; postop, postoperative; preop, preoperative; PRWE, patient-rated wrist evaluation; QDASH, quick disabilities of the arm, shoulder, and hand; RI, radial inclination; ROM, range of motion; UI, ulnar inclination; VAS, visual analog scale.

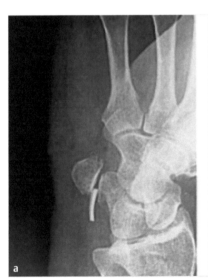
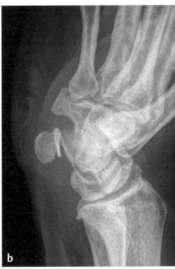

Fig. 29.12 (a) Early subluxation of a Pyrocardan implant. (b) Repositioned Pyrocardan after 2 years follow up.

29

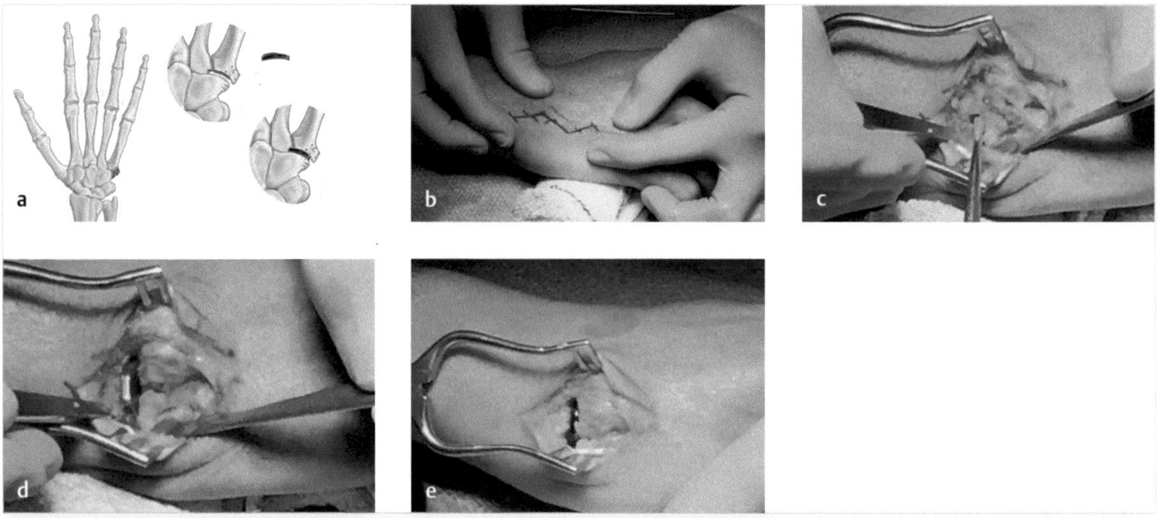

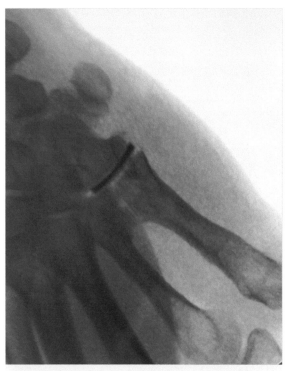

Fig. 29.13 **(a)** Drawings of treatment of little finger carpometacarpal joint arthroplasty with a Pyrocardan implant. **(b)** Surgical approach. **(c)** Joint preparation. **(d)** Trial implantation. **(e)** Final implantation and joint capsule closure.

Fig. 29.14 Perioperative fluoroscopic assessment.

29.5 Conclusion

Although the indications are infrequent, the use of pyrocarbon implants for partial wrist arthroplasties has been very encouraging in our practice. Moreover, in case of failure, they do not exclude revision by traditional techniques. Mostly these implants are not fixed directly to the bone so there are no issues with bone implant stabilization. As well as use of a good technique, appropriate indications are very important. In addition, there are appreciable learning curves with all these techniques.

References

[1] Bellemère P. Medium- and long-term outcomes for hand and wrist pyrocarbon implants. J Hand Surg Eur Vol. 2019; 44(9):887–897

[2] Pequignot JP, Lussiez B, Allieu Y. A adaptive proximal scaphoid implant. Chir Main. 2000; 19(5):276–285

[3] Grandis C, Berzero GF, Bassi F, Allieu Y. Prime esperienze di utilizzo in Italia della protesi parziale di scafoide APSI. Riv Chir Mano. 2004; 41:36–42

[4] Grandis C, Berzero GF. Partial scaphoid pyrocarbon implant: personal series review [abstract]. J Hand Surg Eur Vol. 2007; 32:S95

[5] Daruwalla ZJ, Davies K, Shafighian A, Gillham NR. An alternative treatment option for scaphoid nonunion advanced collapse (SNAC) and radioscaphoid osteoarthritis: early results of a prospective study on the pyrocarbon adaptive proximal scaphoid implant (APSI). Ann Acad Med Singapore. 2013; 42(6):278–284

[6] Bellemère P, Bouju Y, Chaise F, et al. Pseudarthrose du scaphoïde: résection proximale et interposition d'un implant en pyrocarbone, à propos de 20 cas. Chir Main. 2011; 30:429–430

[7] Lima Santos F, Oliveira M, Santos Pereira R, Frias M, Ferreira A, Canela P. Proximal scaphoid hemiarthroplasty for the treatment of post-fracture avascular necrosis of the proximal pole. Chir Main. 2015; 34: 353

[8] Dreant N, Pequignot JP, Fernadez J. L'implant APSI: indications et résultats. Chir Main. 2015; 34:353

[9] Pequinot JP, Allieu Y. Pyrocarbon proximal scaphoid implant allowing adaptive mobility (APSI) in proximal scaphoid pseudarthrosis. In: Driver M, ed. Coating for biomedical applications. Woodhead Publishing; 2012:298–306

[10] Gras M, Wahegaonkar AL, Mathoulin C. Treatment of avascular necrosis of the proximal pole of the scaphoid by arthroscopic resection and prosthetic semi-replacement arthroplasty using the pyrocarbon Adaptive Proximal Scaphoid Implant (APSI): long-term functional outcomes. J Wrist Surg. 2012; 1(2):159–164

[11] Aribert M, Bouju Y, Chaise F, Loubersac T, Gaisne E, Bellemère P. Adaptive Proximal Scaphoid Implant (APSI): 10-year outcomes in patients with SNAC wrists. Hand Surg Rehab. 2019; 38(1):34:43

29

[12] Stanley J, Klawitter J, More R. Replacing joints with pyrolytic carbon. In: Revell PA, ed. Joint replacement technology. Woodhead Publishing; 2008:631–656

[13] Garcia-Elias M, Goubier JN. Arthrodèse radioscapholunaire avec excision du scaphoïde. Chir Main. 2008; 27(5):227–231

[14] Vinnars B, Adamsson L, af Ekenstam F, Wadin K, Gerdin B. Patient-rating of long term results of silicone implant arthroplasty of the scaphoid. Scand J Plast Reconstr Surg Hand Surg. 2002; 36(1):39–45

[15] Smeraglia F, Ciaramella G, Cerbasi S, Balato G, Mariconda M. Treatment of proximal scaphoid non-union by resection of the proximal pole and palmaris longus interposition arthroplasty. Handchir Mikrochir Plast Chir. 2015; 47(3):171–174

[16] Bain GI, Watts AC. The outcome of scaphoid excision and four-corner arthrodesis for advanced carpal collapse at a minimum of ten years. J Hand Surg Am. 2010; 35(5):719–725

[17] Neubrech F, Mühldorfer-Fodor M, Pillukat T, Schoonhoven Jv, Prommersberger KJ. Long-term results after midcarpal arthrodesis. J Wrist Surg. 2012; 1(2):123–128

[18] Richou J, Chuinard C, Moineau G, Hanouz N, Hu W, Le Nen D. Proximal row carpectomy: long-term results. Chir Main. 2010; 29(1):10–15

[19] Wagner ER, Bravo D, Elhassan B, Moran SL. Factors associated with improved outcomes following proximal row carpectomy: a long-term outcome study of 144 patients. J Hand Surg Eur Vol. 2016; 41(5):484–491

[20] Rothe M, Rudolf KD, Partecke BD. Langzeitergebnisse nach Handgelenkdenervation bei fortgeschrittenem karpalem Kollaps (SLAC-/SNAC-Wrist Stadium II und III). Handchir Mikrochir Plast Chir. 2006; 38(4):261–266

[21] Simon E, Zemirline A, Richou J, Hu W, Le Nen D. La dénervation totale du poignet : une étude rétrospective de 27 cas au recul moyen de 77 mois. Chir Main. 2012; 31(6):306–310

[22] Hohendorff B, Mühldorfer-Fodor M, Kalb K, von Schoonhoven J, Prommersberger KJ. Langzeitergebnisse nach Handgelenkdenervation. Unfallchirurg. 2012; 115(4):343–352

[23] Lepage D, Obert L, Clappaz P, Hampel C, Garbuio P, Tropet Y. Arthrose radio-scaphoïdienne traitée par autogreffe ostéocartilagineuse après résection proximale du scaphoïde. Rev Chir Orthop Repar Appar Mot. 2005; 91:307–313

[24] Obert L, Lepage D, Ferrier M, Tropet Y. Rib cartilage graft for posttraumatic or degenerative arthritis at wrist level: 10-year results. J Wrist Surg. 2013; 2(3):234–238

[25] Dereudre G, Kaba A, Pansard E, Mathevon H, Mares O. Avascular necrosis of the capitate: a case report and a review of the literature. Chir Main. 2010; 29(3):203–206

[26] Jagodzinski NA, Taylor CF, Al-Shawi AK. Pyrocarbon interposition arthroplasty for proximal capitate avascular necrosis. Hand (N Y). 2015; 10(2):239–242

[27] Ferrand M, Bellemère P. Pyrocarbon interposition after capitate head resection. J Wrist Surg. 2013; 2(4):351–354

[28] Marcuzzi A, Ozben H, Russomando A, Petit A. Chronic transscaphoid, transcapitate perilunate fracture dislocation of the wrist: Fenton's syndrome. Chir Main. 2013; 32(2):100–103

[29] Bellemère P, Aribert M, Choughri H, Leroy M, Gaisne E. Treatment of piso-triquetral arthritis by pyrocarbon interposition arthroplasty. J Wrist Surg. 2018; 7(1):2–10

[30] Clendenin MB, Smith RJ. Fifth metacarpal/hamate arthrodesis for posttraumatic osteoarthritis. J Hand Surg Am. 1984; 9(3):374–378

[31] Dubert TP, Khalifa H. "Stabilized arthroplasty" for old fracture dislocations of the fifth carpometacarpal joint. Tech Hand Up Extrem Surg. 2009; 13(3):134–136

[32] Gainor BJ, Stark HH, Ashworth CR, Zemel NP, Rickard TA. Tendon arthroplasty of the fifth carpometacarpal joint for treatment of posttraumatic arthritis. J Hand Surg Am. 1991; 16(3):520–524

[33] Black DM, Watson HK, Vender MI. Arthroplasty of the ulnar carpometacarpal joints. J Hand Surg Am. 1987; 12(6):1071–1074

[34] Green WL, Kilgore ES, Jr. Treatment of fifth digit carpometacarpal arthritis with Silastic prosthesis. J Hand Surg Am. 1981; 6(5):510–514

[35] Proubasta IR, Lamas CG, Ibañez NA, Lluch A. Treatment of little finger carpometacarpal posttraumatic arthritis with a silicone implant. J Hand Surg Am. 2013; 38(10):1960–1964

[36] Pruzansky JS, Goljan P, Bachoura A, Jacoby SM, Culp RW. Little finger carpometacarpal arthroplasty technique and result in 3 cases. J Hand Surg Am. 2014; 39(9):1734–1738

29

30 Revision Wrist Arthroplasty

Sumedh C. Talwalkar, Matthew Ricks, and Ian Trail

Abstract

The management of a failed wrist replacement represents a significant challenge. Revision arthroplasty of the wrist has the theoretical advantage of preserving motion in comparison to a wrist arthrodesis in the management of a failed TWA. The long-term results of revision total wrist arthroplasty are currently unknown with loosening, instability and other complications a significant concern. Wrist fusion can be difficult to perform in the absence of adequate bone stock and resection arthroplasties perform poorly in all but the most low demand patient. Although it is reasonable to offer revision wrist arthroplasty in a selective cohort of patients a regular clinical and radiological follow-up is recommended.

Keywords: revision wrist arthroplasty; revision wrist replacement; wrist replacement survival; impaction bone grafting

30.1 Introduction

It has been predicted that the demand for upper limb arthroplasty will outstrip hip and knee arthroplasties in the future.[1] In the absence of a joint registry, it is difficult to estimate how many primary arthroplasties are performed in the United Kingdom or in most other European countries. Currently, there are many fewer upper limb arthroplasties performed each year, than lower limb arthroplasties. There are likely to be a number of surgeons performing low numbers of a complex procedure bringing with it an increasing revision burden with its own challenges. A failed total wrist replacement is very difficult to manage and patients may be elderly with systemic issues.

Treatment options for a failed total wrist arthroplasty (TWA) include a salvage wrist arthrodesis, resection arthroplasty, or revision arthroplasty. Wrist fusion following a failed TWA is technically difficult to perform due to the loss of bone stock. Resection arthroplasties do poorly except in the lowest demand individuals due to the loss of stability resulting in a weak grip. It has been shown in the literature that revision to another wrist replacement has similar results to a wrist fusion in the short term and patients value the range of movement that you get from a replacement over a fusion.[2] Ryu et al showed that 70% of maximal range of movement of the wrist is required to accomplish all tasks in the 40 patients in their study.[3]

30.2 Causes of Failure of a Wrist Arthroplasty

30.2.1 Infection

As with any failed arthroplasty, there has to be a high level of suspicion of an infection. It has been shown that low-grade infection can be difficult to diagnose, particularly with the prevalence of *Propionibacterium*[4] in failed shoulder arthroplasty. Studies have shown that infection has been the cause of some failed TWA but it does not seem to be as much common as in the shoulder.[5] The highest concentration of *P. acnes* has been demonstrated around the shoulder girdle and axilla and not over the wrist; however, it remains a potential source.[6,7] Perioperative tests for infection in revision arthroplasty can be challenging with high sensitivity but low specificity.[4] Common practice to exclude/diagnose infection is the combination of clinical suspicion, blood markers, and in some situations an aspiration or tissue biopsy for microbiological culture. If there is a suspicion of infection and loosening, then similar to other arthroplasties a revision can be performed as a two-stage process rather than a simple reimplantation. The two-stage process involves the removal of the suspected infected implant with the placement of a temporary antibiotic-loaded spacer. Following a period of time typically 6 to 8 weeks depending upon the organism present and antibiotic sensitivity, a second stage is performed with a reimplantation of the prosthesis.

30.2.2 Aseptic Loosening

Implant loosening in the absence of infection can be the result of inadequate initial fixation, mechanical loss of fixation over time, or secondary to a particle-induced osteolysis resulting in biologic loss of fixation. Loosening or bone reabsorption can be due to the forces exerted by the implant on the surrounding bone. Loosening of a TWA can cause pain and instability which may require a revision arthroplasty (▶ Fig. 30.1, ▶ Fig. 30.2).

At our institution we reviewed 220 TWA, predominantly patients with rheumatoid arthritis (92%). Twenty-five wrists were identified as requiring revision surgery. The most common cause of revision after a TWA is implant loosening of the distal component in our series.[8] Work done by Retting and Beckenbaugh showed a comparable pattern of loosening, with the majority needing revision for loosening of the distal component.[9]

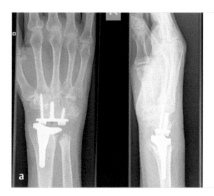

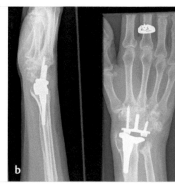

Fig. 30.1 (a, b) Aseptic loosening of the Universal II prosthesis at 10 years. Presenting with increasing pain and loss of range of movement.

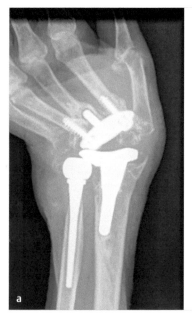

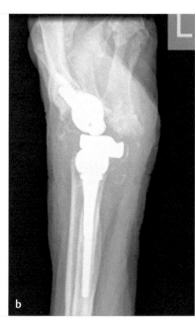

Fig. 30.2 (a, b) Aseptic Loosening in a patient with polyarticular rheumatoid at 9 years with periprosthetic osteolysis (ulnar head replacement). The ulnar head replacement was difficult to remove and needed an osteotomy.

Boeckstyns and Herzberg looked at 44 consecutive cases of Re-Motion TWA (Small Bone Innovations Inc.). They found periprosthetic radiolucency (more than 2 mm) around the radial component in 16 cases and on the carpal side in 7 cases (▶ Fig. 30.3, ▶ Fig. 30.4). These developed gradually, adjacent to the prosthetic components regardless of the primary diagnosis, and seemed to stabilize in most patients over a period of 1 to 3 years. They found that in a small percentage of patients the periprosthetic area of bone was significantly larger. In their study they were able to show that the radiolucency was not necessarily related to loosening of the implants; only five carpal components and one radial component subsided or tilted. They recommended close and continued observation of TWA and especially radiolucency. A similar phenomenon has been demonstrated in ulnar head replacements in which no artificial components articulate with each other. This resorption seems to stabilize after a period of 6 months to 1 year and is attributed to stress shielding.[10]

Packer et al have published promising intermediate results using the Motec TWA which is a cementless modular metal-on-metal ball-and-socket wrist arthroplasty. Rokkum et al using the same arthroplasty reviewed 57 patients with end-stage arthritis. They report survivorship of 86% at 10 years, suggesting that the Motec TWA can provide long-lasting unrestricted hand function in young active patients. Recently, Reito et al reported early catastrophic failure in two cases. In one case, the failure was secondary to metal debris (▶ Fig. 30.5) and in the other it was thought to be due to an adverse reaction to polyether ether ketone. The first patient showed elevated levels of blood cobalt and chrome levels and magnetic resonance imaging (MRI) imaging showed clear signs of a pseudotumor. The other patient had an extensive release of polyether ether ketone particles into the surrounding synovia due to adverse wear conditions in the cup, leading to the formation of a fluid-filled cystic sac with a black lining and diffuse lymphocytic dominated inflammation in the synovia. The authors recommended regular follow-up including radiographs and monitoring of cobalt and chrome ion levels and a low threshold for cross-sectional imaging in patients who underwent TWA with a Motec TWA.

30

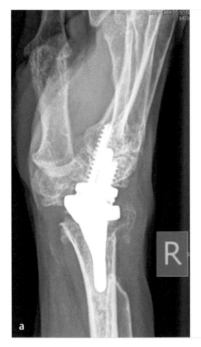

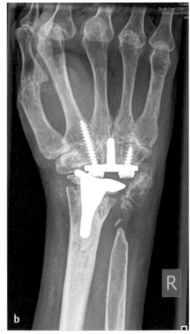

Fig. 30.3 (a, b) Periprosthetic radial component radiolucency at 2 years in an otherwise asymptomatic patient.

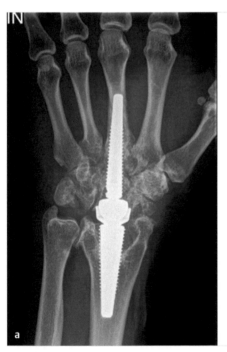

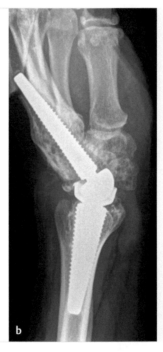

Fig. 30.4 (a, b) Aseptic loosening at 5 years. Courtesy Dr Toni Luokkala.

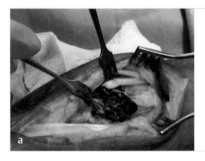

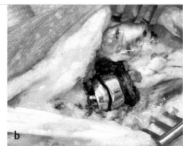

Fig. 30.5 (a, b) Metal debris on exploration of the loose prosthesis. Courtesy Dr Toni Luokkala.

30

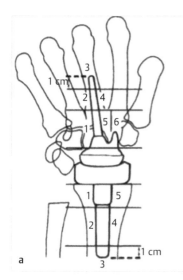
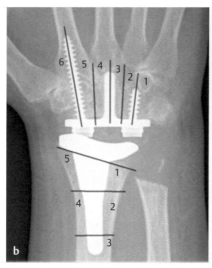

Fig. 30.6 Zones of loosening for (a) biaxial and (b) Universal II implant. Reproduced from Pinder E. M., Chee K. G., Hayton M. et al. Survivorship of Revision Wrist Replacement. Journal of Wrist Surgery 2018; 07(01): 018–023.

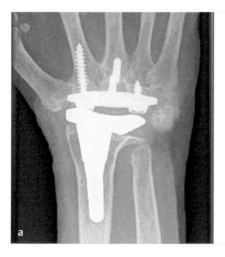
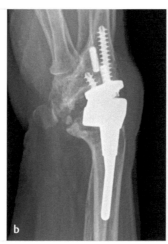

Fig. 30.7 (a, b) Broken peg (Universal II).

The biaxial and Universal II implant has five zones described in the distal radial area and six zones in the metacarpal and carpal areas (▶ Fig. 30.6).

30.2.3 Implant Fracture

This is an uncommon presentation secondary to implant loosening. In our series we had three implant fractures: two with breakage of the screws used to fix the distal component, and one component a fracture of the peg at its junction with the baseplate (▶ Fig. 30.7). All of the prostheses could be salvaged with revision TWA.[2]

30.2.4 Biomechanical Mismatch

Like all unconstrained prostheses, the success of a TWA is dependent on the remaining bone stock. Conservation of bone stock is particularly important in patients with rheumatoid arthritis and adequate soft tissue releases are

crucial to ensuring an adequate exposure and to help balance the prosthesis. In our experience, volar capsular releases and tendon transfers are typically required in the presence of a severely deformed wrist. This is based on our knowledge in dealing with severe deformities in primary wrist replacements, although our experience with revision surgery is limited in this respect. In our series of patients, one patient underwent revision at 4 months postoperatively due to inadequate distal radial resection.[12] Vogelin and Nagy reviewed a series of failed Meuli TWA. They reported the failures occurred due to a combination of mechanical failure and soft tissue problems.[11] Stringer et al in his series of 23 Swanson silicone rubber implants used in patients with rheumatoid arthritis published an implant fracture rate greater that 50% with a revision rate of 30%. Particulate tenosynovitis and instability with radiologic deterioration were reasons for revision surgery. The Swanson wrist arthroplasty is largely of historical significance.

30

30.3 Managing Bone Loss

30.3.1 Bone Grafting

At revision TWA there may be a considerable bone loss particularly around an otherwise well-fixed implant. A large bone defect makes replanting a prosthesis challenging. Gaining stability of an implant in the absence of a solid bone fixation is likely to lead to early failure. The options available for filling of the defect include autograft and allograft bone augmentation. Autograft bone stock has limited supply whilst allograft bone stock has a much larger volume available but has a low risk of infection and is biologically inert. Bone grafting of the defect can be carried out in a single- or two-stage process. Stability can be a challenge with a single-stage bone grafting in large defects. In a two-stage procedure, bone is impacted into the defect and allowed to incorporate, and then the reimplantation is performed at a later stage typically 8 to 12 weeks when the bone is thought to have incorporated. Incorporation is assessed radiologically when the graft appears to merge with the adjacent cancellous bone.

30.3.2 Wrist Arthrodesis

Wrist fusion is a recognized and recently more popular salvage procedure for failed TWA. A fused wrist provides a stable wrist joint but it can be challenging due to the difficulties in restoring wrist height, obtaining a stable fixation, and achieving bony fusion. The fusion procedure is routinely augmented with bone graft to promote healing. The remaining articular cartilage is prepared to allow bony union. During this osteointegration phase, stability is commonly maintained with a dorsal plate running between the base of a metacarpal and the distal radius. Carlson and Simmons showed that in their series of 12 failed wrist arthroplasties they were able to achieve fusion in all patients. They combined a bulk allograft from a femoral head and iliac crest autograft and were able to achieve a largely pain-free fusion.[14] Although these results are promising, the sacrifice is the loss of wrist movement (► Fig. 30.8). Interposition bone graft is a useful technique to regain wrist length to optimize the function of the flexors and extensor tendons, thereby restoring grip strength. However, in the presence of extensive bone loss overlengthening can cause issues with the median nerve and loss of tendon excursion due to a fixed length phenomenon, not dissimilar to what occurs in a chronic compartment syndrome.

30.3.3 Resection Arthroplasty

Resection arthroplasty of the wrist can result in an unstable joint with significant deformity and consequently poor hand function. We only recommend this in patients with significant comorbidities or with overwhelming evidence of active infection in whom fusion or revision surgery is contraindicated (► Fig. 30.9).

30.3.4 Summary of Options for Revision of a Wrist Arthroplasty

Surgical options following removal of a total wrist replacement are limited to revision arthroplasty, resection arthroplasty, and wrist arthrodesis. The goal is to provide a stable joint in order to restore function.

30.4 Revision Arthroplasty Technique

30.4.1 Technique

At Wrightington the (typical) original dorsal incision is used to approach the wrist through the third dorsal com-

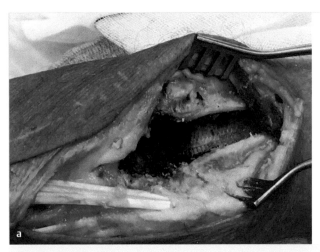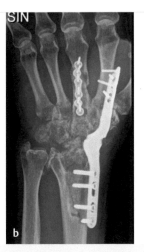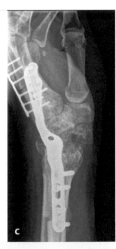

Fig. 30.8 (a–c) Extensive bone loss following removal of total wrist components and subsequent fusion. Courtesy Dr Toni Luokkala.

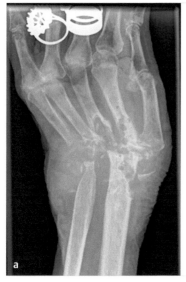
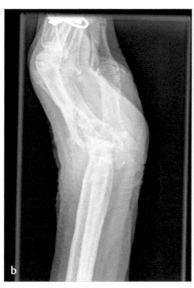

Fig. 30.9 (a, b) Extensive bone loss patient left with a resection arthroplasty.

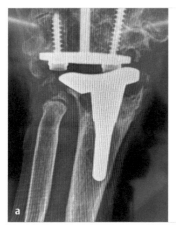
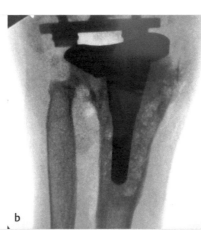

Fig. 30.10 (a, b) Loose radial component for impaction bone grafting.

partment. This allows for Z lengthening of the extensor retinaculum if required with the joint being opened with an inverted-T-shaped incision exposing the prosthesis. During removal of the prosthesis, we pay particular attention to the preservation of bone stock as noted above. We use a femoral head allograft to supplement fixation with the judicious use of bone cement to compensate for any gaps following implantation of the prosthesis. ▶ Fig. 30.10 demonstrates the use of morselized bone graft and cement used to fill the large void left behind after removal of the prosthesis.

There are several techniques described for surgical management of bone loss with cortical destruction. Methods range from long-stem custom implants to bypassing the defect, cortical structural allografts, allograft-prosthesis composites, to impaction bone grafting. The severity of bone loss proportionately increases the challenge of the revision surgery. The surgical objective should serve a dual purpose of conferring mechanical stability to the revision implant and a biological aid to

restore bone stock. In the absence of long-stemmed or custom implants, the impaction bone grafting technique has been used in our institution.

30.4.2 The Technique Steps

Step 1: Preparing the Graft

A fresh frozen unprocessed femoral head is used for the allograft. This is decorticated with cartilage removed using a rongeur. Pea-sized morsels of cancellous bone are created with bone nibblers instead of a bone mill. This is done to create a wide range of particle size for graft impaction (▶ Fig. 30.11).

Step 2: Graft Rinsing

The graft material is then rinsed several times in warm saline to wash away the marrow fat. The prepared graft then assumes a porous texture which is felt to allow for better incorporation of the graft into the host bone.

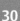

30

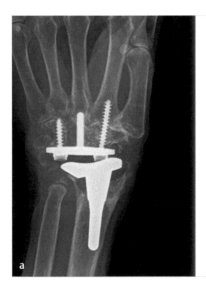
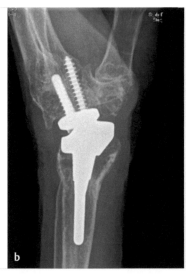

Fig. 30.11 (a, b) Loose radial component for impaction bone grafting.

Step 3: Preparation of the Medullary Cavity

All debris is removed from the joint and medullary cavity using a combination of curette and scalpel dissection.

Step 4: Graft Impaction

The medullary cavity is turned into a rigid but porous containment area by using a cement plug. The trial implants are inserted to assess the size of the defect and are left in the cavity temporarily to serve as a template. The graft material is impacted with a high-energy impaction technique and cyclical loading around the trial stem. Effective impaction leaves the graft-stem interface rigid enough to allow removal of the trial stem leaving a stable mantle of bone graft that will act as a scaffold for the prosthesis (▶ Fig. 30.12).

Step 5: Cementing the Implant

Cementing of the actual prosthesis is done in usual manner using a cement gun and pressurization. Care is taken to remove any excess cement and waiting until the cement and bone graft "mixture" is partially set to prevent the cement from being pushed down the canal. This can be quite tricky and each case is different due to varying amounts of bone loss (▶ Fig. 30.13, ▶ Fig. 30.14).

30.5 Unit Experience at Wrightington Hospital

30.5.1 Unit Experience Background

We looked at our 5-year survivorship of revision TWA in 2016. We reviewed the midterm clinical and radiological outcomes of the revision wrist arthroplasties performed between 1997 and 2010. Clinical notes were reviewed and outcome scoring was collected including quick disabilities of the arm, shoulder, and hand (QuickDASH), patient evaluation method (PEM), patient-related wrist evaluation (PRWE), the ranges of movement, and the visual analog scores (VAS). Radiographic loosening was assessed using two projections including posteroanterior and lateral radiographs of the wrist. The carpal and radial components were divided into zones with gross loosening being defined as radiolucency in all zones of the implant.[12]

30.5.2 Survivorship of the Revision TWA in Our Series

Eighteen patients underwent revision wrist arthroplasty between 1997 and 2010. All these patients had rheumatoid arthritis. The mean time from primary arthroplasty to revision was 6.7 (range: 4 months to 20.5) years. The one revision that was revised at 4 months was due to insufficient bone resection which led to stiffness and pain. The radial component was revised and further bone was resected. Ten of the 18 patients did not require bone grafting while six patients required impaction bone grafting and one had an iliac cress autograft. Three of the patients required further soft tissue procedures including soft tissue releases, flexor tenolysis, and centralization of the extensor carpi radialis longus.[12,15]

There was an 83% cumulative 5-year implant revision survival rate. All 12 of the wrist revisions that were followed up had some radiological evidence of carpal loosening. Seven of the implants demonstrated gross carpal component loosening (60%) and six had radial component (50%) loosening.

30.5.3 Comparison with Other Units

Other investigators have published similar work looking at revision TWA. A Swedish study by Fischer et al

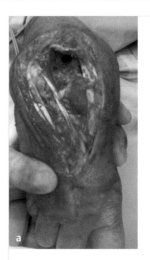
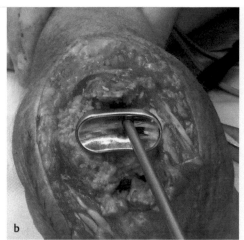

Fig. 30.12 (a–c) Impaction bone grafting using trial prosthesis as template.

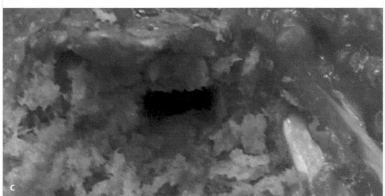

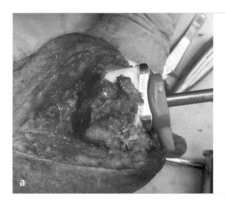
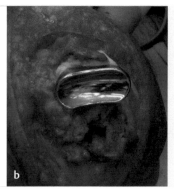

Fig. 30.13 (a, b) Cement used to augment fixation of radial component.

published their work in patients with rheumatoid arthritis with a mean follow-up of 6.6 years.[13] They looked at a retrospective cohort of 16 revision TWAs. The indication for surgery was a failed TWA. They used synthetic allograft, corticocancellous bone graft, and cement. Four of the 16 revision TWAs were re-revised; one to another TWA related to infection; and three others underwent total wrist arthrodesis due to a lack of adequate bone stock. In the 12 cases that were not re-revised the preoperative ranges of wrist motion and grip strength were preserved, i.e., there is no improvement in grip strength despite revision to a (theoretically) more stable implant.

Although the VAS pain score in activity was found to be improved this was not statistically significant. The Canadian occupational performance measure and satisfaction as well as the PRWE scores improved significantly at 1 year but not significantly at 5 year follow-up. The authors concluded that although revision TWA is a valid motion preserving strategy in the management of the failed TWA, outcomes were uncertain and as many as 25 % patients needed additional surgery.[13]

Retting and Beckenbaugh published their experience from the Mayo clinic in 1993.[9] They used the biaxial wrist replacement to salvage 13 failed TWA of various designs.

30

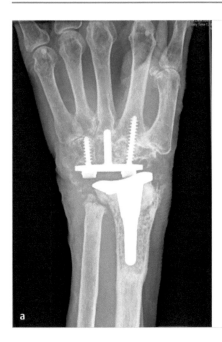
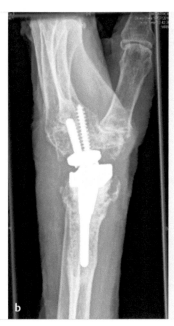

Fig. 30.14 (a, b) Postoperative radiographs at 6 months follow-up.

After a follow-up of 31 months, two wrists had undergone further revision TWA for loosening and one wrist was arthrodesed. In the remaining ten wrists, eight had no pain, one had mild pain, and one had moderate pain. Eight patients reported to be feeling much better while one patient was reported as feeling better and one patient had no difference. Follow-up radiological evaluations showed two patients had significant loosening. They felt that loosening of the revision TWA was a significant problem. It is important to note that the biaxial wrist replacement was withdrawn from the market due to a very high rate of loosening of the distal component. The article indicates that loosening of the prosthesis was related to the length of follow-up as all the failed implants were in place at least 2 years before loosening. They found that none of the implants that have been followed up for less than 2 years were loose. All five of the wrists that failed or had asymptomatic loosening were in patients with rheumatoid arthritis. They noted that none of the three revision TWAs in patients treated for post-traumatic arthritis failed or were radiologically loose.[9]

In a study from the Netherlands, Berkhout et al investigated the role of the Universal II implants as an alternative to total wrist arthrodesis for the salvage of failed biaxial TWA.[15] They assessed 40 Universal II revision TWA retrospectively. Fourteen of these wrists were converted to total wrist arthrodeses and two wrists had a third total TWA after a mean period of 5.5 years. Twenty-four of the Universal II implants that remained in situ after a mean follow-up of 9 (range 4–13) years were re-examined. Sixteen functioned satisfactorily. The PRWE and quickDASH scores were 53 and 47, respectively. In a satisfaction study, 29 patients preferred the Universal II and would also recommend it to other patients. The survival of the revision implants was 60% at a mean follow-up of 9 years.[16]

30.6 Summary

The decision about how to revise a failed primary TWA is challenging. It depends upon patient factors and the bone stock left after removal of the primary implant. Although wrist fusion allows a predictable outcome, it sacrifices the range of movement that can be achieved with the wrist replacement.[14] The long-term results of a TWA is uncertain and loosening and subsequent instability is an issue. Based on the evidence, an arthrodesis gives a more predictable outcome with lower revision rates when compared to a revision TWA.[12,14] However, if a patient "requires" movement and better function the revision TWA is an option with a survival rate between 60 and 83% at greater than 5 years.[12,13,16]

References

[1] Day JS, Lau E, Ong KL, Williams GR, Ramsey ML, Kurtz SM. Prevalence and projections of total shoulder and elbow arthroplasty in the United States to 2015. J Shoulder Elbow Surg. 2010; 19(8):1115–1120

[2] Talwalkar SC, Hayton MJ, Trail IA, Stanley JK. Management of the failed biaxial wrist replacement. J Hand Surg [Br]. 2005; 30(3):248–251

[3] Ryu JY, Cooney WP, III, Askew LJ, An KN, Chao EY. Functional ranges of motion of the wrist joint. J Hand Surg Am. 1991; 16(3):409–419

[4] Ahmadi S, Lawrence TM, Sahota S, et al. Significance of perioperative tests to diagnose the infection in revision total shoulder arthroplasty. Arch Bone Jt Surg. 2018; 6(5):359–364

[5] Lorei MP, Figgie MP, Ranawat CS, Inglis AE. Failed total wrist arthroplasty: analysis of failures and results of operative management. Clin Orthop Relat Res. 1997(342):84–93

30

[6] Patel A, Calfee RP, Plante M, Fischer SA, Green A. Propionibacterium acnes colonization of the human shoulder. J Shoulder Elbow Surg. 2009; 18(6):897–902

[7] Levy O, Iyer S, Atoun E, et al. Propionibacterium acnes: an underestimated etiology in the pathogenesis of osteoarthritis? J Shoulder Elbow Surg. 2013; 22(4):505–511

[8] Mohil R, Nwachuku I, Talwalkar S, Hearnden A, Hayton M, Trail I. The management of the failed total wrist replacement: the Wrightington experience: level 4 evidence. J Hand Surg Am. 2010; 35(10)(Suppl):47

[9] Rettig ME, Beckenbaugh RD. Revision total wrist arthroplasty. J Hand Surg Am. 1993; 18(5):798–804

[10] Boeckstyns ME, Herzberg G. Periprosthetic osteolysis after total wrist arthroplasty. J Wrist Surg. 2014; 3(2):101–106

[11] Vogelin E, Nagy L. Fate of failed Meuli total wrist arthroplasty. J Hand Surg [Br]. 2003; 28(1):61–68

[12] Pinder EM, Chee KG, Hayton M, Murali SR, Talwalkar SC, Trail IA. Survivorship of revision wrist replacements. J Wrist Surg. 2018; 7(1):18–23

[13] Fischer P, Sagerfors M, Brus O, Pettersson K. Revision arthroplasty of the wrist in patients with rheumatoid arthritis, mean follow-up 6.6 years. J Hand Surg Am. 2018; 43(5):489.e1–489.e7

[14] Takwale VJ, Nuttall D, Trail IA, Stanley JK. Biaxial total wrist replacement in patients with rheumatoid arthritis: clinical review, survivorship and radiological analysis. J Bone Joint Surg Br. 2002; 84(5):692–699

[15] Zijlker HJA, Berkhout MJ, Ritt MJPF, van Leeuwen N, IJsselstein CB. Universal 2 total wrist arthroplasty for the salvage of failed biaxial total wrist arthroplasty. J Hand Surg Eur Vol. 2019; 44(6):614–619

[16] Adams BD, Kleinhenz BP, Guan JJ. Wrist arthrodesis for failed total wrist arthroplasty. J Hand Surg Am. 2016; 41(6):673–679

30

Section 5

Arthroplasty of the DRUJ

31 Systematic Review of Distal Radioulnar Joint (DRUJ) Arthroplasty

Lawrence Stephen Moulton and Grey Giddins

Abstract

The distal radioulnar joint (DRUJ) is important for normal function and load bearing of the forearm. A number of surgical procedures have been developed to try to treat painful DRUJ disorders; however, these alter forearm biomechanics and can cause painful ulna stump impingement.

The use of DRUJ arthroplasties is increasing in the treatment of DRUJ disorders in primary, revision, and salvage settings. We have undertaken a systematic review of the literature looking at their use. This has been performed using the Preferred Reporting Items for Systematic Reviews and Meta-Analyses (PRISMA) guidelines. Papers were assessed for outcomes, implant survival, and methodological quality.

Nineteen papers assessed ulna head replacements. The implant survival rate was 92 % at a mean follow-up of 74 months. Twenty papers assessed total DRUJ replacements; all but two used the Aptis prosthesis. These implants had a survival rate of 96 % at a mean of 47 months. There were two studies that assessed partial ulna head replacements. No implant revisions were reported in these two small papers. Complications were low with all implant types.

These results are similar to those in a systematic review we previously undertook. Although these data are impressive, this systematic review demonstrates that implant arthroplasty for the DRUJ has produced acceptable results but is mostly only reported in small numbers of patients. These procedures are a good salvage option in patients with ongoing DRUJ symptoms and appear to provide good longevity. More research is still needed to further evaluate these implants in larger numbers and over the longer term.

Keywords: distal radioulnar joint, arthroplasty, outcomes, ulna head replacement, distal radioulnar joint replacement

31.1 Introduction

The distal radioulnar joint (DRUJ) is important for normal function and load bearing of the forearm.[1] The DRUJ is important for forearm pronation and supination. It also bears weight; when holding a weight in an extended arm, forces are transferred across the DRUJ, sharing the load across the forearm bones.

The DRUJ can be affected by a number of pathologies, including trauma and following osteo- or rheumatoid arthritis. A number of surgical procedures have been developed for treating painful DRUJ disorders. These include: the Sauvé-Kapandji procedure, Darrach resection, or various hemiresection interposition procedures (Bower's, Watson, etc.).[2,3,4,5]

Any procedure that excises part of the distal ulna will alter forearm biomechanics as the load transfer that normally occurs from the radius to ulna at the DRUJ when carrying a weight is no longer possible.[6] As the forearm is suspended from the ulna because this is the bone fixed at the elbow, both the ulna and radius are unstable following its resection, and painful ulna stump impingement can occur.[5] This may be a particular problem in younger, more active patients who wish to undertake heavier manual activities. Patients with these problems will develop pain in the distal forearm with activity and often with forearm rotation.

Due to the disabling nature of these symptoms, attempts have been made to replace the excised portion of bone, primarily the ulnar head, with implants to restore more forearm stability. Initial attempts with silicone implants were unsuccessful.[7,8,9] Recently, hard-bearing DRUJ implant arthroplasties have been developed. These fall into two broad groups: isolated replacements of the ulna head (complete or partial),[10] and implants that replace the entire DRUJ articulation.[11]

The use of these implants is increasing. We had previously undertaken one systematic review assessing outcomes[12]; further results have been published. We, therefore, undertook an updated systematic review to assess the outcomes of DRUJ replacement.

31.2 Methods

31.2.1 Inclusion Criteria

We performed this systematic review in line with the Preferred Reporting Items for Systematic Reviews and Meta-Analyses (PRISMA) statement, although without formally registering the review.[13] Articles were included in this review using the following criteria:
- Patients had undergone an implant arthroplasty of the DRUJ joint either to the ulna head or a complete DRUJ replacement.
- Studies had to include a minimum of four implants in four wrists.
- The ranges of movement, pain, strength, complications, or failure rates were reported as outcomes.
- A minimum follow-up of at least 1 year.

31.2.2 Exclusion Criteria

The exclusion criteria were:
- Case reports of fewer than four cases.
- Cadaver studies.
- Biomechanical studies.
- Studies of nonimplant arthroplasties.
- Reviews.
- Follow-up less than 1 year.
- Soft, i. e., silicone arthroplasties, as they are no longer used.

31.2.3 Literature Search

The literature review was performed using Medline, with the most recent literature search being performed on May 27, 2019. The PubMed database was searched using the following search criteria: ((Distal radioulnar joint) OR (DRUJ) OR (Distal radio ulnar joint) OR (Ulna head)) AND ((Arthroplasty) OR (replacement) OR (implant) OR (prosthesis) OR (ulnar head replacement)). MEDLINE and Embase were also searched using similar strategies. The Cochrane database was also searched.

The abstracts of these articles were then reviewed to select appropriate papers, and these papers were then obtained. If during the review of these papers, further papers were identified from the referenced literature then those papers were also obtained. We tabulated the results based on implant type to assist analysis.

31.2.4 Outcome Measures

We assessed the studies for the following outcome parameters: numbers of implants; mean follow-up; Patient-Rated Wrist Evaluation (PRWE) or Disability of the Arm, Shoulder, and Hand (DASH) scores; pain scores; ranges of movement; grip strength; complications; and survivorship. If individual patient data were presented within a paper then the mean values were calculated manually as part of the review.

31.2.5 Assessment of the Level of Evidence

We used a design classification of levels, developed by Jovell and Navarro-Rubio, to characterize the quality and consistency of the studies.[14] Using this taxonomy, we determined the quality of the evidence for the included studies and generated the strength of recommendation.

31.2.6 Assessment of Methodological Quality

Both reviewers independently assessed the methodological quality of the reported studies using the Coleman methodology.[15] If there were any discrepancies then a further discussion was undertaken until a consensus score was achieved for each study.

31.2.7 Assessment of Survivorship

Implant survivorship is important when comparing different types of implant. Reported survivorship or specific implant failures were recorded for the studies.

31.3 Results

31.3.1 Studies Identified

The final database search produced 902 records, of which 417 were duplicates. We also identified ten records from other sources but these were all duplicate entries. This left 485 records to be screened; 433 were excluded as they did not meet the inclusion criteria, leaving 52 full text studies to review. The studies by De Smet and Peeters[16] and Garcia-Elias[17] were excluded as they have few patients (three), and three more studies were removed as they involved the use of silicone prostheses. A further study by Cooney and Berger[18] was excluded as the results were the same as those published in another paper published by the same authors at the same time.[10] The other studies were excluded as the abstracts were not clear initially and on review of the full text they were found to be review articles. Hence, a total of 41 studies were included in the final analysis (▶ Fig. 31.1).

31.3.2 Implant Types

During the course of the literature search, three main types of implant were identified: ulnar head replacements; partial ulnar head replacements; and total DRUJ replacements. We will consider each in turn.

Ulnar Head Replacement

There were 19 studies that reported 430 uniquely implanted ulnar head replacements (▶ Table 31.1, ▶ Table 31.2, and ▶ Table 31.3). One study by van Schoonhoven et al is a long-term follow-up study of patients reported in a previously identified study.[19] The study by Willis et al[20] originates from the same unit of that of Berger et al[10]; it is not clear whether this is a new series of patients or whether this is a longer follow-up of the previously reported series. We have attempted to contact the authors to clarify this but without success. We have included this paper in our analysis and tables.

The implants used were predominantly the Herbert (KLS Martin Group) or the Avanta uHead (Small Bone Innovations) designs. Other implants (First Choice Ulnar Head replacement, Integra) were also used. In one study the implant was not stated.[30] We attempted to contact the authors directly for clarification but without success. In six of the studies, a mixture of implants was used. One

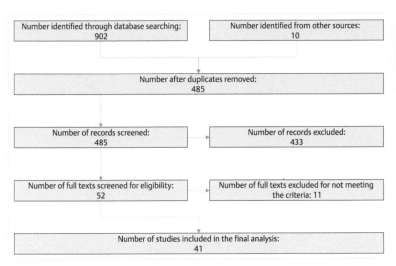

Fig. 31.1 Preferred Reporting Items for Systematic Reviews and Meta-Analyses (PRISMA) flowchart for the review.

Table 31.1 Herbert ulna head prosthesis

Author	Implant	Indications for surgery	Number of implants	Mean follow-up (mo)	Mean pain score after treatment	Mean forearm pronation (degrees)	Mean forearm supination (degrees)	Mean wrist extension (degrees)	Mean wrist flexion (degrees)	Grip strength (vs. opposite)
Van Schoonhoven et al[21]	Herbert	Failed resection arthroplasty	23	27	1.9	76	82	NR	NR	68%
Fernandez et al[22]	Herbert	Failed resection arthroplasty	10	31.2	NR	73	69	NR	NR	55%
van Groningen et al[23]	Herbert	Associated with radio-scapho-lunate fusion for post-traumatic arthritis	6	24	VAS 25	69	38	28	19	59%
Van Schoonhoven et al[19]	Herbert	Failed resection arthroplasty	16	132	1.7	83	81	NR	NR	81%
Axelsson et al[24]	Herbert	Mixture of primary and revision cases	22	90	1.7	65	70	50	35	83%
Fok et al[25]	Herbert	Failed Sauvé-Kapandji	17	72	NR	74	76	66	64	66%

Abbreviation: NR, not reported.
Note: Originator studies in **bold**.

of these studies included the results of both ulnar head replacement and partial ulnar head replacement without separating the results by partial and total implant type.[35] When assessing these papers, it was not always possible to identify separate results for each individual implant as they were reported as one dataset.[29,31,32,33,35,36]

There is considerable heterogeneity within the study populations. The study groups included patients with rheumatoid arthritis, other forms of inflammatory arthritis disease, primary osteoarthritis, posttraumatic arthritis, and patients who had had previous surgery, i.e., salvage procedures. For studies with a homogenous

patient group, the most common indication was for failed prior resection arthroplasty.

Details of the reported results are variable. While some studies present detailed results of postoperative ranges of movement, grip strength, pain and function scores, 15 of the studies did not report one or more of these parameters. A number of the papers used their own outcome parameters. All of the papers stated that the majority of patients were happy with the results and described the outcomes as good.

The reported complication rates in these series are low (▶ Table 31.4). These include residual instability of the

Table 31.2 Avanta ulna head prosthesis

Author	Implant	Indications for surgery	Number of implants	Mean follow-up (mo)	Mean pain score after treatment	Mean fore-arm pro-nation (degrees)	Mean fore-arm supi-nation (degrees)	Mean wrist extension (degrees)	Mean wrist flexion (degrees)	Grip strength (vs. opposite)
Berger et al[10]	Avanta U Head	Mixture of RA, trauma, and failed resection	22	24	Excellent results reported in 18 out of 22 cases but no discreet results reported					
Willis et al[20]	Avanta uHead	Mixture of RA, trauma, and failed resection	19	32	NR	75	60	NR	NR	83%
Kaiser et al[26]	Avanta uHead	Multiple indications	8	17.94	0.8	75	70	53	51	69%
Kakar et al[27]	Avanta uHead	Mixed indications	47	56	2	71	59	43	47	NR
Baring et al[28]	Avanta uHead	Mixed indications	10	48	2.7	86	70	51	54	NR

Abbreviation: NR, not reported.
Note: Originator studies in **bold**.

distal ulna, infection, implant loosening, bone resorption, tendon rupture, and implant failure. Only two papers reported implant survival rates; these are stated as 83% at 6 years of follow-up using the Avanta implant and 90% at 15 years of follow-up using a mixture of implant types.[27,33] Overall 34 implant failures (removal or revision) were reported, giving an implant survival rate of 92% at a mean follow-up of 74 (range 17–132) months.

Total DRUJ Replacement

We identified 20 studies with a total of 448 implants (▶ Table 31.5 and ▶ Table 31.6). All but two of these studies used the Aptis implant (Aptis Medical); the others used a prototype implant. Seven of the studies using the Aptis implant originate from the unit of the implant designer. It is stated that the senior author in one of these papers has treated more than 231 patients with this prosthesis.[11,37,38] We contacted Dr. Scheker directly to clarify how many of these papers report individual cases and how many were duplicates. He confirmed that the only paper in this series that includes previously published patients is that of Rampazzo et al.[39] Therefore, this paper has been excluded from the survival analysis. There are other papers with crossover of patients; however, these did not meet the inclusion criteria for the review as they had too few implants, etc.

There is a considerable range of indications for total DRUJ replacement in these studies. While the majority had undergone previous surgery, there were some patients who had undergone primary DRUJ replacement and two papers where the indications were not stated. In those papers where there is a single indication for surgery this was most commonly salvage surgery following previous ulnar head excision.

The reported results are again variable. Only four of the papers report ranges of movement in all planes of movement, grip strength, pain and function scores. One paper uses its own scoring system. All papers report satisfactory or good outcomes with good patient satisfaction.

The reported complication rates are low. Complications include: infection (deep and superficial); heterotopic bone formation; tendonitis; bone resorption; implant fracture; screw irritation; loosening; and stress responses in the bones (▶ Table 31.7). Twenty-five implant failures are reported in these studies; seven of these were in the series of prototype implants reported by Schuurman.[54] There were no implant failures in the paper using the Stability implant (Small Bone Innovations).[53] In the papers using the Aptis implants (381 implants), there were 16 revisions, i.e., an implant survival rate of 95.8% at a mean of 47.1 months (range 24–75 mo).

Partial Ulnar Head Replacement

We identified two studies reporting the outcomes of partial ulnar head replacement alone (▶ Table 31.8 and ▶ Table 31.9). In addition, there was one further study that included the results of partial and total ulnar head replacements in the same paper without differentiating

Table 31.3 Other or mixed ulna head prosthesis

Author	Implant	Indications for surgery	Number of implants	Mean follow-up (mo)	Mean pain score after treatment	Mean forearm pronation (degrees)	Mean forearm supination (degrees)	Mean wrist extension (degrees)	Mean wrist flexion (degrees)	Grip strength (vs. opposite)
Shipley et al[29]	14 Herbert 7 Avanta	Mixture of primary and revision cases	22	54.3	1.73	Primary procedures: 60% reported as good, 40% excellent Salvage: 25% poor, 50% good, and 23% excellent These terms not defined				NR
Herzberg[30]	Not stated	Mixture of primary and salvage cases	17	36	2	146-degree arc		NR	NR	NR
Sauerbier et al[31]	20 uHead 5 Herbert	Mixture of primary and salvage cases	25	30	2.4	124-degree arc		77-degree arc		NR
Warwick et al[32]	52 Herbert 3 uHead 1 Martin spherical	49 primary, 7 salvage	56	60	2.15	NR	NR	NR	NR	NR
Sabo et al[33]	53 Herbert 6 First choice 21 unclear	Broad range of indications, traumatic, inflammatory and others	79	Minimum 24	NR	80	53	39	44	NR
Aita et al[34]	First Choice	Posttraumatic	10	16.8	2.3	174.5-degree arc		NR		90/7%
Adams et al[35]	18 partial ulna head 10 total ulna head	Mixed indications	28	55	NR	71	55	52	55	85%
Poujade et al[36]	7 Herbert 2 uHead	Instability following Darrach's procedure	9	78.5	0	70	50	60	60	60%

Abbreviation: NR, not reported.
Note: Originator studies in **bold**.

between the different implants.[35] The results of this paper are included in the ulnar head replacement section.

In the two papers reporting solely on partial ulnar head replacements, there were nine implants. One paper used these implants in patients with rheumatoid arthritis and the other was for osteoarthritis of the DRUJ. There were good postoperative ranges of movement and pain scores. No complications were reported and no revisions performed.

31.3.3 Literature Quality and Risk of Bias

The included studies were all low level (IV and V) studies. All included studies were case series without any controls. In addition, there was considerable heterogeneity even within the studies. This is confirmed when assessing the Coleman scores for these studies (▶ Table 31.10). While there is a wide range of scores, the highest score was only 67, demonstrating the low level of these studies.

Table 31.4 Complications of ulna head replacement listed by study

Study	Number of implants	Complications	Number of revisions
Van Schoonhoven et al[21]	23	2 recurrent instability requiring further surgery Remodeling of sigmoid fossa in all cases 1 stem loosening (revised) 1 deep infection requiring removal	4
Berger et al[10]	22	2 revisions for loosening 1 revision for malpositioning 2 required further soft tissue procedures 1 residual instability	3
Fernandez et al[22]	10	4 radiographic calcifications (1 requiring removal) 2 fractures	1
Willis et al[20]	19	1 dorsal ulna instability 1 revision for persistent pain 2 loosening requiring revision 5 bone resorption 1 ulna fracture 1 painful neuroma	3
Kaiser et al[26]	8	Not reported	0
Shipley et al[29]	22	Recurrent instability (2 revisions) Implant fracture (1 revision) Continued pain	3
Herzberg[30]	17	1 removal of implant due to persistent pain 1 dorsal shortening capsuloplasty for implant instability Bone resorption at collar in 10 cases Radial erosion in 30 %	0
van Groningen et al[23]	6	1 revision of prosthesis to smaller size 1 triquetrumectomy 1 PIN division required	1
Van Schoonhoven et al[19]	16	Long-term follow-up from previous paper None further after previous report	0
Kakar et al[27]	47	8 implant failures 3 soft tissue stabilization procedures 2 screw removals 1 capsule reconstruction Implant survival 83 %	8
Sauerbier et al[31]	25	None reported	0
Warwick et al[32]	56	1 delayed tendon rupture 1 infected loosening (revised) 1 aseptic loosening 1 fracture 1 unstable	1
Sabo et al[33]	79	6 aseptic revisions 1 revision for infection 7 ECU tendon operations 4 notch plasties 5 releases 6 wrist fusions/arthroplasties 1 ulna shortening 1 distal radius osteotomy 90 % survivorship at 15 years	6

(Continued)

Table 31.4 (*Continued*) Complications of ulna head replacement listed by study

Study	Number of implants	Complications	Number of revisions
Axelsson et al[24]	22	Seroma Ulna sensory nerve deficit Little finger stiffness DRUJ instability requiring capsuloplasty	0
Aita et al[34]	10	Dorsal ulna instability and pain	0
Baring et al[28]	10	1 aseptic loosening 1 oversized implant 2 sensory deficit	0
Adams et al[35]	28	2 DRUJ pain and instability (one revised, one removed) Bone resorption Stress shielding	2
Poujade et al[36]	9	1 scar dysesthesia	0
Fok et al[25]	17	2 osteolysis (revised) 2 dorsal subluxation of prosthesis 1 fracture of SK requiring fixation	2
Total	430 unique cases	142 (33%)	34 (8%)

Abbreviations: DRUJ, distal radioulnar joint; ECU, extensor carpi ulnaris; SK.
Note: Originator studies in **bold**.

Table 31.5 Aptis total joint prosthesis

Author	Implant	Indications for surgery	Number of implants	Mean follow-up (mo)	Mean pain score after treatment	Mean forearm prona-tion (degrees)	Mean forearm supination (degrees)	Mean wrist extension (degrees)	Mean wrist flexion (degrees)	Grip strength (vs. opposite)
Laurentin-Perez et al[37]	Aptis	Mixed including salvage	31	42 (clinical) 75 (phone)	1	79	72	56	52	61%
Scheker[11]	Aptis	Mixed indications	49	24	1.3	79	72	NR	NR	63%
Zimmerman et al[40]	Aptis	Prior excision arthroplasty	6	28	NR	87	80	NR	NR	59%
Savvidou et al[38]	Aptis	92% salvage	27	60	2.71	81	75	NR	NR	90%
Scheker et al[41]	Aptis first generation	NR	31	70	1	79	72	56	52	NR
	Aptis second generation	NR	35	60	NR	83	75	NR	NR	NR
Axelsson et al[42]	Aptis	All salvage	9	45	0.3	70	80	NR	NR	NR
Bizimungu et al[43]	Aptis	Primary implantations	10	60	3.6	70	73	45	32	NR
Galvis et al[44]	Aptis	Rheumatoid arthritis	19	39	2.2	78	72	NR	NR	NR
Kakar et al[45]	Aptis	Failed previous surgery	10	48	NR	137-degree arc		81.6-degree arc		52%

(Continued)

Table 31.5 (*Continued*) Aptis total joint prosthesis

Author	Implant	Indications for surgery	Number of implants	Mean follow-up (mo)	Mean pain score after treatment	Mean forearm pronation (degrees)	Mean forearm supination (degrees)	Mean wrist extension (degrees)	Mean wrist flexion (degrees)	Grip strength (vs. opposite)
Kachooei et al[46]	Aptis	Failed previous surgery	14	60	0	64	51	62	54	47%
Martinez-Villen et al[47]	Aptis	Failed previous surgery	5	52	6.22	127-degree arc		127-degree arc		NR
Rampazzo et al[39]	Aptis	Mixed including salvage	46	61	2	77	73	56	56	NR
Reissner et al[48]	Aptis	Mixed	10	32	2.9	88	84	52	53	20.2 kg
Wimalawansa et al[49]	Aptis	Failed tendon interposition	7	25.9	2.3	86	86	46	56	24 kg
Bellevue et al[50]	Aptis	Mixed including salvage	52	19	NR	NR	NR	NR	NR	NR
Lans et al[51]	Aptis	Previous wrist arthrodesis	14	67	1.3	76.1	76.1	NA	NA	8.5 kg
DeGeorge et al[52]	Aptis	Salvage	50	35.8	1.5	73.4	69	51.6	49.9	18.3 kg

Abbreviation: NR, not reported.
Note: Originator studies in **bold**.

Table 31.6 Other total joint prosthesis

Author	Implant	Indications for surgery	Number of implants	Mean follow-up (mo)	Mean pain score after treatment	Mean forearm pronation (degrees)	Mean forearm supination (degrees)	Mean wrist extension (degrees)	Mean wrist flexion (degrees)	Grip strength (vs. opposite)
Ewald et al[53]	Stability	Posttraumatic	4	46	2.5	80	64	NR	NR	73%
Schuurman[54]	Not reported (3 different prototypes)	17 salvage 2 primary	19	49	3.5	79	70	59	46	NR

Abbreviation: NR, not reported.
Note: Originator studies in **bold**.

31.4 Discussion

This updated systematic review demonstrates that in small numbers of patients with a range of indications, implant arthroplasty of the DRUJ gives good results. In the small numbers of published series, there are good short-term implant survival rates.

The strengths of this review are that we have been able to identify and access all the relevant studies in the literature. In addition, we have been able to access new data available since our previous systematic review on this subject.[12] This has enabled us to collate and tabulate all of the published data and calculate implant survival rates for the relevant implants where possible.

The small number of published studies with relatively short-term follow-up limits this review. When we previously reviewed the literature, there were 690 reported implants. Two years later, there are 887 reported implants. It is unclear if some of these are duplicates. It is reassuring that more centers are publishing their experience with these implants; however, the overall numbers

Table 31.7 Complications of total joint arthroplasty listed by study

Study	Number of implants	Complications	Number of revisions
Laurentin-Perez et al[37]	31	1 infection requiring two-stage revision 2 implant fractures after high-energy trauma (revised) 1 heterotopic ossification	3
Scheker[11]	49	2 soft tissue infection 2 ECU tendonitis 1 ectopic bone formation 1 bone resorption	0
Zimmerman et al[40]	6	2 continued pain 1 screw irritation requiring downsizing 1 chronic pain syndrome	0
Ewald et al[53]	4	None reported	0
Savvidou et al[38]	27	2 soft tissue infections 6 ECU tendonitis 5 ectopic bone formation 1 screw/cap loosening 1 revision 2 loosening on X-ray	1
Scheker et al[41]	31	None reported	0
	35	2 soft tissue infection 6 ECU tendonitis 5 ectopic bone formation 1 screw loosening 2 stem loosening 1 revision 100% 5-year survival reported	1
Axelsson et al[42]	9	1 carpal tunnel syndrome 1 De Quervain's 2 elbow pain 1 resorption around a screw	0
Schuurman[54]	17	7 removed for loosening	7
Bizimungu et al[43]	10	None reported	0
Galvis et al[44]	19	1 loosening (revised) ECU tendon irritation requiring surgery	1
Kakar et al[45]	10	1 revision for aseptic loosening Extensor tendon irritation Screw exchange Median neuropathy	1
Kachooei et al[46]	14	2 debridement of screw tip No revisions	0
Martinez-Villen et al[47]	5	1 heterotopic ossification 1 stress response in distal ulna	0
Rampazzo et al[39]	46	9 ECU tendonitis 2 revisions 3 Ectopic bone formation Implant clinking Implant malposition Implant failure Lunate implant impingement	2 NB duplicate from previous papers
Reissner et al[48]	10	1 radiological loosening (revised) 2 ectopic bone growth 2 superficial radial nerve irritation	1

(Continued)

Table 31.7 (*Continued*) Complications of total joint arthroplasty listed by study

Study	Number of implants	Complications	Number of revisions
Wimalawansa et al[49]	7	2 ECU synovitis (requiring further surgery)	0
Bellevue et al[50]	52	4 periprosthetic fracture 3 infection 2 aseptic loosening 2 implant failures Screw loosening 3 neuromas 2 finger stiffness needing tenolysis 2 heterotopic ossification 5 revisions/explants 1 conversion to one-bone forearm NB only reported complications requiring surgical intervention	5
Lans et al[51]	14	1 deep infection (revision) 1 heterotopic ossification 5 ulna-sided wrist pain 3 pisiform excision 1 triquetrum excision 2 superficial infections	1
DeGeorge et al[52]	50	11 wound complications 9 paresthesia 5 tendonopathy 1 symptomatic scar 5 symptomatic hardwear 3 periprosthetic fracture (2 x ORIF) 2 periprosthetic infections (both removed)	2
Total	448	169 (38%)	25 (6%)
Total-Aptis only:	381	144 (38%)	16 (4%)

Abbreviations: ECU, extensor carpi ulnaris; NB,; ORIF, open reduction internal fixation.
Note: Originator studies in **bold**.

Table 31.8 Partial ulna head replacements

Author	Implant	Indications for surgery	Number of implants	Mean follow-up (mo)	Mean pain score after treatment	Mean forearm pronation (degrees)	Mean forearm supination (degrees)	Mean wrist extension (degrees)	Mean wrist flexion (degrees)	Grip strength (vs. opposite)
Bigorre et al[55]	Eclypse	RA	5	64	1.5	70	80	NR	NR	148%
Kakar et al[56]	Integra with meniscal allograft	DRUJ OA	4	NR	NR	156-degree arc		125-degree arc		92%

Abbreviations: DRUJ, distal radioulnar joint; NR, not reported; OA, osteoarthritis; RA, rheumatoid arthritis.
Note: Originator studies in **bold**.

are still very low, limiting our ability to give robust recommendations on their use.

We have to be cautious that the implant survival rates used in this paper may not be a true representation of the actual implant survival rates. The majority of the papers report short-term results only without longer term results. If this were a major lower limb implant, we would expect much longer follow-up to make definitive statements on survival. Even in those centers that perform large numbers of these implants, there are not very large numbers of implants compared to lower limb arthroplasty. Dr. Scheker has reported to us that between 2005 and 2015 he performed 357 Aptis (personal communication).

Table 31.9 Complications of partial ulna head replacement listed by study

Study	Number of implants	Complications	Number of revisions
Bigorre et al[55]	5	None reported	0
Kakar et al[56]	4	None reported	0
Total	9	0	0

Note: Originator studies in **bold**.

Table 31.10 Coleman scores listed by study

Study	Coleman score
Ulna head replacement	
Van Schoonhoven et al[21]	67
Berger et al[10]	36
Fernandez et al[22]	34
Willis et al[20]	35
Kaiser et al[26]	36
Shipley et al[29]	33
Herzberg[30]	19
van Groningen et al[23]	28
Van Schoonhoven et al[19]	63
Kakar et al[27]	35
Sauerbier et al[31]	42
Warwick et al[32]	49
Sabo et al[33]	40
Axelsson et al[24]	54
Aita et al[34]	48
Baring et al[28]	43
Adams et al[35]	45
Poujade et al[36]	34
Fok et al[25]	51
Total joint replacement	
Laurentin-Perez et al[37]	44

Table 31.10 (*Continued*) Coleman scores listed by study

Study	Coleman score
Scheker[11]	31
Zimmerman et al[40]	41
Savvidou et al[38]	52
Scheker et al[41]	45
Axelsson et al[42]	43
Bizimungu et al[43]	41
Galvis et al[44]	41
Kakar et al[45]	39
Kachooei et al[46]	40
Rampazzo et al[39]	62
Martinez-Villen et al[47]	33
Reissner et al[48]	33
Wimalawansa et al[49]	39
Bellevue et al[50]	34
Lans et al[51]	41
DeGeorge et al[52]	52
Ewald et al[53]	46
Schuurman[54]	31
Partial ulna head replacement	
Bigorre et al[55]	45
Kakar et al[56]	35

Note: Originator studies in bold.

As with all newly emerging technologies and implants, identification of problems and failures is important. While the number of papers reporting outcomes following these surgeries is increasing, it is important that any units performing these implants report their short- and long-term results. This is particularly important for surgeons not involved in the design of these implants. These reports need to contain as many outcomes as possible to allow independent assessment. We have seen that in many of the studies identified, there are a number of important outcome measures that are not reported.

Finally, with the increasing success of joint registries around the world identifying well and poorly performing implants, it may be beneficial to include these types of implant either in the existing registries or alternately in a specific multinational registry for these implants. This will help to provide better outcome data.

31.5 Conclusions

DRUJ implant arthroplasty provides good outcomes for function and survival in the small numbers of reported cases in the literature. The indications for their use are variable and often they are used in the salvage situation. There is still a need for further studies to assess these implants further. Nonetheless, DRUJ arthroplasty seems to be a successful intervention for a range of conditions affecting the DRUJ.

Overall for the typical patient with pain and stiffness centered on the DRUJ suitable for an arthroplasty, we would recommend using a hemiarthroplasty, i. e., an ulna head replacement, rather than a total DRUJ replacement. A partial or full ulnar head replacement is an appreciably smaller operation than a total DRUJ arthroplasty which is relatively straightforward to revise. Total DRUJ replacements seem more suitable for salvage procedures particularly with damage to the sigmoid notch of the distal radius or marked instability as well as pain.

References

[1] Shaaban H, Giakas G, Bolton M, Williams R, Scheker LR, Lees VC. The distal radioulnar joint as a load-bearing mechanism: a biomechanical study. J Hand Surg Am. 2004; 29(1):85–95

[2] Bowers WH. Distal radioulnar joint arthroplasty: the hemiresection-interposition technique. J Hand Surg Am. 1985; 10(2):169–178

[3] Darrach W. Partial excision of the lower shaft of the ulna for deformity following Colles' fracture. Ann Surg. 1913; 57(5):764–765

[4] Sauvé L, Kapandji M. Nouvelle technique de traitement chirurgical des luxations récidivantes isolées de l'extrémité inférieure du cubitus. J Chir (Paris). 1936; 47:589–594

[5] Zimmerman RM, Jupiter JB. Instability of the distal radioulnar joint. J Hand Surg Eur Vol. 2014; 39(7):727–738

[6] Douglas KC, Parks BG, Tsai MA, Meals CG, Means KR, Jr. The biomechanical stability of salvage procedures for distal radioulnar joint arthritis. J Hand Surg Am. 2014; 39(7):1274–1279

[7] Sagerman SD, Seiler JG, Fleming LL, Lockerman E. Silicone rubber distal ulnar replacement arthroplasty. J Hand Surg [Br]. 1992; 17 (6):689–693

[8] Stanley D, Herbert TJ. The Swanson ulnar head prosthesis for post-traumatic disorders of the distal radio-ulnar joint. J Hand Surg [Br]. 1992; 17(6):682–688

[9] Swanson AB. Implant arthroplasty for disabilities of the distal radio-ulnar joint. Use of a silicone rubber capping implant following resection of the ulnar head. Orthop Clin North Am. 1973; 4(2):373–382

[10] Berger RA, Cooney WP, III. Use of an ulnar head endoprosthesis for treatment of an unstable distal ulnar resection: review of mechanics, indications, and surgical technique. Hand Clin. 2005; 21(4):603–620, vii

[11] Scheker LR. Implant arthroplasty for the distal radioulnar joint. J Hand Surg Am. 2008; 33(9):1639–1644

[12] Moulton LS, Giddins GEB. Distal radio-ulnar implant arthroplasty: a systematic review. J Hand Surg Eur Vol. 2017; 42(8):827–838

[13] Liberati A, Altman DG, Tetzlaff J, et al. The PRISMA statement for reporting systematic reviews and meta-analyses of studies that evaluate healthcare interventions: explanation and elaboration. BMJ (Clinical research ed). 2009;339(jul21 1):b2700–b2700

[14] Jovell AJ, Navarro-Rubio MD. Evaluation of scientific evidence. Med Clin (Barc). 1995; 105(19):740–743

[15] Coleman BD, Khan KM, Maffulli N, Cook JL, Wark JD, Victorian Institute of Sport Tendon Study Group. Studies of surgical outcome after patellar tendinopathy: clinical significance of methodological deficiencies and guidelines for future studies. Scand J Med Sci Sports. 2000; 10(1):2–11

[16] De Smet L, Peeters T. Salvage of failed Sauvé-Kapandji procedure with an ulnar head prosthesis: report of three cases. J Hand Surg [Br]. 2003; 28(3):271–273

[17] Garcia-Elias M. Eclypse: partial ulnar head replacement for the isolated distal radio-ulnar joint arthrosis. Tech Hand Up Extrem Surg. 2007; 11(1):121–128

[18] Cooney WP, III, Berger RA. Distal radioulnar joint implant arthroplasty. J Am Soc Surg Hand. 2005; 5(4):217–231

[19] van Schoonhoven J, Mühldorfer-Fodor M, Fernandez DL, Herbert TJ. Salvage of failed resection arthroplasties of the distal radioulnar joint using an ulnar head prosthesis: long-term results. J Hand Surg Am. 2012; 37(7):1372–1380

[20] Willis AA, Berger RA, Cooney WP, III, Cooney WP. Arthroplasty of the distal radioulnar joint using a new ulnar head endoprosthesis: preliminary report. J Hand Surg Am. 2007; 32(2):177–189

[21] van Schoonhoven J, Fernandez DL, Bowers WH, Herbert TJ. Salvage of failed resection arthroplasties of the distal radioulnar joint using a new ulnar head prosthesis. J Hand Surg Am. 2000; 25(3):438–446

[22] Fernandez DL, Joneschild ES, Abella DM. Treatment of failed Sauvé-Kapandji procedures with a spherical ulnar head prosthesis. Clin Orthop Relat Res. 2006; 445(445):100–107

[23] van Groningen JM, Schuurman AH. Treatment of post-traumatic degenerative changes of the radio-carpal and distal radio-ulnar joints by combining radius, scaphoid, and lunate (RSL) fusion with ulnar head replacement. Eur J Plast Surg. 2011; 34(6):465–469

[24] Axelsson P, Sollerman C, Kärrholm J. Ulnar head replacement: 21 cases; mean follow-up, 7.5 years. J Hand Surg Am. 2015; 40(9):1731–1738

[25] Fok MWM, Fernandez DL, van Schoonhoven J. Midterm outcomes of the use of a spherical ulnar head prosthesis for failed Sauvé-Kapandji procedures. J Hand Surg Am. 2019; 44(1):66.e1–66.e9

[26] Kaiser GL, Bodell LS, Berger RA. Functional outcomes after arthroplasty of the distal radioulnar joint and hand therapy: a case series. J Hand Ther. 2008; 21(4):398–409

[27] Kakar S, Swann RP, Perry KI, Wood-Wentz CM, Shin AY, Moran SL. Functional and radiographic outcomes following distal ulna implant arthroplasty. J Hand Surg Am. 2012; 37(7):1364–1371

[28] Baring TKA, Popat R, Abdelwahab A, Ferris B. Short- to mid-term results of ulna head replacement as both a primary and revision implant. J Clin Orthop Trauma. 2016; 7(4):292–295

[29] Yen Shipley N, Dion GR, Bowers WH. Ulnar head implant arthroplasty: an intermediate term review of 1 surgeon's experience. Tech Hand Up Extrem Surg. 2009; 13(3):160–164

[30] Herzberg G. Periprosthetic bone resorption and sigmoid notch erosion around ulnar head implants: a concern? Hand Clin. 2010; 26 (4):573–577

[31] Sauerbier M, Arsalan-Werner A, Enderle E, Vetter M, Vonier D. Ulnar head replacement and related biomechanics. J Wrist Surg. 2013; 2 (1):27–32

[32] Warwick D, Shyamalan G, Balabanidou E. Indications and early to mid-term results of ulnar head replacement. Ann R Coll Surg Engl. 2013; 95(6):427–432

[33] Sabo MT, Talwalkar S, Hayton M, Watts A, Trail IA, Stanley JK. Intermediate outcomes of ulnar head arthroplasty. J Hand Surg Am. 2014; 39(12):2405–11.e1

[34] Aita MA, Ibanez DS, Saheb GCB, Alves RS. Arthroplasty of the distal ulna distal in managing patients with post-traumatic disorders of the distal radioulnar joint: measurement of quality of life. Rev Bras Ortop. 2015; 50(6):666–672

[35] Adams BD, Gaffey JL. Non-constrained implant arthroplasty for the distal radioulnar joint. J Hand Surg Eur Vol. 2017; 42(4):415–421

[36] Poujade T, Balagué N, Beaulieu J-Y. Unipolar ulnar head replacement for treatment of post-Darrach procedure instability. Hand Surg Rehabil. 2018; 37(4):225–230

[37] Laurentin-Pérez LA, Goodwin AN, Babb BA, Scheker LR. A study of functional outcomes following implantation of a total distal radioulnar joint prosthesis. J Hand Surg Eur Vol. 2008; 33(1):18–28

[38] Savvidou C, Murphy E, Mailhot E, Jacob S, Scheker LR. Semiconstrained distal radioulnar joint prosthesis. J Wrist Surg. 2013; 2 (1):41–48

[39] Rampazzo A, Gharb BB, Brock G, Scheker LR. Functional outcomes of the Aptis-Scheker distal radioulnar joint replacement in patients under 40 years old. J Hand Surg Am. 2015; 40(7):1397–1403.e3

[40] Zimmerman RM, Jupiter JB. Outcomes of a self-constrained distal radioulnar joint arthroplasty: a case series of six patients. Hand (N Y). 2011; 6(4):460–465

[41] Scheker LR, Martineau DW. Distal radioulnar joint constrained arthroplasty. Hand Clin. 2013; 29(1):113–121

[42] Axelsson P, Sollerman C. Constrained implant arthroplasty as a secondary procedure at the distal radioulnar joint: early outcomes. J Hand Surg Am. 2013; 38(6):1111–1118

[43] Bizimungu RS, Dodds SD. Objective outcomes following semi-constrained total distal radioulnar joint arthroplasty. J Wrist Surg. 2013; 2(4):319–323

[44] Galvis EJ, Pessa J, Scheker LR. Total joint arthroplasty of the distal radioulnar joint for rheumatoid arthritis. J Hand Surg Am. 2014; 39 (9):1699–1704

[45] Kakar S, Fox T, Wagner E, Berger R. Linked distal radioulnar joint arthroplasty: an analysis of the APTIS prosthesis. J Hand Surg Eur Vol. 2014; 39(7):739–744

[46] Kachooei AR, Chase SM, Jupiter JB. Outcome assessment after Aptis distal radioulnar joint (DRUJ) implant arthroplasty. Arch Bone Jt Surg. 2014; 2(3):180–184

[47] Martínez Villén G, García Martínez B, Aso Vizán A. Total distal radioulnar joint prosthesis as salvage surgery in multioperated patients. Chir Main. 2014; 33(6):390–395

[48] Reissner L, Böttger K, Klein HJ, Calcagni M, Giesen T. Midterm results of semiconstrained distal radioulnar joint arthroplasty and analysis of complications. J Wrist Surg. 2016; 5(4):290–296

[49] Wimalawansa SM, Lopez RR, de Lucas FG, et al. Salvage of failed Achilles tendon interposition arthroplasty for DRUJ instability after ulnar head resection with Aptis prosthesis. Hand (N Y). 2017; 12 (5):476–483

[50] Bellevue KD, Thayer MK, Pouliot M, Huang JI, Hanel DP. Complications of semiconstrained distal radioulnar joint arthroplasty. J Hand Surg Am. 2018; 43(6):566.e1–566.e9

[51] Lans J, Chen S-H, Jupiter JB, Scheker LR. Distal radioulnar joint replacement in the scarred wrist. J Wrist Surg. 2019; 8(1):55–60

[52] DeGeorge BR, Jr, Berger RA, Shin AY. Constrained implant arthroplasty for distal radioulnar joint arthrosis: evaluation and management of soft tissue complications. J Hand Surg Am. 2019; 44(7):614. e1–614.e9

[53] Ewald TJ, Skeete K, Moran SL. Preliminary experience with a new total distal radioulnar joint replacement. J Wrist Surg. 2012; 1(1):23–30

[54] Schuurman AH. A new distal radioulnar joint prosthesis. J Wrist Surg. 2013; 2(4):359–362

[55] Bigorre N, Saint Cast Y, Cesari B, Rabarin F, Raimbeau G. Intermediate term evaluation of the Eclypse distal radio-ulnar prosthesis for rheumatoid arthritis: a report of five cases. Orthop Traumatol Surg Res. 2016; 102(3):345–349

[56] Kakar S, Noureldin M, Elhassan B. Ulnar head replacement and sigmoid notch resurfacing arthroplasty with a lateral meniscal allograft: "calamari procedure". J Hand Surg Eur Vol. 2017; 42(6):567–572

32 First Choice Distal Radioulnar Joint Arthroplasty

Ladislav Nagy

Abstract

The "first choice" partial ulnar head prosthesis has been designed to match as best as possible to the shape and the biomechanical properties of the native ulnar head. In contrast to the total ulnar head implants, it requires only minimal bone resection and hereby preserves the soft tissue stabilizers of the distal radioulnar joint (DRUJ). On the other hand, the indication is limited to primary salvage procedures of the DRUJ. The surgical technique for the insertion of this one-piece implant is less forgiving than that for the total head prostheses as it requires an oblique and curved osteotomy at a predetermined level and, more importantly, at the anatomically correct rotatory orientation. This defines the position of the prosthesis and its biomechanical behavior. The results of this procedure compare favorably with total ulnar head replacements. Our experience in 21 cases has been free of complications and shows better pain relief and strength than that with ulnar head replacements, probably due to the improved stability of the DRUJ, however, at the expense of some of the range of motion, namely supination. This needs further attention in future, but we consider the benefits of this prosthesis outweigh the disadvantages.

Keywords: distal radioulnar joint, arthroplasty, prosthesis, resurfacing

32.1 Introduction

Most salvage procedures of the distal radioulnar joint (DRUJ) include the ablation of the ulnar head, e.g., the Darrach's procedure, hemiresection arthroplasty, or Sauvé-Kapandji. With the absence of the ulnar head or part of it, and due to the complete absence of separating forces, the residual distal end of the ulna will press upon the radius—this convergence may be markedly symptomatic, but in most patients it is not. Moreover, this convergence will lead to laxity of the radioulnar ligaments causing sagittal as well as coronal instability.

Replacement of the ulnar head was designed to address this and provide a more anatomical reconstruction of the DRUJ. Following failure of silicone ulnar head replacements,[1] metallic or ceramic replacements were introduced.[2] Biomechanical testing confirmed the prevention of convergence of the distal radius and ulna[3] and clinical testing showed reliable outcomes.[2] Nonetheless ulnar head replacements are not designed anatomically: prosthetic ulna heads are effectively spheres with the ends removed, designed to lie along the axis of the ulna. Ulna head prostheses are not stabilized by ligaments attaching to them, but by encapsulation creating a soft tissue envelope around the implant. If the soft tissue envelope is inadequate there may be symptomatic DRUJ instability. In contrast, in normal anatomy the sphere of the ulnar head lies eccentric to the long axis of the ulna.[4,5] This is necessary to correctly tension the radioulnar ligaments and the interosseous membrane in order to maintain the stability of the DRUJ and the forearm unit. The First Choice replacement is an "anatomic" ulnar head designed to lie eccentric to the axis of the ulna and preserve the insertion of the radioulnar ligaments in order to ensure greater DRUJ stability[6,7] although in my experience the "critical" foveal attachment of the triangular fibrocartilage complex (TFCC) cannot be preserved during the operative procedure.

32.2 Implant Characteristics

The "First Choice" partial ulnar head prosthesis is a one-piece implant constructed of Cobalt-Chromium alloy. The distal articulating surface is highly polished while the proximal stem surface is roughened with an aluminum oxide grit blast to optimize the chance of bone ingrowth following press-fit fixation (▶ Fig. 32.1). There are four different head sizes (145, 160, 175, 190 mm diameter) and three different stem diameters (45, 55, 65 mm), giving 12 different implants. The head corresponds to 220° (of 360°) of the head circumference with an oblique collar orientation. This sits on an eccentrically placed 5.5 cm long slightly conical stem. The aim of the design is to replace the articulating surface only, sparing the ulnar styloid and its ligament attachment and the sulcus for the extensor carpi ulnaris tendon.

For salvage procedures, there is also a modular standard total head implant with the same stem-design and

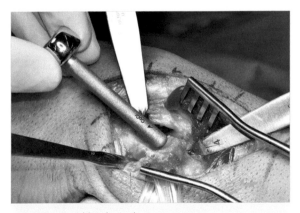

Fig. 32.1 Partial head prosthesis.

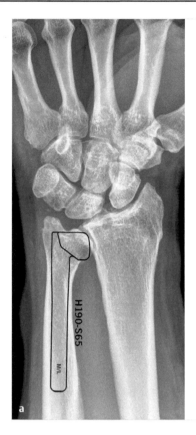
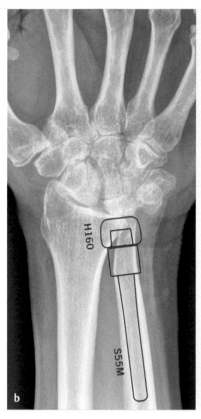

Fig. 32.2 (a, b) Use of template for the partial head and the total modular head prostheses.

sizes meaning the same reamers can be used. There are three different collar heights (3, 11, 20 mm), and three differently sized heads (160, 175, 190 mm) with a conical Morse taper coupling. The heads, as in the uHead ulnar head system introduced by Small Bone Innovations (now Stryker), feature holes for the attachment of local soft tissues.

32.3 Surgical Technique

Preoperatively transparent templates are used to assess the appropriate size of the stem and the head (▶ Fig. 32.2). For the latter, if available, axial CT-scan sections can be used for potentially more precise measurement. It is particularly important to measure ulnar variance as this will determine the amount of resection. The surgical aim is for a slightly more negative ulnar variance than normal for the patient.

We prefer to expose the DRUJ capsule through the fifth extensor tendon compartment. A dorsal rectangular capsulotomy is performed proximal to the dorsal radioulnar ligament preserving the TFC insertion to the ulnar styloid and leaving a capsular rim on the dorsum of the sigmoid notch of the radius for later closure. We have found that sparing the foveal attachment of the TFC is not possible: with this structure intact, adequate dislocation of the ulnar head is mostly impossible, and in any case the reamer would damage/destroy this attachment. The ulnar

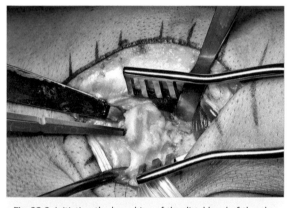

Fig. 32.3 Initiating the broaching of the distal head of the ulna with the awl almost at the fovea.

head is dislocated dorsally with the forearm pronated and the wrist flexed. The ulnar head is held displaced with one or two Hohman retractors. When starting to prepare the medullary canal it is important to remember the eccentricity of the ulnar head relative to the medullary canal. In particular, the entrance of the awl should not be in the center of the ulnar head, but more ulnar, almost at the fovea (▶ Fig. 32.3). Care must be given not to advance the correctly sized reamer deeper than based upon the measurements of the preoperative ulnar variance (▶ Fig. 32.4). Next, and in my opinion the most

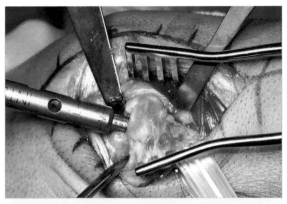

Fig. 32.4 Position of the reamer for placement of the prosthesis at 0 mm.

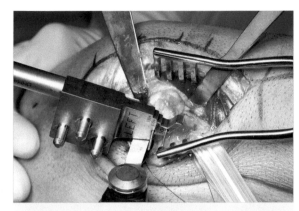

Fig. 32.5 Cutting off of the articular part of the ulnar head along the resection guide.

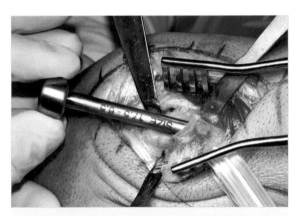

Fig. 32.6 Insertion of the trial implant.

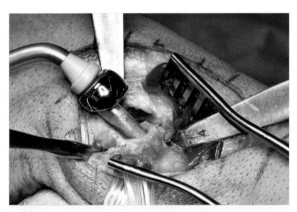

Fig. 32.7 Replacing trial implant with the definitive prosthesis.

important step is to make a correctly oriented, oblique, incomplete bone cut relative to the long axis of the ulna in contrast to the complete, perpendicular bone cut made for total ulnar head replacements. The resection guide clips onto the reamer in one single position, so the reamer handle needs to be aligned precisely with the long axis of the ulna, which is not that easy to determine; the location of the ulnar styloid to guide the bone cut is critical. The resection guide is secured into the native ulnar head with K-wires and the angled osteotomy is performed paying attention not to overcut the corners, as this risks a distal ulna fracture (▶ Fig. 32.5). After completion of the osteotomy with a longitudinal bone cut preserving the ulnar styloid, the hemiresected section of the ulnar head is removed and used to determine the optimal prosthetic head size. Next, the trial stem and ulnar head are inserted (▶ Fig. 32.6). Following reduction of the joint, check the congruity of the head in the sigmoid fossa of the distal radius and the stability of the DRUJ. Sometimes, especially with preoperative positive ulnar variance, the sigmoid fossa needs to be leveled with a large spherical burr. Then the correct position and fit of the trial implant is verified. Once the trial is deemed correct, the trial

implant is replaced by the definitive prosthesis (▶ Fig. 32.7, ▶ Fig. 32.8); this needs careful positioning and rotational control while hammering it in until there is a good tight fit between the prosthetic head and the ulna. The capsule and the fifth extensor tendon compartment are closed separately with interrupted 3–0 resorbable sutures. Postoperatively, the forearm rotation is held in an above elbow plaster cast in neutral/slight supination for 3 weeks. After this, the plaster cast is removed and the forearm and wrist are mobilized nonweight bearing for another 3 weeks. At 6 weeks if the implant appears stable clinically and radiologically, strengthening and progressive weight bearing are initiated with hand therapy support. Further clinical and radiological follow-up is undertaken at 6 months and 1 year, then 2, 5, and 10 years postoperatively.

32.4 Indications

The prime indication is symptomatic DRUJ arthritis unresponsive to nonoperative treatment. Major deformities of the distal radius, especially after fractures, must be corrected beforehand or simultaneously. The particular

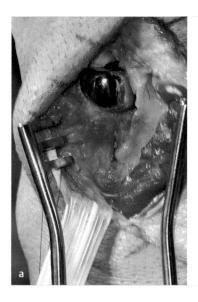 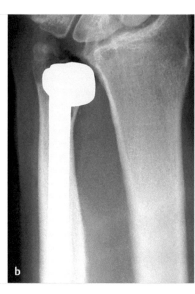

Fig. 32.8 (a, b) Final presentation intraoperatively.

contraindication of the partial head implant is ulnar variance of ≥ 4 mm as there is limited potential for correcting length with the First Choice implant.

32.5 Results in the Literature

There are only three published reports on the first choice partial ulnar head prosthesis. Unfortunately, in these published series several different ulnar head replacements were used but the results of each implant were not reported separately.

Santos et al[8] reported on three patients, two of them treated with a partial head implant and the third with a modular total head prosthesis. At 1 year, all three were reported to have good pain relief and increased motion and strength.

Sabo et al[9] reviewed 74 patients with 79 ulna head implants at a mean of 7±4 (minimum 2) years. Among these, there were six First Choice implants (whether they were hemi or total arthroplasties was not stated). Overall there were six revisions; none was a First Choice implant.

Adams and Gaffey[10] treated 18 patients with a partial and 10 with a total ulnar head prosthesis. Twenty-one (of 28) were followed-up for a mean of 4.6 (range 1–10) years; they were reported to have similar results. The mean ranges of motion were pronation 71 degrees, supination 55 degrees, and grip strength of 35 kgf (85% of contralateral hand). Two patients reported no change or worse pain than preoperatively, 17 improved reporting no or minimal pain with regular activities, but pain with strenuous activities, which was tolerable and resolved within hours, and 2 patients were pain-free. Radiographs showed bone resorption under the partial ulnar head implant of a mean of 1.7 (range 0–9) mm and mean sigmoid notch erosion of 2 (range 0–7) mm. One prosthesis had to be removed due to pain and another one was unstable; the latter was successfully changed to an implant with a smaller head size.

32.6 Author's Own Experience

Between 2007 and 2018 we have treated 24 patients with a First Choice ulnar head prosthesis. In 21 wrists, a partial head implant was used and in 3 cases a total modular head.

One partial head implant had to be removed 1.3 years after implantation due to persistent dorsal subluxation blocking supination; it was replaced by an Aptis total implant with an excellent result. There were no infections and no implant loosening at a mean follow-up of 3.4 (range 0.3–10, SD 2.7) years but three fractures occurred at the proximal end of the prosthetic stem after direct trauma. All these were treated with open reduction and plate fixation leading to bone union without reported functional loss.

The remaining 20 patients treated with a partial head implant had a mean age of 56 (range 30–77, SD 12.9) years. The follow-up was a mean of 3.4 (range 0.3–10, SD 2.7) years. Pronation was unchanged at a mean of 66 degrees (range 40–90 degrees, SD 16 degrees), while supination reduced from a mean of 67 degrees (range 10–95 degrees, SD 19 degrees) to 49 degrees (range 0–85 degrees, SD 22 degrees). Grip strength increased from a mean of 19 (range 7–31, SD 7) kgf to 25 (range 8–45, SD 11) kgf, respectively, 60 to 87% of the opposite side. The mean pain score (on a scale 0–4) reduced from 3.0 (range 1–4, SD 0.9) to 1.2 (range 0–4, SD 1.3); nine patients were completely pain-free, seven reported improved pain levels, and four reported no change; none reported worse pain. Apart from pronation the other objective changes were statistically significant ($p < 0.05$). Radiographic analysis at 1 year showed bone resorption under the partial ulnar head implant of 1.3 (range 0–2.5) mm and sigmoid notch erosion of 0.5 (range 0–2) mm without subsequent progression.

The three patients with a total modular head prosthesis had a mean age of 50 (range 45–55, SD 4.7) years and

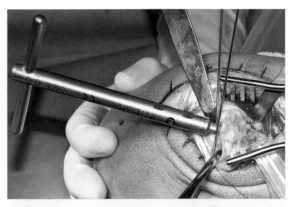

Fig. 32.9 Locate ulnar styloid with needles or pins to align the reamer handle for proper rotational orientation.

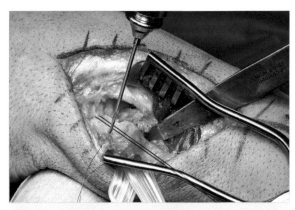

Fig. 32.10 Prepare drill holes in the outer cortex of the ulna for the triangular fibrocartilaginous complex (TFCC) attachment.

were reviewed at a mean of 2 (range 1–2.6, SD 0.9) years postoperatively. Pronation increased from a mean of 62 to 77 degrees and supination from a mean of 45 to 78 degrees. Grip strength increased from a mean of 11 to 14 kgf. The mean pain (on a scale 0–4) reduced from 3.3 point to 1.7; one patient was completely pain-free, another one improved, and one was unchanged.

In our experience the partial ulnar head prosthesis offers better DRUJ stability based upon clinical assessment and a greater increase in strength; it is therefore our preferred implant. The loss of supination is a concern but we consider it is an acceptable limitation. If this is symptomatically important we would recommend a palmar capsulectomy of the DRUJ[11]; we have performed it in three cases, improving forearm supination from a mean of 18 (range 5–30 degrees) to a mean of 35 degrees (range 20–50 degrees).

The loss of supination may increase stability due to increased soft tissue tension. The loss of supination may also be due to incorrect positioning of the implant; it can be difficult to assess the correct orientation of the original ulnar head. We recommend determining the position of the ulnar styloid with respect to the ulnar head intraoperatively with needles and aligning the handle of the reamer accordingly (▶ Fig. 32.9). In addition, when inserting the definitive prosthesis, attention must be paid to the rotation of the implant and inserting it in the same orientation as the resection. This can be particularly difficult, because the definitive prosthesis does not have any holding device unlike the trial implant. A theoretical advantage of the partial ulnar head implant is

preservation of the ulnar styloid which permits reinsertion of the TFCC to live bone (▶ Fig. 32.10).

References

[1] Sagerman SD, Seiler JG, Fleming LL, Lockerman E. Silicone rubber distal ulnar replacement arthroplasty. J Hand Surg [Br]. 1992; 17(6): 689–693

[2] van Schoonhoven J, Fernandez DL, Bowers WH, Herbert TJ. Salvage of failed resection arthroplasties of the distal radioulnar joint using a new ulnar head prosthesis. J Hand Surg Am. 2000; 25(3):438–446

[3] Sauerbier M, Hahn ME, Fujita M, Neale PG, Berglund LJ, Berger RA. Analysis of dynamic distal radioulnar convergence after ulnar head resection and endoprosthesis implantation. J Hand Surg Am. 2002; 27(3):425–434

[4] Conaway DA, Kuhl TL, Adams BD. Comparison of the native ulnar head and a partial ulnar head resurfacing implant. J Hand Surg Am. 2009; 34(6):1056–1062

[5] Gordon KD, Dunning CE, Johnson JA, King GJW. Kinematics of ulnar head arthroplasty. J Hand Surg [Br]. 2003; 28(6):551–558

[6] Sauder DJ, King GJ. Hemiarthroplasty of the distal ulna with an eccentric prosthesis. Tech Hand Up Extrem Surg. 2007; 11(1):115–120

[7] Kopylov P, Tägil M. Distal radioulnar joint replacement. Tech Hand Up Extrem Surg. 2007; 11(1):109–114

[8] Santos C, Pereira A, Sousa M, Trigueiros M, Silva C. Indications for distal radioulnar arthroplasty: report on three clinical cases. Rev Bras Ortop. 2015; 46(3):321–324

[9] Sabo MT, Talwalkar S, Hayton M, Watts A, Trail IA, Stanley JK. Intermediate outcomes of ulnar head arthroplasty. J Hand Surg Am. 2014; 39(12):2405–11.e1

[10] Adams BC, Gaffey JL. Non-constrained implant arthroplasty of the distal radioulnar joint. J Hand Surg Am. 2017; 42E:415–421

[11] Kleinman WB, Graham TJ. The distal radioulnar joint capsule: clinical anatomy and role in posttraumatic limitation of forearm rotation. J Hand Surg Am. 1998; 23(4):588–599

33 UHP DRUJ Arthroplasty

Jörg van Schoonhoven

Abstract

Arthritic destruction of the distal radioulnar joint (DRUJ) leads to painful restriction of forearm rotation. Partial or complete resection of the ulnar head as well as the Kapandji procedure restore the rotation but may result in forearm instability and painful radioulnar impingement between the ulnar stump and the radius. Biomechanically, replacement of the ulnar head using an ulnar head prosthesis combined with a soft tissue procedure will restore the stability of the forearm. Clinically, this procedure has been investigated in several studies demonstrating good and long lasting results not only as a revision procedure in failed resection arthroplasties but as a primary procedure in the painfully destroyed DRUJ as well. Contraindications consist of insufficient soft tissues for stabilization of the hemiarthroplasty, insufficient bone quality to allow primary press fit stabilization and osseous integration of the stem of the prosthesis within the ulna and longitudinal instability of the forearm following radial head resection or Essex Lopresti injuries. In my opinion, hemiarthroplasty using the ulnar head prosthesis is the primary option in failed resection arthroplasties of the DRUJ and in the symptomatic painfully destroyed DRUJ in the young and active patient. In the rare cases of failure, removal of the prosthesis creating an ulnar head resection situation or constrained complete radioulnar joint replacement remain revision options.

Keywords: ulnar head, prosthesis, hemiresection arthroplasty, distal radioulnar joint, instability, radioulnar impingement, Kapandji

33.1 Introduction

Arthritic destruction of the distal radioulnar joint (DRUJ) is frequently associated with painful limitation of forearm rotation and a reduction of grip strength. Multiple pathologies may cause the arthritic degeneration of the joint including chronic instability of the DRUJ, rheumatoid, or primary osteoarthritis and Madelung's deformity. Primary osteoarthritis is rare. Posttraumatic arthritis is common especially following distal radius fractures, that is, both malunited extra-articular distal radius fractures and intra-articular fractures involving the sigmoid notch or the ulnar head.

Traditional treatment options for symptomatic degeneration of the DRUJ have included resection of the ulnar head, hemiresection +/− interposition arthroplasties, and the Sauvé-Kapandji procedure. All these procedures can restore forearm rotation and often give satisfactory clinical results. But some patients have persisting or new pain and functional impairment following these procedures. This is typically due to painful instability of the forearm bones especially under loading. The loss of the ulnar support of the wrist may lead to a carpal supination deformity. The loss of the bony support for the radius may lead to painful radioulnar impingement with the distal radius abutting the distal end of the ulna under transverse loading called the "ulnar impingement syndrome."[1] This can be shown with stress radiographs as proposed by Lees and Scheker[2] (▶ Fig. 33.1).

To treat this secondary forearm instability, Timothy Herbert reported reconstruction of the original DRUJ using a silicone ulnar head spacer. The concept included the realignment of the radius relative to the ulna using the spacer and an ulnar-based local soft tissue flap to stabilize the forearm complex. The initial results were good but did not last due to failure of the silicone with loading.[3] Based on this experience, Schoonhoven and Herbert developed a more biocompatible and lasting ulnar head replacement, called the ulna head prosthesis (UHP).

The primary goal of the new technique was to relieve pain and restore stability and function in patients with painful instability of the forearm following previous resection arthroplasties of the DRUJ. The reported biomechanical[4] and clinical studies[5,6,7,8] have demonstrated good restoration of DRUJ stability and improved clinical outcomes which are maintained into the long-term. This has led to increasing use of the UHP as the primary operation to treat patients with painful arthritis of the DRUJ.

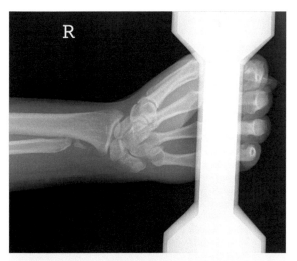

Fig. 33.1 Radiograph with transverse loading of the wrist demonstrating radioulnar impingement following ulnar head resection.

33.2 Herbert Ulnar Head Prosthesis

Following anatomical and radiological investigations assessing the diameter of the intramedullary canal of the distal ulna, the diameter and shape of the ulnar head, and the geometry of the DRUJ, an interchangeable, modular ulnar head prosthesis was developed. The anatomical shape of the stem of the prosthesis is designed to achieve primary fit-press stability within the intramedullary canal of the ulna. The titanium coating of the stem allows for osseointegration for long-term stability. There are three different stem designs. The standard stem with a collar length of 2 mm was developed for primary reconstruction of the distal radioulnar joint. The stem with a collar length of 4 mm allows for accurate length reconstruction following mild previous resection of the distal ulna, whereas the revision stem with a collar length of 17 mm allows reconstruction following larger previous resections.

Due to its elasticity and biocompatibility, zirconium ceramic was chosen as the material for the head of the prosthesis. It is also available in three sizes, and all stems and heads are interchangeable (▶ Fig. 33.2).

33.3 Operative Technique

The operative technique depends in part upon how much distal ulna is remaining and the local soft tissue structures/damage. Principally, it consists of bony and soft tissue elements.

The bone cut is primarily determined by preoperative templating. If the ulnar head is still in place it is removed by cutting the distal ulna at the predetermined level. It is better to start cutting the distal ulna too long as it can easily be cut further proximal. The sigmoid notch of the radius is inspected and any osteophytes are removed or steps within the joint line are smoothed with a burr. Using the appropriate rasps (standard or revision), the intramedullary canal of the ulna is prepared and the trial stem is inserted into the ulna. A trial head is used and intraoperative fluoroscopy is performed to check the correct stem size and fit within the intramedullary canal of the ulna. The trial head is chosen based upon the size of the excised ulnar head or if already excised by preoperative templating against the opposite side. The trial head needs to be

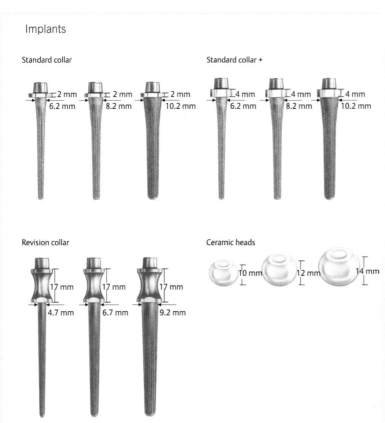

Fig. 33.2 Designs and sizes of the different stems and heads of the Herbert ulna head prosthesis.

matched against the sigmoid notch of the distal radius. The correct alignment of the head within the sigmoid notch of the radius and the correct length of the implant aims to achieve an ulna-minus variance of 2 mm to avoid ulnar impaction syndrome. This is the time to make adjustments prior to insertion of the definitive implant.

Stabilization of the restored DRUJ following ulnar head replacement is achieved using an ulnar-based local soft tissue flap consisting of the joint capsule, the extensor retinaculum, the sixth extensor compartment with the extensor carpi ulnaris tendon, and the triangular fibrocartilaginous complex (TFCC).

Following a longitudinal incision over the dorsal aspect of the DRUJ, the fifth extensor compartment is identified, opened longitudinally, and the extensor digiti minimi tendon is mobilized and retracted radially. A soft tissue flap is incised through the floor of the fifth extensor compartment and the dorsal capsule of the joint overlying the DRUJ. This flap is extended proximally about 3 cm to expose the neck of the distal ulna (▶ Fig. 33.3). It is then raised ulnarly in one layer and extended distally along the dorsal radioulnar ligament. Following osteotomy of the ulna, the ulnar head or its remains are excised. We recommend that any deficiencies of the floor of the sixth extensor compartment or the TFCC should be repaired. At this stage, two or three holes are drilled through the dorsal rim of the sigmoid notch using a small drill or K-wire (0.8 mm). Nonabsorbable (2–0) sutures are inserted through these drill holes to allow fixation of the ulnar flap following insertion of the prosthesis. The definitive implant is inserted and the ulnar-based soft tissue flap is sutured to the dorsal radioulnar ligament and the dorsal rim of the sigmoid notch (▶ Fig. 33.4). Prior to the final reattachment, the forearm rotation and stability of the DRUJ are checked to estimate the correct tension of the flap. This dorsal reattachment may be further supported with a longitudinal suture of the ulnar remains of the extensor retinaculum of the fifth extensor compartment onto the dorsal part of the flap using 3–0 absorbable suture material, leaving the extensor digiti minimi tendon subcutaneously. We recommend inserting a drain into the wound, although there is no evidence to establish its use and the skin is closed. A sterile dressing and a long arm plaster are applied, with the elbow in about 70 degrees of flexion, supination of about 30 degrees, and the wrist in 20 degrees of extension to minimize tension on the ulnar-based soft tissue flap.

This approach and the operative technique have been published previously.[9,10,11]

Postoperative immobilization depends on the quality of soft tissues and the stability that has been achieved with the procedure and varies from 2 to 4 weeks of immobilization in the above elbow plaster followed by 2 to 4 weeks of immobilization in an ulnar gutter splint. Unrestricted movement is allowed between 6 and 8

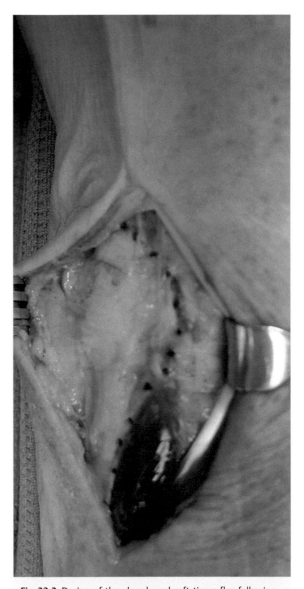

Fig. 33.3 Design of the ulnar-based soft tissue flap following opening of the fifth extensor compartment and radial retraction of the extensor digiti minimi tendon.

weeks and unrestricted use and loading 12 weeks following the procedure.

33.4 Indications

- Painful primary and posttraumatic arthritis of the DRUJ.
- Painful DRUJ instability and impingement following resection arthroplasties of the DRUJ or the Sauvé-Kapandji procedure.
- Destruction of the ulnar head due to a tumor or trauma.

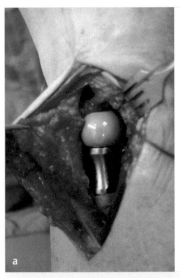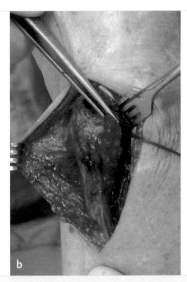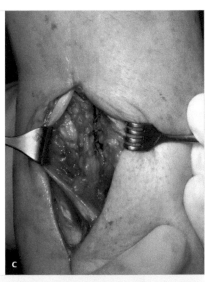

Fig. 33.4 **(a)** Reconstruction of the distal radioulnar joint (DRUJ) following implantation of the ulna head prosthesis under the triangular fibrocartilaginous complex (TFCC) lined up distally, with the ulnar-based soft tissue flap grasped with the forceps on the ulnar side and the intraosseous sutures lined up radially to suture the flap to the dorsal rim of the sigmoid notch. **(b)** Testing the tension prior to suturing the flap to the sigmoid notch. **(c)** Final result following suturing of the flap.

33.5 Contraindications

- Insufficient soft tissue for adequate soft tissue stabilization such as following several previous operations or soft tissue insufficiency due to rheumatoid arthritis.
- Insufficient ulnar bone to allow for primary press-fit stability and osseous integration.
- Longitudinal instability of the forearm following an Essex-Lopresti injury or previous radial head resection.
- A relative contraindication is malalignment of the radius or the ulna as these should be corrected prior to or simultaneously with the reconstruction of the DRUJ.

33.6 Results

33.6.1 Results in the Literature

This prosthesis and the connected soft tissue procedure have been subject to a prospective long-term trial in three steps. Following an initial trial of three patients with good clinical results,[12] a prospective, international, multicenter study was performed including an additional 20 patients. These 23 patients were followed up and the short-term results were assessed after a mean of 28 (10–43) months and published.[13] Finally, and as the last step of the intended trial, 16 of the original 23 patients could be examined after a mean of 11 (range 97–158 mo) years postoperatively. These long-term results were compared to the preoperative and short-term clinical and radiological data. No patients reported DRUJ instability. The mean visual analog scale (VAS) pain scores improved from 3.7 preoperatively to 1.7 in the short and the long term. The mean VAS patient satisfaction improved from 2.2 (out of

10) to 8.2 and 8.9, respectively. The ranges of motion improved from mean pronation of 73 degrees to 86 and 83 degrees, and mean supination of 52 degrees to 77 and 81 degrees. The mean grip strength improved from 42% to 72 and 81% of the unaffected side. All clinical parameters improved significantly from preoperatively to the short-term follow-up with no further statistically significant change between the short- and long-term follow-up. Radiographs demonstrated no signs of stem loosening or DRUJ incongruity.[14] As a result of the press-fit impaction of the stem of the prosthesis within the intramedullary canal of the ulna, signs of stress shielding may occur with resorption of bone directly under the collar of the prosthesis. This had not yet led to any instability or loosening of the prosthesis; the process appears to stop progressing within 8 to 12 months.[7] In a number of patients (not specified in the publications) remodeling of the sigmoid fossa around the ceramic head was noticed on short-term follow-up radiographs with no further progress long-term. These radiological findings have been noted by other experts. They appear not to cause clinical problems.[15]

Complications have been reported including infection and in cases of deep infection the prosthesis had to be removed. Recurrent or persisting instability is typically due to insufficient soft tissues. This procedure relies on the existence and durability of the original soft tissue structures stabilizing the DRUJ. Therefore, insufficient soft tissue structures due to several previous operations at the DRUJ, destruction by means of inflammation, e.g., in rheumatoid arthritis, a complex longitudinal instability of the forearm following an Essex-Lopresti injury or resection of the radial head are contraindications for this

33

procedure. In these cases a constrained system should be considered. Loosening of the implant within the ulna has been reported. Other than due to infection it appears to be due to bony malalignment of the radius or the ulna typically following fractures. The reconstruction of the DRUJ using an implant is only indicated in patients with anatomical longitudinal alignment of the two forearm bones and the sigmoid notch of the radius. Any malalignment will lead to increased forces onto the prosthesis and potentially secondary loosening or symptomatic DRUJ instability. Malalignment is not an absolute contraindication for reconstruction of the DRUJ using an implant but has to be corrected either prior to or simultaneously with the DRUJ reconstruction.

33.6.2 Patient Example

This male truck driver had sustained bilateral intra-articular fractures of the distal radius aged 28 years, treated conservatively. He developed bilateral posttraumatic radiocarpal arthrosis and DRUJ arthritis. Despite denervations and a right wrist radioscapholunate arthrodesis he presented in 2007, aged 46, with increasing left wrist and forearm pain and stiffness (▶ Fig. 33.5a). A radioscapholunate fusion combined with a hemiresection interposition arthroplasty of the DRUJ of the left wrist was performed (▶ Fig. 33.5b). Due to persisting pain of the left wrist joint and secondary painful radioulnar impingement syndrome, he had a

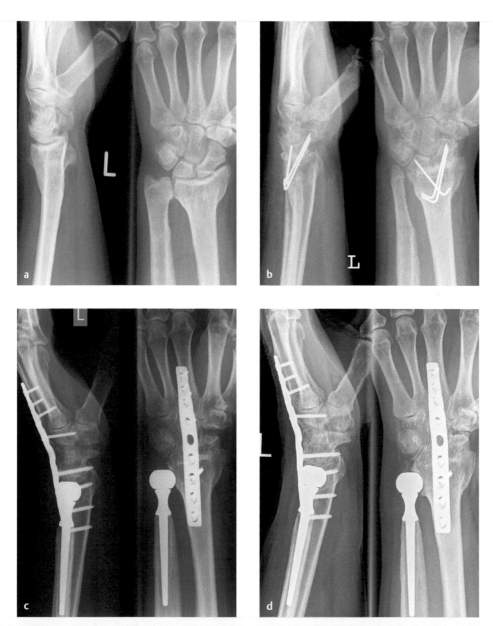

Fig. 33.5 (a–d) Patient example.

33

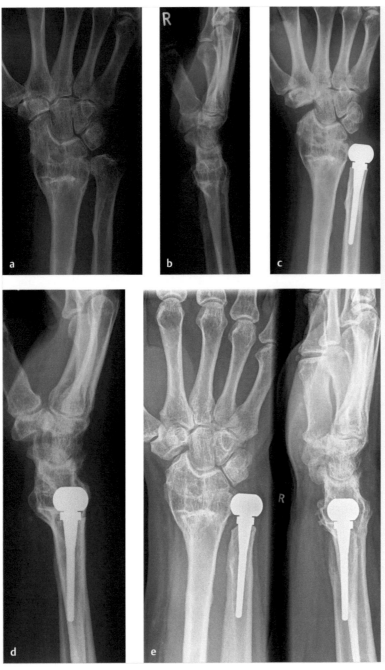

Fig. 33.6 (a–e) Patient example.

wrist arthrodesis and reconstruction of the DRUJ with the UHP prosthesis in 2008 (▶ Fig. 33.5c).

As he complained about persisting symptoms in his right wrist and forearm (▶ Fig. 33.6a, b), he received a primary right UHP ulnar head replacement and resection of the distal pole of the scaphoid in 2011 (▶ Fig. 33.6c, d).

At the latest review in 2017 (aged 56) he reported no left wrist pain with a stable DRUJ, pronation, and supination of 70 degrees each and grip strength of 32 kgf. On the right side he reported pain with loading (4 of 10 on a VAS). He had wrist extension of 40 degrees and flexion of 30 degrees, a stable DRUJ, forearm pronation and supination each of 80 degrees, and a grip strength of 28 kgf. Radiographs showed stable implants with some mild resorption under the neck of the right ulnar collar but no signs of loosening or other problems (▶ Fig. 33.5d, ▶ Fig. 33.6e).

33.7 Conclusion

In my experience ulnar head replacement leads to very reliable, functionally good, and long-lasting clinical results, provided the contraindications are remembered. In the last review of my own 89 patients treated with this prosthesis between 1995 and 2012, the 15-year survival rate was 90% (unpublished data). Therefore, in my opinion this procedure is the procedure of choice in failed resection arthroplasties of the DRUJ and represents the first treatment option in the young and active patient with a painfully destroyed DRUJ. If this procedure fails due to any reason, revision using a constrained prosthesis is possible.

References

[1] Bell MJ, Hill RJ, McMurtry RY. Ulnar impingement syndrome. J Bone Joint Surg Br. 1985; 67(1):126–129

[2] Lees VC, Scheker LR. The radiologic demonstration of dynamic ulnar impingement. J Hand Surg Am. 1997; 22B:448–450

[3] Stanley D, Herbert TJ. The Swanson ulnar head prosthesis for posttraumatic disorders of the distal radio-ulnar joint. J Hand Surg [Br]. 1992; 17(6):682–688

[4] Sauerbier M, Hahn ME, Fujita M, Neale PG, Berglund LJ, Berger RA. Analysis of dynamic distal radioulnar convergence after ulnar head resection and endoprosthesis implantation. J Hand Surg Am. 2002; 27(3):425–434

[5] V Schoonhoven J, Herbert TJ, Fernandez DL, Prommersberger KJ, Krimmer H. Ulnar head prosthesis. Orthopade. 2003; 32(9):809–815

[6] Yen Shipley N, Dion GR, Bowers WH. Ulnar head implant arthroplasty: an intermediate term review of 1 surgeon's experience. Tech Hand Up Extrem Surg. 2009; 13(3):160–164

[7] Sauerbier M, Arsalan-Werner A, Enderle E, Vetter M, Vonier D. Ulnar head replacement and related biomechanics. J Wrist Surg. 2013; 2 (1):27–32

[8] Axelsson P, Sollerman C, Kärrholm J. Ulnar head replacement: 21 cases; mean follow-up, 7.5 years. J Hand Surg Am. 2015; 40(9):1731–1738

[9] van Schoonhoven J, Herbert T. The dorsal approach to the distal radioulnar joint. Tech Hand Up Extrem Surg. 2004; 8(1):11–15

[10] Herbert TJ, van Schoonhoven J. Ulnar head replacement. Tech Hand Up Extrem Surg. 2007; 11(1):98–108

[11] Mühldorfer-Fodor M, Pillukat T, Pausch T, Prommersberger KJ, van Schoonhoven J. Reconstruction of the distal radioulnar joint using the Herbert ulnar head prosthesis. Oper Orthop Traumatol. 2011; 23 (2):86–97

[12] van Schoonhoven J, Herbert TH, Krimmer H. New concepts for endoprostheses of the distal radio-ulnar joint. Handchir Mikrochir Plast Chir. 1998; 30(6):387–392

[13] van Schoonhoven J, Fernandez DL, Bowers WH, Herbert TJ. Salvage of failed resection arthroplasties of the distal radioulnar joint using a new ulnar head prosthesis. J Hand Surg Am. 2000; 25(3):438–446

[14] van Schoonhoven J, Mühldorfer-Fodor M, Fernandez DL, Herbert TJ. Salvage of failed resection arthroplasties of the distal radioulnar joint using an ulnar head prosthesis: long-term results. J Hand Surg Am. 2012; 37(7):1372–1380

[15] Herzberg G. Periprosthetic bone resorption and sigmoid notch erosion around ulnar head implants: a concern? Hand Clin. 2010; 26 (4):573–577

33

34 Eclypse Distal Radioulnar Joint Arthroplasty

Dirck Ananos Flores and Marc Garcia-Elias

Abstract

Distal radioulnar joint (DRUJ) arthropathy is relatively uncommon but problematic when present. Surgical options to address this condition are divided into nonanatomical procedures and prosthetic reconstruction. Nonanatomical procedures (Sauve-Kapandji, Darrach's, etc.) have widespread use among hand surgeons but patients can develop impingement syndrome which can be debilitating.

The Eclypse prosthesis was designed as an alternative to these procedures with the intention of avoiding this rather common complication. The implant consists of a pyrocarbon head and a stem. The insertion technique should be meticulous and is thoroughly described in this chapter.

This prosthesis is indicated in mono arthropathy of the DRUJ as long as there is no major instability of the said joint. It is not indicated in patients who have had a previous Darrach's or Sauve-Kapandji.

Published literature suggests that good results are achieved early with reliable stability over time. Complications so far have been minimal but we have witnessed one case of molybdenum allergy requiring explantation.

Keywords: eclypse, distal radioulnar joint (DRUJ) arthroplasty, DRUJ arthropathy, pyrocarbon prosthesis

34.1 Introduction

An intact distal radioulnar joint (DRUJ) is critical to stability and load transmission during forearm and wrist motion.[1] The DRUJ is the keystone in coordination of forearm rotation and wrist circumduction.[2] Arthropathy of the DRUJ is an uncommon problem but when present can cause severe limitations.

Current treatment options for DRUJ arthropathy can be divided into nonanatomical procedures and prosthetic reconstruction.

Salvage nonanatomical procedures (Darrach's, Bowers', matched distal ulnar resection, or the Sauvé-Kapandji procedure) fail to restore normal joint anatomy and can carry complications of their own, including instability, subluxation, clicks, and translocations.[3]

The most common complication is ulna impingement syndrome. Described by Bell et al[4] as a radioulnar convergence with subsequent impingement, patients present with pain, clicking, and a weak grip. Clinical signs include narrowing of the wrist and pain on compression of the forearm bones and on forced supination. Radiographs may demonstrate scalloping of the radius metaphysis at the site of contact.

The Eclypse prosthesis was designed as an alternative to nonanatomical surgical excisions with the intention of avoiding ulnar impingement syndrome. The goal is to re-establish the distal pivot point necessary for adequate tension of the soft tissue such as the interosseus membrane, thus allowing optimal transfer of loads between the radius and ulna.

34.2 Characteristics of the Implant and Technique

The Eclypse prosthesis is a pyrocarbon spacer developed to replace the articular portion of the damaged ulnar head in patients with isolated DRUJ arthropathy.[2] It can be implanted without major disruption to the foveal insertion of the triangular fibrocartilage complex (TFCC) or to the extensor carpi ulnaris (ECU) sheath, i.e., preserving the physiological DRUJ stabilizers.

It has two components: a titanium four-pronged stem and a pyrocarbon ulnar head. The purpose of the stem is to prevent dislocation of the spacer at extremes of motion. The pyrocarbon head "replaces" the native ulnar head restoring more normal DRUJ kinematics. It is better able to resist compression and shear stress than a tendon "anchovy" or scarring of an excision arthroplasty.

34.2.1 Technique

Via a dorsoulnar skin incision centered on the ulnar head, the dorsal cutaneous branches of the ulnar nerve are identified and preserved. The fifth extensor compartment is released longitudinally and an ulnarly based extensor retinacular flap is elevated avoiding opening the DRUJ and without disrupting the ECU sheath. This will expose the underlying DRUJ capsule (▶ Fig. 34.1a, b).

A dorsal capsulotomy is designed to allow access to the ulnocarpal space, the dorsal edge of the TFCC, and the ulnar head.[5] This is obtained by raising an ulnarly based capsular flap using the following anatomical landmarks (▶ Fig. 34.2): the dorsal border of the triquetrum; the retinacular septum between the fourth and fifth compartments; and the neck of the ulnar head. The most distal component of this flap design will involve an incision along the most proximal fibers of the dorsal radiotriquetral ligament. The flap is raised and if necessary, the TFCC meniscoid can be excised to aid visualization of the ulnocarpal space.

The ulnar head is subluxed for full exposure. This is achieved with full pronation of the forearm and some dorsal translation force onto the ulna. The TFCC should remain attached during this maneuver.

The osteotomy should be regarded as the most important step of the procedure. Accurate orientation of the excision osteotomy is essential. Two cuts are designed with the aid of an osteotomy guide: (1) Transverse: at the proximal end of the DRUJ articular surface of the ulnar head,

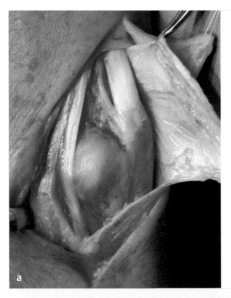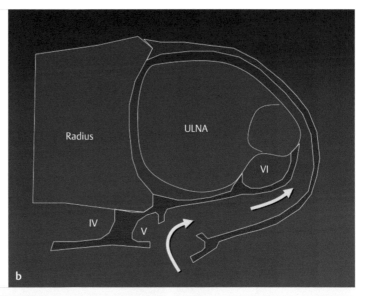

Fig. 34.1 (a, b) Ulnarly based extensor retinacular flap with preservation of underlying distal radioulnar joint (DRUJ) capsule and extensor carpi ulnaris (ECU) sheath.

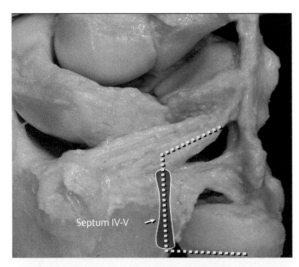

Fig. 34.2 Landmarks for ulnarly based capsular flap.

perpendicular to the longitudinal axis of the ulna; and (2) Longitudinal: through the cartilage of the ulnar head, parallel to the longitudinal axis of the ulna, without breaching the fovea to allow for preservation of the radio-ulnar ligament (RUL) insertion (▶ Fig. 34.3). In addition, the longitudinal osteotomy needs to be perpendicular to the flexion/extension plane of the elbow. The aim is for the osteotomy to direct the implant so that it will lie parallel to the ground with the elbow flexed at 90 degrees, irrespective of the position of forearm rotation.

After removal of the damaged articular surface, the forearm is fully pronated and the ulna dorsally translated. This will allow for the introduction of an awl into the medullary cavity. The entry point should be set adjacent

to the base of the ulnar styloid while avoiding damage to the radioulnar ligament at the fovea. The awl should be aimed toward the center of the ulnar medullary canal in the direction of the ulnar diaphysis. With a 3.5-mm drill bit, a 4-cm long tunnel is created into the ulna. Drilling permits simultaneous sizing: if the drill makes contact with the inner cortex a small stem should be selected. If drilling is performed with no cortical contact (wider bone cavity), a 4.5-mm drill bit should be used next and a medium-sized stem subsequently inserted. In large patients a 5.5-mm drill and a large stem will be necessary. The stem should be inserted with a tight press-fit.

The four legs of the stem should be held together during insertion with a rubber band around the stem distal to the head (anatomically proximal) prior to final insertion. The band will roll distally as the stem is inserted and can later be cut away. Once inside the bone the four legs will spread apart creating an inherently stable construct that will prevent spontaneous extrusion. It is expected that new bone will grow around the legs within 6 weeks; therefore, some protection against extremes of pronation or supination should be enforced during that period.

Three trial heads are available: small, medium, and large. The head should match the diameter of the excised portion of the ulnar head. If the original head is too deformed for a reliable assessment, the small size is tried first and checked for stability and full mobility of the joint. With the trial in situ the construct should be neither too loose nor too tight based upon experience (▶ Fig. 34.4).

Careful closure in layers is recommended. The first step is to repair the dorsal connection between the TFCC and the dorsal capsule fibers on the capsular flap with a 3–0 Vicryl suture (▶ Fig. 34.5). This should not be overlooked as it will help ensure implant stability. The distal portion

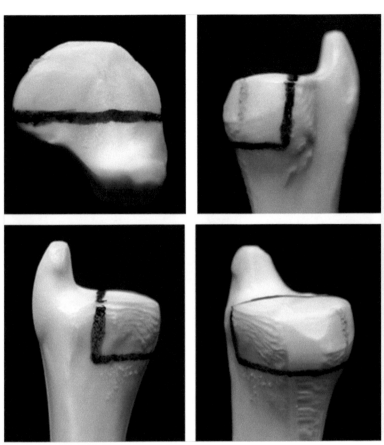

Fig. 34.3 Osteotomies.

of the capsulotomy is closed via interrupted sutures connecting parallel fibers of the dorsal radiotriquetral ligament. The vertical portion can be reinforced by suturing the capsule to the septum between fourth and fifth compartments. This septum will be also used to reinsert the retinacular flap. Finally, subcutaneous tissue and skin closure are performed.

Postoperatively an above-elbow plaster cast is worn for 3 weeks with the forearm slightly supinated. Then a removable wrist splint is applied, which is removed three times a day for active forearm rotation performed within the limits of pain. Passive forearm mobilization should be avoided for at least until 6 weeks postoperatively to prevent damage to the bone ingrowth around the legs of the stem. At this point muscle strengthening of both the brachioradialis (the only muscle able to dynamically unload the DRUJ) and the ECU muscle (an effective dynamic DRUJ stabilizer) is begun. We recommend that contact sports should be avoided for 6 months.

34.3 Indications and Contraindications

The prime indication for the Eclypse prosthesis is isolated arthropathy of the DRUJ of various causes, provided there is no major DRUJ instability (▶ Fig. 34.6, ▶ Fig. 34.7). The

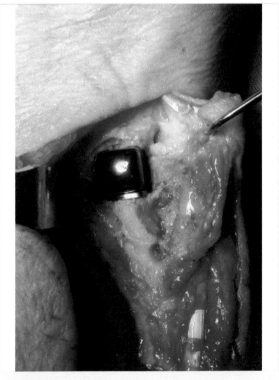

Fig. 34.4 Implant in situ.

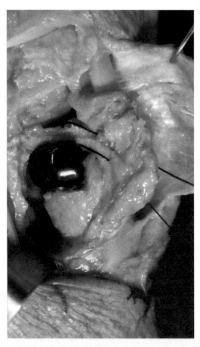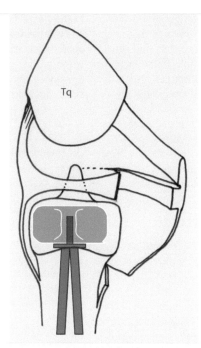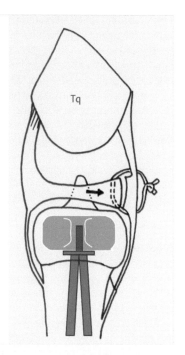

34

Fig. 34.5 Capsule repair.

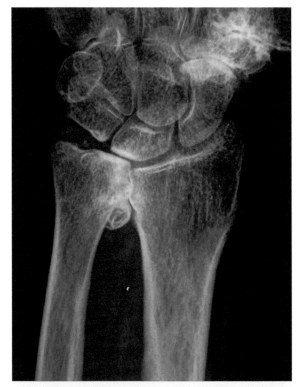

Fig. 34.6 Distal radioulnar joint (DRUJ) arthropathy.

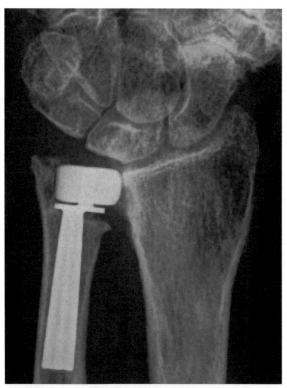

Fig. 34.7 Wrist radiograph with an implant in situ.

typical causes include idiopathic osteoarthritis (OA), post-traumatic incongruency of the joint surface of the ulnar head with preservation of the sigmoid notch, and ulnar head degeneration secondary to chronic inflammatory disease (pseudogout, rheumatoid arthritis, etc.). It is also indicated in patients who have had a symptomatic hemi-resection interposition arthroplasty of the DRUJ.

It is contraindicated in patients who have had a previous Darrach's or Sauvé-Kapandji procedure, in marked DRUJ instability secondary to TFCC insufficiency, in the presence of an incongruent sigmoid notch, and in significant malalignment of the distal radius such as following a fracture.

34.4 Results in the Literature

Bigorre et al[6] reported their mid-term results on five patients who underwent Eclypse DRUJ hemiarthroplasty over a period of 6 years. The sole indication was DRUJ arthropathy secondary to rheumatoid arthritis. One patient was lost to follow-up; the remaining four were assessed at a mean of 64 (range 43–90) months postoperatively. The mean range of motion was 70 degrees of pronation and 80 degrees of supination. The mean grip strength was 148% compared to the contralateral hand. The mean DASH score was 55.9 points. No intra- or post-operative complications were reported. The authors concluded that there is good early benefit and the prosthesis remains stable over time.

Mesquida[7] reviewed 27 patients who underwent Eclypse implantation in his thesis with a mean follow-up of 30 (range 12–69) months. He reported 100% pronation and 84% supination compared to the opposite side. Grip strength was also > 100% of the opposite hand. The mean DASH score was 26.3. The complications included: one revision (incomplete removal of a portion of the ulnar head with limitation of supination); one patient with symptomatic instability of the DRUJ; and one implant causing ulnocarpal impaction. Radiographs revealed bone resorption under the metal platform in ten patients (38%) and sigmoid notch remodeling in nine patients (33%); these did not seem to be associated with any adverse symptoms. There was no radiological evidence of implant loosening.

34.5 Author's Experience and Preferred Technique (Tips and Tricks)

Since its introduction to the market we have implanted seven Eclypse prosthesis in seven patients. Six prosthesis have been successful in improving symptoms; one had to be removed due to molybdenum allergy after 35 months.

The indications for surgery included DRUJ OA of various causes (5), pseudogout (1), and both ulnocarpal impaction and pseudogout (1).

The mean follow-up was 97 (range 35–147) months. The pre- and postoperative assessments included a visual analog pain score (EVA), forearm ranges of motion (measured with a goniometer), grip strength (using a Jamar dynamometer), functional and radiographic examinations, and the patient-rated wrist evaluation (PRWE).

34.5.1 Results

On review the mean pronation was 70 degrees (range 55–80 degrees) and mean supination 54 degrees (range 30–70 degrees). The mean percentage of motion compared to the contralateral side was 73% (range 44–89%). The mean grip strength was 17.4 (range 0–35) kgf, 74.8% (range 0–100%) of the opposite side. The patient with 0 kgf grip strength is the one with the molybdenum allergy. The mean PRWE score was 26.7%. All DRUJs were clinically stable based on a ballottement test. One revision occurred at 35 months postoperatively because of ongoing pain; the prosthesis was removed and a matched ulna procedure was performed. It was later identified that the patient was allergic to molybdenum. No other revision surgery has been required.

34.5.2 Tips and Tricks

- If there are any limitations in supination once the trial ulnar head spacer has been inserted, attention needs to be drawn toward the volar joint capsule and the pronator quadratus (PQ) muscle. Proximal extension of the incision and flexion of the wrist will allow for exploration and release of these structures as required.
- The Eclypse is not indicated if the DRUJ is unstable.

Acknowledgment

The authors thank Juana Medina MD for her contribution to this chapter.

References

[1] Garcia-Elias M. Failed ulnar head resection: prevention and treatment. J Hand Surg [Br]. 2002; 27(5):470–480

[2] Garcia-Elias M. Eclypse: partial ulnar head replacement for the isolated distal radio-ulnar joint arthrosis. Tech Hand Up Extrem Surg. 2007; 11(1):121–128

[3] Minami A, Iwasaki N, Ishikawa J, Suenaga N, Yasuda K, Kato H. Treatments of osteoarthritis of the distal radioulnar joint: long-term results of three procedures. Hand Surg. 2005; 10(2–3):243–248

[4] Bell MJ, Hill RJ, McMurtry RY. Ulnar impingement syndrome. J Bone Joint Surg Br. 1985; 67(1):126–129

[5] Garcia-Elias M, Smith DE, Llusá M. Surgical approach to the triangular fibrocartilage complex. Tech Hand Up Extrem Surg. 2003; 7(4):134–140

[6] Bigorre N, Saint Cast Y, Cesari B, Rabarin F, Raimbeau G. Intermediate term evaluation of the Eclypse distal radio-ulnar prosthesis for rheumatoid arthritis: a report of five cases. Orthop Traumatol Surg Res. 2016; 102(3):345–349

[7] Mesquida V. Partial ulnar head replacement: Eclypse prosthesis: a multicentric review of 27 patients. Médecine humaine et pathologie 2011. ffdumas-00658822f

35 Salvage Distal Radioulnar Joint Arthroplasty with the Aptis Implant

Maurizio Calcagni, Thomas Giesen, Marco Guidi, Lisa Reissner, and Florian S. Frueh

Abstract

When lifting an object by flexing the elbow with the forearm in neutral rotation, the force is transferred from the ulnar insertion of the brachialis muscle up to the head of the ulna, the sigmoid notch, and eventually the hand. When the distal radioulnar joint (DRUJ) is damaged or unstable, weight lifting can be difficult or even painful. Most surgical procedures to treat this problem aim at removing the ulnar head, failing to maintain the key anatomical structures necessary for force transfer from the hand to the forearm.

The Aptis implant is a total joint arthroplasty able to replace not only the two joint components of the DRUJ, but also the function of the triangular fibrocartilage complex (TFCC). In our experience, this implant is a safe and very effective solution for painful and unstable osteoarthritis of the DRUJ. Moreover, it is indicated as salvage procedure for unstable and painful ulna stumps or ulnar head replacements. The published results reveal a statistically significant reduction in pain as well as improvement in grip strength. Forearm rotation normally improves but to a lesser extent. The most common complications of tendon and nerve irritation can be prevented with an accurate technique, and a survival rate of 97 % at 5 years is reported.

Keywords: DRUJ arthroplasty, DRUJ implant, DRUJ instability, DRUJ osteoarthritis, joint replacement, semiconstrained implant

35.1 Introduction

The radioulnar joint is a bicondylar joint made up of the proximal (PRUJ) and distal radioulnar joints (DRUJ).[1] When lifting an object by flexing the elbow with the forearm in neutral rotation, the force is transferred from the ulnar insertion of the brachialis muscle up to the head of the ulna, the sigmoid notch, and eventually the hand.

When the DRUJ is damaged or unstable, weight lifting can be difficult or even painful.[2] Typically, patients with DRUJ conditions experience ulnar-sided wrist pain, exacerbated by lifting objects.[3,4]

Different surgical strategies have been proposed to treat these problems. The majority of these aims at removing the ulnar head, partially[5] or totally.[6] The success of these arthroplasties relies on the integrity of the capsule and ligament that maintain the joint congruency. However, they fail to maintain the key anatomical structures necessary for force transfer from the hand to the forearm. Arthrodesis of the DRUJ together with the interruption of the diaphysis (i. e., Sauvé-Kapandji procedure) results in the same uncoupling of the two forearm bones and can lead to loss of function.[7] Another approach is the replacement of the ulnar head with[8] or without ligament reinsertion.[9] Finally, interposition arthroplasty with Achilles tendon has been proposed to avoid the painful impingement of the distal ulnar stump with the radius.[10] Importantly, the function of the DRUJ remains often limited after this procedure and may be associated with pain, residual symptomatic instability, or stiffness, particularly under load.[11]

All these operations may result in limited functional recovery, mainly due to residual instability of the ulnar head replacement or the impingement of the ulnar stump with the radius, especially in active patients. In some cases, patients experience a painful snap during forearm rotation that further limits function.

35.2 The Implant and Technique

The semiconstrained DRUJ prosthesis (Aptis Medical) was first proposed in 2001[12] as a total joint arthroplasty able to replace not only the two joint components of the DRUJ, but also the function of the triangular fibrocartilage complex (TFCC).[13]

The prosthesis is completely modular. The radial component is a plate adapted to the anatomical shape of the ulnar aspect of the radius and terminates distally with a hemisocket to receive the ball. It is available in three sizes; it has a peg on the radial side and it is coated with a titanium plasma spray to enhance osteointegration. The plate is secured to the radius by three to five screws depending on the size of the plate. Recently, locking implants have been developed, further improving the quality of the radial fixation. The ulnar stem is also coated with titanium plasma spray and has a distal pin for the ultra-high molecular weight polyethylene ball. The stem is available in different sizes and neck length to allow for loss of the distal ulna at previous operations.

The size of the implant can be planned on posteroanterior and lateral radiographs. The approach is dorsal through an 8-cm long skin incision along the ulnar border of the distal ulna with a 3-cm oblique extension over the wrist. In most cases, scars from previous surgery dictate the skin incision, but it should be as close to the ulnar border of the forearm as possible for an easy positioning and fixation of the plate on the ulnar margin of the radius. The dorsal branch of the ulnar nerve must be identified and carefully protected throughout the whole operation. The extensor retinaculum is then exposed and partially incised at the level of the second dorsal compartment to harvest an ulnar-based flap. At the level of the DRUJ the dorsal capsule is also included in the flap. The extensor carpi ulnaris (ECU) compartment is then incised and the tendon completely freed up to its distal insertion. At this point, the ulnar head, if still present, is removed and the interosseous membrane is cut for 8 to 9 cm to allow for a better mobilization of the ulnar stump and exposure of the sigmoid notch. It is recommended to resect the volar margin of the radius to place the radial plate trial at 90 degrees to the coronal plane and not tilted dorsally. The distal end of the plate should be at least 3 mm below the lunate fossa. The plate is temporarily fixed with K-wires and screws and its position is checked with a fluoroscope. The plate should not overlap the dorsal cortex of the radius to reduce the risk of extensor tendon irritation. The definitive plate is then placed and secured with screws. The most proximal screw should be monocortical to prevent stress fractures.

The forearm is rotated into maximal pronation and a guide used to resect the ulna to the planned length. A 2.4-mm guide is placed in the medullary canal and progressive reamers (4.0–6.0 mm) are inserted up to the 11-cm mark until a tight fit is ensured. The distal part of the ulna is finally prepared with the medullary finish reamer of the corresponding size. At this point, the stem is introduced with a plastic impactor until the coated part is flush with the bone. The distal end of the ulnar peg should be proximal to the distal end of the radial plate. The ball and the closing cover are then placed and secured. The retinaculum flap is passed under the ECU tendon and sutured in its original position over the second dorsal compartment. The wound is closed in layers and a short arm splint is applied to protect the soft tissues.

Hand therapy is started within 1 to 2 days with finger mobilization, active wrist movement, and gentle forearm rotation. After 4 weeks, full rotation of the forearm is allowed and weight-bearing exercises are started 6 weeks after surgery. Full load is allowed after 3 months.

35.3 Indications and Contraindications

The Aptis semiconstrained implant can in theory be used for all cases of pain and instability of the DRUJ.[4] The main indications are adults with symptomatic rheumatoid, degenerative or posttraumatic arthritis of the DRUJ, and after previous surgery.[13]

In our experience most patients had had one or more previous surgical interventions for different DRUJ problems, in particular, partial or total ulnar head excision with instability with the proximal stump impinging with the radius (▶ Fig. 35.1a–c).[14] We have also used the Aptis implant for ulnar head or ulnar stump instability following wrist fusion (▶ Fig. 35.2a–d) and for salvage of painful, unstable ulnar head replacements (▶ Fig. 35.3a–f).

Contraindications are known metal allergy (cobalt-chrome, nickel), an immature skeleton, active infection, or an ulnar stump of less than 11 cm.

35.4 Results in the Literature

There are relatively few reports in the literature; recent reviews[15,16] could identify only 14 studies with a little more of 300 implants. The great majority had been operated in the department of the implant developer.

The mean reported pronation/supination ranged from 167 to 115 degrees with a grip strength between 46 and 90 % of the contralateral DRUJ. There is a reported survival rate of 97 % at a mean follow-up of 56 months (range 24–75)[16] with relatively few major complications.

Another review, however, reported a reoperation rate of up to 21 %[15] mainly because of irritation of the ECU tendon or of the radial nerve.

35.5 Authors' Own Experience and Preferred Technique (Tips and Tricks)

Our experience is based on more than 40 cases operated in the last 10 years. Our results are very similar to those reported by other authors.[14] In our first ten cases we had a high reoperation rate of 21 % due to a number of different complications. The two implant removals we have had to do were in the first ten cases. Strict indications and a very precise technique are the key to avoid complications, as in all other joint replacement procedures, and small details make the difference, making the learning curve quite flat.

The main indication in our patients was an unstable, painful proximal ulnar stump after ulnar head excision. The number of previous operations was variable and we observed that the residual range of forearm rotation was the main factor influencing the final result since this was not improved significantly by surgery[14] (▶ Fig. 35.4). Pain, force, and lifting capability were statistically improved (▶ Fig. 35.5) at a mean follow-up of 5 years (unpublished data). It is our impression that primary replacements for symptomatic DRUJ problems without previous surgery have better results, but numbers are too small for statistical significance.

The original description of the technique is very reliable and only a few changes have been introduced following reports of complications. In our opinion the key elements are: placement of the radial component; the lengths of the screws; and the size of the ulnar stem.

Extensor tendons irritation, especially of the ECU tendon, is the most common complication. Great attention should be paid to the dissection of the adipofascial flap. This should be planned in the right position and wide enough to cover the distal part of the implant to avoid

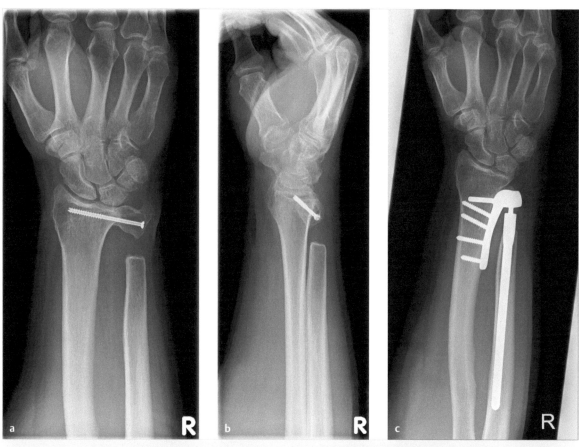

Fig. 35.1 (a, b) Unstable ulna stump after Sauvé-Kapandji procedure. **(c)** Resection of the ulna remnants and implantation of an Aptis implant.

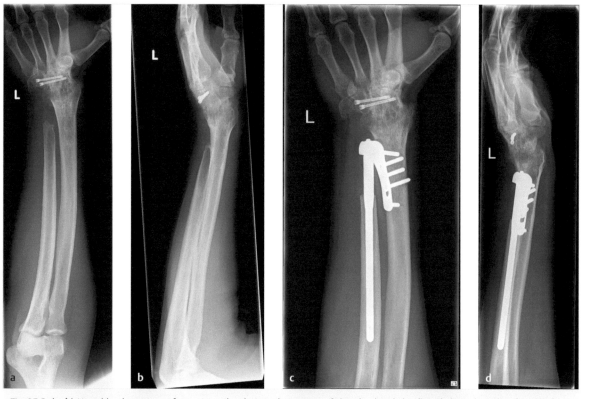

Fig. 35.2 (a, b) Unstable ulna stump after wrist arthrodesis and resection of the ulna head. **(c, d)** Radiological results after distal radioulnar joint (DRUJ) arthroplasty with Aptis implant at 3 months follow-up.

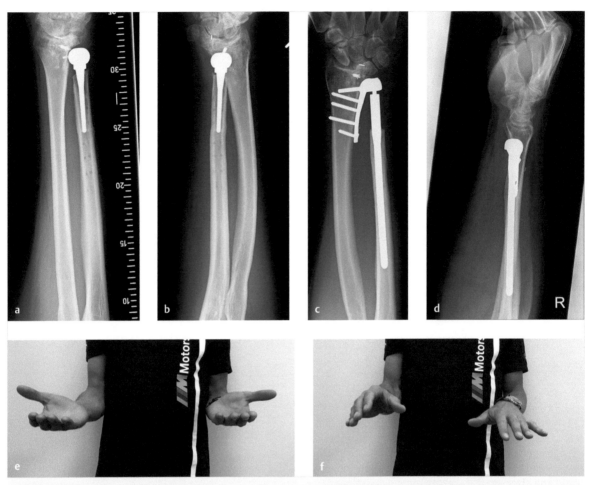

Fig. 35.3 (a, b) Unstable ulna head implant after five previous operations. **(c, d)** Radiological results after distal radioulnar joint (DRUJ) arthroplasty with Aptis implant at 3 months follow-up. **(e, f)** The pronation-supination is only marginally restricted. The range of motion is the same as preoperative.

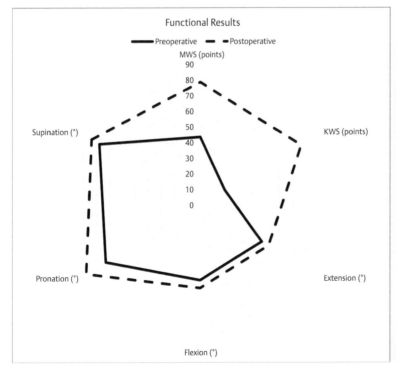

Fig. 35.4 Spider-net diagram of wrist motion (no statistical difference), Mayo wrist score (MWS), and Krimmer wrist score (KWS) are statistically improved (p < .05).

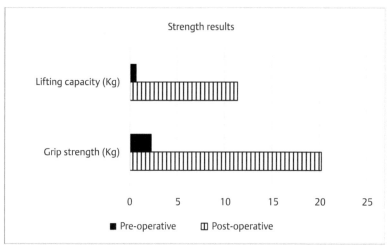

Fig. 35.5 Diagram of grip strength and lifting force pre- and postoperatively (p < .05).

tendon irritation. For the same reason, the ECU tendon sheath should be carefully opened up to the metacarpal insertion. During this maneuver the dorsal branch of the ulnar nerve is at danger; it should be identified and protected throughout the procedure.

Dorsally the radial plate has to be flush with the radius to reduce the risk of tendon irritation.

The radius plate should be placed at least 3 mm proximal to the carpus to avoid impingement. Where possible the TFCC should be preserved if still present, to protect from impingement with the carpal bones. The position of the radial plate should be carefully checked under the fluoroscope in all planes. An easy trick to assess the correct orientation is to observe the position on the radius when the fixation holes of the template are perfectly round, ensuring that the radiographs are perpendicular to the plate.

The length of the screws can also be a source of different complications. The irritation of the superficial radial nerve or of the tendons of the first dorsal compartment by the distal ends of the distal screws is one of the commonest reasons for surgical revision. With this implant, we advise that the tip of the screw should not protrude at all beyond the second cortex. The proximal screw also should be monocortical to reduce the load at the end of the plate which can lead to stress fractures.

Loosening of the radial component has not been reported in the literature and has not been a problem in our experience.

The ulnar stem is available with different extensions to adapt to a wide range of previous ulnar head resections. It has to be noted that the maximal load that can be allowed is inversely proportional to the length of the extension and therefore the shortest possible one should be used. Loosening of the ulnar stem is rare; it has occurred only once in our case series. In our opinion if the largest stem size (6 mm) can be introduced too easily into the canal of the ulna, bone graft or bone cement should be used to strengthen the fixation.

The implant has been modified over time with the introduction of a smaller plate, the locking screw fixation, and an improved radial plate cover. The smaller radial plate has helped to solve many implantation problems in smaller radii. In the first reported cases some periprosthetic calcifications were observed around the distal end of the ulna stem, but the introduction of a minimal extension of 1 cm reduced their occurrence and this was not seen subsequently.

35.6 Conclusions

In our experience, the Aptis implant is a safe and very effective solution for painful and unstable osteoarthritis of the DRUJ. Moreover, it is indicated as salvage procedure for unstable and painful ulna stumps or ulnar head replacements. The published results reveal a statistically significant reduction in pain as well as improvement in grip strength. Forearm rotation normally improves but to a lesser extent. The most common complications of tendon and nerve irritation can be prevented with an accurate technique, and a survival rate of 97 % at 5 years is reported.

References

[1] Markolf KL, Lamey D, Yang S, Meals R, Hotchkiss R. Radioulnar load-sharing in the forearm. A study in cadavera. J Bone Joint Surg Am. 1998; 80(6):879–888
[2] Shaaban H, Giakas G, Bolton M, et al. The load-bearing characteristics of the forearm: pattern of axial and bending force transmitted through ulna and radius. J Hand Surg [Br]. 2006; 31(3):274–279
[3] Savvidou C, Murphy E, Mailhot E, Jacob S, Scheker LR. Semiconstrained distal radioulnar joint prosthesis. J Wrist Surg. 2013; 2(1):41–48
[4] Axelsson P, Sollerman C. Constrained implant arthroplasty as a secondary procedure at the distal radioulnar joint: early outcomes. J Hand Surg Am. 2013; 38(6):1111–1118
[5] Bowers WH. Distal radioulnar joint arthroplasty: the hemiresection-interposition technique. J Hand Surg Am. 1985; 10(2):169–178
[6] Van Schoonhoven J, Lanz U. Salvage operations and their differential indication for the distal radioulnar joint. Orthopade. 2004; 33(6):704–714

[7] Field J, Majkowski RJ, Leslie IJ. Poor results of Darrach's procedure after wrist injuries. J Bone Joint Surg Br. 1993; 75(1):53–57

[8] Willis AA, Berger RA, Cooney WP, III. Arthroplasty of the distal radio-ulnar joint using a new ulnar head endoprosthesis: preliminary report. J Hand Surg Am. 2007; 32(2):177–189

[9] Garcia-Elias M. Eclypse: partial ulnar head replacement for the isolated distal radio-ulnar joint arthrosis. Tech Hand Up Extrem Surg. 2007; 11(1):121–128

[10] Greenberg JA, Sotereanos D. Achilles allograft interposition for failed Darrach distal ulna resections. Tech Hand Up Extrem Surg. 2008; 12(2):121–125

[11] Degreef I, De Smet L. The Scheker distal radioulnar joint arthroplasty to unravel a virtually unsolvable problem. Acta Orthop Belg. 2013; 79(2):141–145

[12] Scheker LR, Martineau DW. Distal radioulnar joint constrained arthroplasty. Hand Clin. 2013; 29(1):113–121

[13] Scheker LR. Implant arthroplasty for the distal radioulnar joint. J Hand Surg Am. 2008; 33(9):1639–1644

[14] Reissner L, Böttger K, Klein HJ, Calcagni M, Giesen T. Midterm results of semiconstrained distal radioulnar joint arthroplasty and analysis of complications. J Wrist Surg. 2016; 5(4):290–296

[15] Calcagni M, Giesen T. Distal radioulnar joint arthroplasty with implants: a systematic review. EFORT Open Rev. 2017; 1(5):191–196

[16] Moulton LS, Giddins GEB. Distal radio-ulnar implant arthroplasty: a systematic review. J Hand Surg Eur Vol. 2017; 42(8):827–838

35

Index

Note: Page numbers set **bold** or *italic* indicate headings or figures, respectively.